A Richard Selzer Reader

A Richard Selzer Reader

Blood and Ink

Edited by
Kevin Kerrane

Introduction by Marie Borroff

UNIVERSITY OF DELAWARE PRESS
Newark

Published by University of Delaware Press
Copublished by The Rowman & Littlefield Publishing Group, Inc.
4501 Forbes Boulevard, Suite 200, Lanham, Maryland 20706
www.rowman.com

Unit A, Whitacre Mews, 26-34 Stannary Street, London SE11 4AB

British Library Cataloguing in Publication Information Available

Library of Congress Cataloging-in-Publication Data Available

ISBN 978-1-61149-642-0 (hardback : alk. paper)
ISBN 978-1-61149-643-7 (electronic)

∞™ The paper used in this publication meets the minimum requirements of American National Standard for Information Sciences Permanence of Paper for Printed Library Materials, ANSI/NISO Z39.48-1992.

Printed in the United States of America

Contents

Preface

With the cooperation of Richard Selzer, *A Richard Selzer Reader: Blood and Ink* has been designed as a career-spanning collection, reflecting the range and depth of the author's work over a period of about forty-five years. When Selzer began writing seriously in the late 1960s, he was practicing as a general surgeon in New Haven, Connecticut, and teaching surgery at the Yale School of Medicine. By the time he retired as a physician in 1985 to devote himself completely to writing, he had already achieved major recognition—a National Magazine Award, a Guggenheim Fellowship, residencies at Yaddo, and acclaim by such literary luminaries as Cynthia Ozick, Denise Levertov, and Tom Wolfe. He had also helped to define the new field of medical humanities, and his influence would later be acknowledged by a younger generation of doctor-writers like Abraham Verghese and Atul Gawande. "Richard Selzer will always be my hero," Verghese has said.

One reason that Selzer's stories and essays have become required reading in many medical programs is that he focuses so thoughtfully on doctor-patient relationships, looking critically at the ways that physicians (including himself) are liable to ignore the full humanity of those under their care. Contrasting examples of medical humility and courtesy highlight the author's portrayals of his father, Julius Louis Selzer, a general practitioner in Troy, New York. Julius died shortly before Richard turned thirteen, and the boy—who was already planning to become a doctor—now had an all-consuming mission. He worked his way through Union College and Albany Medical College, served in postwar Korea as a lieutenant in a medical detachment, returned to a surgical residency at Yale, and then established his own practice. Before being posted to Korea, Selzer had married Janet White, and in New Haven they raised three children in a big house on St. Ronan Terrace.

The birth of his second career is traced out by Selzer himself in "The Pen and the Scalpel," the opening selection in this book—and is then illustrated in the first full unit, which surveys his writing apprenticeship. Subsequent units are arranged topically rather than chronologically, and each grouping is preceded by a brief overview of a theme or trend in Selzer's work.

Limiting the selections was difficult, partly because of the sheer volume of Selzer's work. He is the author of thirteen books—comprising short stories, essays, reportage, memoir, and diary entries—and the co-creator of two others edited by Peter Josyph: *What One Man Said to Another* (Michigan State University Press, 1994) and *Letters to a Best Friend* (State University of New York Press, 2009). Many boxes of additional material, either previously unanthologized or never published, are part of the Richard Selzer Archive in the Moody Medical Library at the University of Texas, Galveston. Selzer has also given dozens of public lectures, and *A Richard Selzer Reader* includes the texts for four of them, each slightly edited according to the author's own recommendations. In addition, for this collection he made available more than a hundred pages of fresh material: new diary entries as well as notes for his writing workshops.

Final decisions about the table of contents gave priority to works that have been difficult, or impossible, for Selzer's readers to find. But *A Richard Selzer Reader* also includes about a dozen pieces whose familiarity makes them even more essential as key texts in Selzer's career, and some stories have been chosen for their sheer brilliance: "Whither Thou Goest" and "Imelda," for example, are likely to be read, and treasured, into the twenty-second century—and beyond. "Imelda" has been mistakenly construed by some readers as a true story even though its fictional premises seem clear. More problematic is "Atrium: October 2001," whose place in the zone between fact and fiction is discussed in the author's explication at the end of the story. And Selzer has always been frank about his embellishments of fact even in "nonfiction" narratives, such as the chronicle of his illness in *Raising the Dead: A Doctor's Encounter with His Own Mortality* (Whittle Communications, 1994). In general, his memoir writing owes as much to imagination as to memory.

In her introduction to this collection, Marie Borroff appraises Richard Selzer's style with an expert eye. She has written major studies of language in medieval and modern literature, from *Sir Gawain and the Green Knight* to works by Wallace Stevens and Robert Frost, and she is an estimable poet in her own right. Her poems in *Stars and Other Signs* (Yale University Press, 2002), written over the course of five decades, remain fresh—with a voice that shifts easily between the formal and the colloquial as it captures moments of splendor amid the details of daily life. It is easy to see why Professor Borroff would appreciate Selzer's prose artistry. But the essential point in her commentary is that his distinctive style is a tool for expressing a distinctive vision: of the human body as holy; of medicine as a compassionate craft; and of the aspiring doctor-writer as a recorder of sacramental moments in the lives of patients and caregivers.

"It is a paradox," Selzer wrote in his published *Diary*, "that I am both a religious writer and a skeptic." In fact, this conundrum is at the heart of his work. His entry continues: "I do not pray in any conventional sense, as I do not believe there is a god to receive prayer. . . . [But] I am attentive to everyone and every living creature, just as a nun includes all humankind in her prayers. That means listening and beholding with all of my might."[1] As this quote suggests, Selzer uses religious language metaphorically—finding "divine" qualities, for example, in purely human acts of profound sensitivity, courtesy, or generosity. His personality on the page is that of a humble searcher, always open to experiences that resist standard scientific explanations. In a 1975 essay, "The Surgeon as Priest," Selzer reported a visit to Yale by the Dalai Lama's personal physician, Yeshi Dhonden, whose astute diagnoses, offered in poetic language, were based on sensitive touching and the discernment of subtle odors. Afterward, in the course of his own hospital rounds, Selzer could sometimes hear the sound of Yeshi Dhonden's voice, "like an ancient Buddhist prayer, its meaning long since forgotten, only the music remaining. Then a jubiliation possesses me, and I feel myself touched by something divine."[2]

Selzer's recent diary entries reveal deeper layers of an atheism that is modest rather than militant—especially when, in reflecting on his voluminous reading, he discovers kindred spirits in the past. One entry from 2011 describes his feeling of fellowship with Robert Louis Stevenson: "I cannot claim a rugged, adventurous experience such as that of RLS, but in a number of ways our two selves were interchangeable. We both shared a skepticism, actually a disbelief in religion, yet found ourselves thanking God for the greatness of the human spirit."

Marie Borroff's commentary suggests two other implications of Selzer's prose style. First, his medical expertise and his metaphorical skill often combine in passages of disturbing vividness, as seen here in "The Corpse" and "Emergency Medicine." The first, a dramatized essay, crystallizes the discomforting details of human mortality and decay; the second, a chapter from the semi-autobiographical novel *Knife Song Korea* (State University of New York Press, 2009), shows a young doctor in a remote outpost making snap decisions as he deals with horrific wounds. Both selections may prove challenging to read. "I would warn off the squeamish," Selzer wrote in a preface to *Mortal Lessons*, "or those who cannot see that the truth is at least as accessible in ugliness as it is in beauty."[3] This aspect of Selzer's work recalls a tribute once paid to the journalist Martha Gellhorn, who was said to write "with a cold eye and a warm heart."[4]

Second, perhaps as a counterweight to his skill in describing ugly truths, Selzer's writing reveals a fine comic sensibility. His unusual word choices and surprising turns of phrase, as noted by Professor Borroff, are often the springboards for elegant wit. In *A Richard Selzer Reader*, that wit is evident in Selzer's lecture on Sherlock Holmes, in his new ending for Dickens' *A Tale of Two Cities*, and even in the digressive style of his essay on the liver. In his memoirs and diary entries, Selzer's humor is usually self-deprecating. In *Down from Troy*, he pictured himself as a spindly and wistful child: "Puny, ill-clothed so as to resemble an ungainly parcel, distracted, I dreamt of building a raft and sailing it all the way down the Hudson to New York Harbor."[5] Seventy years later, as a character in his own diary, Selzer remained spindly and wistful, contending courageously with the travails of aging while enjoying a sense of the absurd. In a 2010 entry, he is joined by another opera-lover in an impromptu performance of a beloved aria from *La Traviata* as both men, described as scrawny octogenarians, stand naked in the locker room of a gym at Yale.

POSTSCRIPT

Richard Selzer died on June 15, 2016, nine days before his eighty-eighth birthday. On July 24, Janet Selzer hosted a celebration of his life for about 120 friends at the Lawn Club in New Haven. Among the highlights were tributes by Richard's three children. Older son Jon honored his father's love of opera by playing several selections on oboe, beginning with "Musetta's Waltz" from *La Bohème*. Larry (nicknamed "Doon") described some of the ways that Richard charmed his children and grandchildren. Gretchen paid homage to her father by reading his own humorous homage to Charles Dickens: "*A Tale of Two Cities* Revisited."

Brief reminiscences were shared by two other doctor-writers: Bernie Siegel, who once shared a surgical practice with Richard; and Lorence Gutterman, a collaborator on writing workshops for medical professionals. Peter Josyph, who edited two Selzer books and provided invaluable assistance on several other projects, read from one of his published conversations with Richard. I also spoke, and told the following story:

Richard Selzer's visit to the University of Delaware in spring 1990 began with a buffet lunch attended by two dozen faculty and students. As Richard was finishing a sandwich, a handsome young man walked over and introduced himself. "I'm majoring in Communication," he said, "and I want to get into television broadcasting. My professor says that I need to practice my interviewing skills, and I wonder if I could do a brief interview with you—maybe for just five minutes."

Richard politely agreed, and the student pulled out a notebook. "OK," the young man said, "my first question is: Who are you?"

I walked away in exasperation. "Who are you?" confirmed a stereotype of TV reporters (or would-be reporters) who seem to think that knowing anything is less important than being photogenic and looking as if they *might* know something. And in this case the question sounded almost insulting. *Who is he?* He's a doctor who turned medical writing into art. He's an innovator who helped to establish medical humanities as a vital field of study. He's a stylist who specializes in brief forms but packs them with language so highly charged that they almost burst at the seams.

When I calmed down, I walked back to find that Richard was interviewing the student! He had encouraged the young man to talk about his various interests, which included eerie movies. Richard was delighted, and proceeded to recommend one of his favorite tales by Poe, "The Facts in the Case of M. Valdemar," describing it as eerier than any film. The student's eyes widened as he heard about the story's premise: a dying man being instructed by a hypnotist to remain alive.

It struck me then that the strongest link between Richard's two careers, doctor and writer, was his ability to *listen*, to attend fully not just to what's said, but to *how* it's said, and to focus intently and amiably on the whole person behind the words.

That evening Richard gave a public reading. The story he chose was one he had recently completed, "Whither Thou Goest." I thought then, and still think, that it stands as one of his finest works. The audience loved it too, especially in Richard's expressive presentation. We laughed at the comic twists of the letters within the story, and teared up at the lyrical beauty of the final paragraphs.

When I left the auditorium, I crossed paths with the young man who had tried to inteview Richard earlier that day. As he looked at me, I saw that his eyes were wet.

"Man," he said, "I *love* him!" And I said: "Me too."

We all did. And we still do.

Kevin Kerrane
Newark, Delaware

NOTES

1. Richard Selzer, *Diary* (New Haven, CT: Yale University Press, 2011), 35–36.
2. Richard Selzer, *Mortal Lessons: Notes on the Art of Surgery*, Touchstone edition (New York: Simon & Schuster, 1987), 35–36.
3. Ibid., 9.
4. James Cameron, quoted in *The Art of Fact: A Historical Anthology of Literary Journalism*, ed. Kevin Kerrane and Ben Yagoda (New York: Scribner, 1997), 422.

5. Richard Selzer, *Down from Troy: A Doctor Comes of Age* (New York: William Morrow, 1992), 131.

Acknowledgments

As I edited this collection, my most helpful reading was Richard Selzer's own brilliant work, including many worthy essays and stories that could not be included here because of space limits. Several scholarly studies also proved valuable—particularly Charles Anderson's *Richard Selzer and the Rhetoric of Surgery* (University of Illinois Press, 1989), as well as essays by Robert Leigh Davis, David B. Morris, Enid Rhodes Peschel, Charles I. Schuster, M. Teresa Tavormina, and Gayle Whittier.

Two other Selzer experts, Mahala Yates Stripling and Peter Josyph, deserve special thanks. Both have been generous in sharing ideas and materials, and their love for Richard Selzer and his writing is infectious. Mahala, who has published thoughtful articles about Selzer and an illuminating interview with him, has now completed a biography with the working title *Doctor of Arts: The Life of Richard Selzer, The Man Who Transformed the Literature of Medicine*. Peter collaborated with Selzer on two books: *What One Man Said to Another* transcribes a series of their lively conversations, including an interview included here in the unit entitled "Being a Writer"; *Letters to a Best Friend* is a record of their steady correspondence over a period of five years, 1988 through 1992. I am also grateful to Peter for suggesting the lecture "The Ivory Crucifixion" as a last-minute addition to this book—and to Kathleen Mylen-Coulombe of the Yale University Art Gallery for helping us to include a photo of that remarkable carving.

Marie Borroff, Sterling Professor of English Emeritus at Yale, has been one of Richard Selzer's dear friends as well as a close reader of his work. This renowned scholar is both genial and incisive, and her introductory essay is a model of appreciative commentary.

A Richard Selzer Reader has been facilitated by two grants: from the Moody Medical Library at the University of Texas, Galveston, and from the

College of Arts and Sciences at the University of Delaware. I owe heartfelt thanks to Bobby Marlin, Sarita Oertling, and Karen Kinney at the Moody Library, and to Matt Kinservik, George Watson, John Ernest, and Kaylee Olney at the University of Delaware. I also appreciate the help and good cheer of colleagues at Delaware—Heyward Brock, James M. Dean, John Ernest, the late Rivers Singleton, Ben Yagoda, Ray Peters, Julia Oestreich, and especially Donald Mell—and of fellow teachers in the Goucher College program in Creative Nonfiction: Tom French, Diana Hume George, Leslie Rubinkowski, Phil Gerard, and Patsy Sims. And I remain grateful to dozens of students over the years, both at Delaware and Goucher, who have shared my appreciation of essays like "Bone" and stories like "Imelda."

Family and friends have been wonderfully supportive, and I extend warm thanks to Barry and Barbara Kerrane, Rosina McDonnell Carter, Billy and Patti Roche, and Dermot and Mary O'Connell. As ever, I am profoundly indebted to my wife, Katharine Carter Kerrane, who is a treasure in every way. Like me, she considers it a privilege to have known Richard Selzer for three decades and to revisit essays and stories that truly improve with age. In particular, I appreciate Katharine's thoughtful suggestions regarding all of the framing material in this collection. In effect, she has been the editor's editor.

Greatest thanks, of course, go to Richard and Janet Selzer for their grace, generosity, and hospitality. This work is dedicated to both of them with deep admiration and affection.

"Risen" (Part Two from *Raising the Dead: A Doctor's Encounter with His Own Mortality*) (Knoxville, TN: Whittle Communications, 1993)
"Flesh Holds the Truth, Mortality," Introduction to Max Aguilera-Hellweg, *The Sacred Heart: An Atlas of the Body Seen through Invasive Surgery* (New York: Bulfinch Press, 1997)
"Five-Finger Exercises" from *The Writer* 112 (September 1999)
"Crimean Vespers" from *Abaton: Des Moines University Literary Review* (Fall 2007)

Reprinted by permission of Peter Josyph: "Wounded with Wonder" from *What One Man Said to Another: Talks with Richard Selzer*, ed. Peter Josyph (East Lansing: Michigan State University Press, 1994).

Reprinted by permission of Counterpoint Press: "The Ivory Crucifixion," "*A Tale of Two Cities* Revisited," and "Atrium: October 2001" from *The Whistlers' Room: Stories and Essays* (Washington, DC: Shoemaker & Hoard, 2004).

Reprinted by permission of State University of New York Press: "Emergency Medicine" (Chapter 12) from *Knife Song Korea: A Novel* (Albany: State University of New York Press, 2009).

Other materials were provided personally by Richard Selzer or were accessed in the Selzer Archive at the University of Texas Medical Library, Galveston (Truman C. Blocker Jr. Collection).

The photograph of "Fragment of a Crucified Christ" appears courtesy of the Yale University Art Gallery, New Haven, Connecticut (Director's Purchase Fund).

Introduction

The Writer Richard Selzer: High, Low, and Mighty

Marie Borroff

Le style, c'est l'homme—"the style, that is the man." So said the eighteenth-century savant the Count de Buffon. I will translate his words more freely here as "the style bespeaks the man," for *bespeaks* points us toward language, the material of which all styles are made.

Richard Selzer once said in an interview, "The language was and still is the most important part of my writing." Reading him, we are led to stretch our vocabularies to the loftiest heights of Latin and Greek derivation in words such as zygomatic, ecchymoses, scaphoid, dyspneic, bosselated, and trabeculations—most of them medical, as is to be expected from a surgeon-turned-writer. And we encounter words of another class, similarly absent from conventional prosaic discourse, such as tiff, dollop, frizzy, chimbly (dialect form of chimney), hefty, muzzy, and waggled. When even the fullest range of the English language does not provide Selzer with a word that suits his purpose, he simply makes up a word that does. Describing himself, for example, as one who habitually takes everything in, he comes up with "receptacular," a lexical item confined to the fine print of *Oxford English* dictionaries and wholly absent from *The American Heritage*.

Words of both kinds glitter in Selzer's prose like tiny chips of mica, setting each other off particularly when the learned and the popular inhabit the same sentence. In an appendix to one of his books, he speaks of "those elongated balloons whose walls . . . are haustrated into incomplete segments, like links of knockwurst." ("Haustrated," like "receptacular," is absent from my dictionaries.) He warns the would-be surgeon that the blood he causes to flow "cannot wait a moment too long lest it become a blob of coagulum." "The sounds of your intestine" are "those gurgles and gaseous pops called borborygmi." And he remembers, in a church in his native city of Troy, New York, "those angels . . . blowing long golden horns, their sweet cheeks puffed in holy insufflation."

We find this same range from the erudite to the homely in figures of speech, when the literal subject is compared with something else. A day is "so hot and humid" that Selzer feels "steamed open like an envelope." Speaking of a woman thought to be retarded, Selzer says "her smile was not the grin of a tickled cretin, but the still, small glee of a saint in full glory." In an exploratory operation, "the peritoneum is snapped open and a giant shining eggplant presents itself. It is the stomach, black from the blood it contains." He and his brother, "pulled by some base and ancient allure" down to the cellar of their house, are "two Orphei descending, and no lyre to pluck . . . no Eurydice waiting to embolden us by her pallor." A young doctor preparing a case for presentation must "rehearse as if [he] were Pavarotti singing *Tosca* at the Met. The Chief who will attempt to destroy you in public is Baron Scarpia. You and your patient are the star-crossed lovers." Nowadays you can buy apes, ivory, and peacocks "out of mail-order catalogues, and Dial-an-Oracle will tell your future over the phone."

This verbal prodigality has its corollary in outpourings of descriptive detail that conjure up the general out of particulars. Observing his doctor father in a rowboat after a flood, he sees, as with X-ray vision, the contents of the black bag "with its rows of pill bottles . . . nitroglycerine; digitalis leaf; phenobarbital, half- and quarter-grain; tincture of opium; rhubarb and soda; glycerine and rosewater." An anesthesiologist is at work, measuring "blood pressure, pulse, heartbeat, flow of urine, loss of blood, temperature, whatever is measurable"; he is also "a titrator, adding a little gas, drug, oxygen, fluid, blood in order to maintain the dynamic equilibrium that is the only state compatible with life." A young doctor, becoming Chief Resident, will predictably attain the privilege of "squiredom" to his ultimate superior, the Professor: "You shall carry his stethoscope, and you shall be to him dresser, clerk, guide, bandage, splint, scissors. You, his scrivener, his scullion, his squirm."

One cannot adequately celebrate this variety without noting something else equally various: its range of allusion. A glance over my notes yields references to, among other authors, Byron, Coleridge, Dickens, Emily Dickinson, Thomas Gray, Gerard Manley Hopkins, Sir Walter Scott, Marlowe, and Rafael Sabatini. The *Odyssey*, the *Iliad*, and the *Aeneid* are recurring presences, as are classical mythology more generally, both testaments of the Bible, and Christian lore such as the sayings of Saint Hildegard and the prayers and letters of Saint Catherine of Siena. Allusion is not necessarily dignified. Imagining himself a wound-dresser in the Civil War, Selzer hears "coonjine songs" chanted by Blacks loading bales of cotton: "Ole roustabout ain' got no home, Makes his livin' by his shoulder bone!" Somewhere, a quotation from *Romeo and Juliet* immediately precedes a quip from the repertoire of Groucho Marx. Selzer's language is a democracy, in which nothing, however lowbrow or highfalutin, is rejected from citizenship.

The man whose language I have described is indeed receptacular, an omnivorous literary consumer storing words and other memorabilia in some boundless inner network. Colorful diction merges with a more general esthetic sensitivity: to visual colors and textures, to the play of light, to the sounds of music and sounds other than music, to pleasant and unpleasant smells. And under all of that lies a kind of meaning that he can describe better than I. Writing a new preface fourteen years after the publication of *Letters to a Young Doctor*, he finds in the book, retrospectively, "a strong note of spirituality . . . only natural for a writer who sees the flesh as the spirit thickened"—a doctor who, contemplating the worst of deformity and disease, comes "to perceive the body as a primal mystery and therefore sacred." In the course of a dissection described in the most dispassionate of technical terms, when the dome of the dead man's skull is at last lifted and the brain revealed, he is moved to cry "O holy, holy, holy!" This in a writer who elsewhere professes skepticism regarding the myths of "revealed religion."

For Richard Selzer, M.D., all bodies are holy and beautiful. His experience while performing a surgical procedure merges the compassionate desire to cure and save with esthetic responsiveness, as the inner shapes and colors of the abdominal organs, and their secrets of tumor and lesion—all "the truth lying curtained in the Ark of the body"—are exposed for the first time by the knife. The loving reverence with which this doctor practices his craft accounts for the fact that so many of the stories he tells deal with actions prompted by compassion: a husband tenderly feeding his dying wife through a stomach tube; a famous plastic surgeon secretly operating in the night on the deformed lip of a girl who had died on the operating table, so that her mother will see her daughter's face in its new comeliness. What other surgeon would, after the departure of the patient, hold to the light the nail he has excised from his big toe, and see that "at the margins, where it is reddened by the boy's blood, there is a glow, as of stained glass"?

The style is the man. I have tried to do justice to both. I will have succeeded if you, the reader, are moved to read on.

Chronology

1928 Richard Selzer is born June 24 in Troy, New York, as "Allen Richard Selzer": the second child of Julius Louis Selzer, M.D., a general practitioner, and Gertrude Schneider Selzer, a singer who performed in local productions of musicals and operas

1941 Loses his beloved father when Julius Selzer succumbs to a heart attack at age 47

1945 Graduates from Troy High School

1948 Graduates from Union College (Schenectady, New York) with a B.S. in biology and extensive course work in literature and history

1953 Receives M.D. from Albany Medical College

Begins internship/surgical residency at Grace-New Haven Hospital

1955 Marries Janet White in New Haven, Connecticut

1955–57 Drafted into the army and serves in Korea as a lieutenant with a medical detachment south of the demilitarized zone (secures permission from his commanding officer to provide medical treatment for Korean civilians as well as American servicemen)

1957 Resumes surgical residency at Grace-New Haven Hospital (which became Yale-New Haven Medical Center in 1965)

1960 Appointed associate professor of surgery at Yale (as a Fellow of Ezra Stiles College) and begins private practice as a general surgeon in New Haven

1968 At age 40 writes his first short story (unpublished until 1985) recasting the narrative of Jonah and the Whale

Begins a regimen of writing from 1:00 to 3:00 every morning

1970 First published fiction, "A Single Minute of Fear," in *Ellery Queen's Mystery Magazine*

1974 *Rituals of Surgery* (Harper's Magazine Press): macabre stories that had appeared in such magazines as *Antaeus*, *New American Review*, and *Esquire*

"Drinking Man's Liver" published in *Esquire* (April), beginning a series of essays about the body, including "Kidney Stone," "Bone," and "Skin"

1975 Receives National Magazine Award from the Columbia School of Journalism for his essays about the body

1976 *Mortal Lessons: Notes on the Art of Surgery* (Simon & Schuster): literary essays

1977 First visit to Yaddo as Artist in Residence (followed by nine more residencies through 1992)

1979 *Confessions of a Knife* (Simon & Schuster): essays and fiction

Resident Scholar at Rockeller Foundation's Bellagio Study Center on Lake Como in Italy

1981 Participates in Interplast surgical expedition to Arequipa, Peru

1982 *Letters to a Young Doctor* (Simon & Schuster): essays and fiction

1983 Receives American Medical Writers Association Book Award for *Letters to a Young Doctor*

1985 Retires from medicine and begins writing full-time

Teaches at Rangers' School, Yellowstone National Park

Receives John Simon Guggenheim Award (Creative Arts, General Nonfiction)

1986 *Taking the World in for Repairs* (William Morrow): essays and fiction

1988 Receives National Endowment for the Arts Fellowship

1990 *Imagine a Woman and Other Tales* (Random House): fiction

1991 In a coma for twenty-three days, followed by a slow recovery, after contracting Legionnaires' disease

1992 *Down from Troy: A Doctor Comes of Age* (William Morrow): memoir

1993 *Raising the Dead: A Doctor's Encounter with His Own Mortality* (Whittle Communications): imaginative treatment of the severe illness of 1991

1994 *What One Man Said to Another: Talks with Richard Selzer*, ed. Peter Josyph (Michigan State University Press): journeys and interviews

1998 *The Doctor Stories* (Picador): twenty-five earlier short stories, and a new novella

1999 Richard Selzer Archive established at the University of Texas Medical Branch, Galveston, in the Moody Medical Library (Truman G. Blocker Jr. Collection)

2001 *The Exact Location of the Soul* (Picador): selected essays

2004 *The Whistlers' Room: Stories and Essays* (Shoemaker & Hoard): fiction, memoir, diary entries, and lectures on art

2005 The Richard Selzer Lecture Series established by Yale's Program for Humanities in Medicine

2009 *Knife Song Korea: A Novel* (State University of New York Press)

Letters to a Best Friend, ed. Peter Josyph (State University of New York Press): correspondence from 1988 through 1992

2010 First annual Richard Selzer Prize for Writing awarded by *Abaton*, a medical humanities literary and arts journal at Des Moines University

2011 *Diary* (Yale University Press): entries from 1997 to 2008, with some earlier undated material, thoughts on writing, and "Memories of Troy"

2013 After forty-eight years in their home on St. Ronan Terrace in New Haven, the Selzers move to a retirement community in North Branford, Connecticut

2016 Richard Selzer dies on June 15 in North Branford

Prologue

Two Vocations

"The Pen and the Scalpel" is one of several efforts by Richard Selzer to provide perspective on his double life. Another thoughtful overview appears in "The Making of a Doctor/Writer," his introduction to essays collected in *The Exact Location of the Soul* (Picador, 2001). Written in mid-career, "The Pen and the Scalpel" offers an implicit justification of Selzer's decision in 1985 to retire from his surgical practice.[1]

When he was still working as a surgeon, Selzer wrote for two hours in the middle of the night, and he has often attributed the dark and dreamlike aspects of his early compositions to this strange schedule. But as he explains here, it was not fatigue that led to his retirement from surgery; it was a psychological disjunction between the walling off of feeling—a steeliness necessary for any person who would cut into the body of another—and the emotional openness required in the creation of literature.

In practicing his second vocation, Selzer says, "I have tried to make use of the poetic potential in scientific language." That effort is clear in his comparison of writing to the medical procedure called "transillumination," and in the diary entry that ends the essay. It will also be clear throughout this collection, because every selection displays the power of metaphor as a tool of enlightenment and empathy. In this respect, Richard Selzer uses his pen as precisely as if it were a scalpel.

NOTE

1. Selzer's essay appeared in the *New York Times* on August 21, 1988. He discussed his decision to retire from medicine in several later interviews—for example, with Dale Flynn in "Rituals of Writing: An Interview with Richard Selzer," *Writing on the Edge* 2, no. 1 (Fall 1990), 57–68.

The Pen and the Scalpel

I had been a general surgeon for 15 years when, at the age of 40, the psychic energy for writing inexplicably appeared. It was an appearance that was to knock over my life. For 15 years I had studied, practiced, and taught surgery at the Yale School of Medicine, all the while enjoying the usefulness and the handsomeness of the craft. For the next 16 years, until my retirement, I would practice both surgery and writing. But where to fit in the writing when all of my days and half of my nights were fully engaged? Certainly not evenings. In the evening one visits with one's next-of-kin; in the evening one helps with homework; in the evening, if one is so inclined, one has a martini. Instead, I became the first adult in the state of Connecticut to go to bed in the evening. Having slept from 8:30 P.M. to 1:00 in the morning, I rose, wrote in longhand (a typewriter would disturb the household) until precisely 3 o'clock. Then it was back upstairs and to sleep until 6:00 in the morning, when I began the day's doctoring. Plenty of sleep, only divided by two hours, when I was alone with my pen, and all the light in the world gathered upon a sheet of paper. In this way, I wrote three collections of stories, essays, and memoirs.

Time was when in the professions—medicine and law—to patronize the arts was respectable; to practice them was not. For a surgeon it was even more questionable. Who wants to know, after all, what a surgeon does in his spare time? When it became known how I was spending my wild nights, my colleagues at the hospital were distressed. "Come, come" they coaxed in (more or less) the words of the poet Richard Wilbur, "Forsake those roses of the mind, and tend the true, the moral flower." But because the subject of my writings was my work as a doctor, the two seemed inseparable. The one fertilized the other. Why, I wondered, doesn't every surgeon write? A doctor walks in and out of a dozen short stories a day. It is irresistible to write them down. When, at last, the time came to make a choice between my two passions, it had already been made for me. Listen:

In the operating room, the patient must be anesthetized in order that he feel no pain. The surgeon too must be "anesthetized" in order to remain at some distance from the event: when he cuts the patient, his own flesh must not bleed. It is this seeming lack of feeling that gives the surgeon the image of someone who is out of touch with his humanity, a person wanting only to cut, to perform. I assure you that it is the image only. A measure of insulation against the laying open of the bodies of his fellow human beings is necessary for the well-being of both patient and doctor. In surgery, if nowhere else, dispassion is an attribute. But the surgeon-writer is not anesthetized. He remains awake; sees everything; censors nothing. It is his dual role to open and repair the body of his patient and to report back to the waiting world in the keenest language he can find. By becoming a writer, I had stripped off the protective carapace. It was time to go. A surgeon can unmake himself; a writer cannot.

A Faustian bargain, you say? Perhaps, but, truth to tell, New Haven had begun to seem rather like The Beast with a Thousand Gallbladders. And where is it graven in stone that, once having been ordained, a surgeon must remain at the operating table until the scalpel slips from his lifeless fingers? Nor had I any wish to become like the old lion whose claws are long since blunt but not the desire to use them. Still, one does not walk away from the workbench of one's life with a cheery wave of the hand. In the beginning, I felt a strange sense of dislocation. As though I were standing near a river whose banks were flowing while the stream itself stood still. Only after two years did I cease to have attacks of longing for the labor that so satisfied and uplifted my spirit. Then, too, there was the risk that by withdrawing from the hospital, with its rich cargo of patients and those who tend them, I would be punished as a writer, suffer from impotence of the pen. A writer turns his back upon his native land at his own peril. Besides, to begin the life of a writer at the age of 56 is to toil under the very dart of death. As did another doctor-writer, John Keats, I too "have fears that I may cease to be before my pen has gleaned my teeming brain."

In medicine, there is a procedure called transillumination. If, in a darkened room, a doctor holds a bright light against a hollow part of the body, he will see through the outer tissues to the structures within that cavity—arteries, veins, projecting shelves of bone. In such a ruby gloom he can distinguish among a hernia, a hydrocele of the scrotum, and a tumor of the testicle. Or he can light up a sinus behind the brow. Unlike surgery, which opens the body to direct examination, transillumination gives an indirect vision, calling into play the simplest perceptions of the doctor. To write about a patient is like transillumination. You hold the lamp of language against his body and gaze through the covering layers at the truths within.

At first glance, it would appear that surgery and writing have little in common, but I think that is not so. For one thing, they are both sub-celestial arts; as far as I know, the angels disdain to perform either one. In each of them you hold a slender instrument that leaves a trail wherever it is applied. In one there is the shedding of blood; in the other it is ink that is spilled upon a page. In one the scalpel is restrained; in the other the pen is given rein. The surgeon sutures together the tissues of the body to make whole what is sick or injured; the writer sews words into sentences to fashion a new version of human experience. A surgical operation is rather like a short story. You make the incision, rummage around inside for a bit, then stitch up. It has a beginning, a middle, and an end. If I were to choose a medical specialist to write a novel, it would be a psychiatrist. They tend to go on and on. And on.

Despite that I did not begin to write until the middle of my life, I think I must always have been a writer. Like my father who was a general practitioner during the Depression in Troy, New York, and who wrote a novel. It was all about a prostitute with a heart of gold (her name was Goldie!) and the doctor who first saves her life, then falls in love with her. Mother read it and told him: "Keep it away from the children."

Father's office was on the ground floor of an old brownstone, and we lived upstairs. At night, after office hours, my brother Billy and I (we were ten and nine years old) would sneak downstairs to Father's darkened consultation room and there, shamefaced, by the light of a candle stub, we would take down from the shelves his medical textbooks. Our favorite was "The Textbook of Obstetrics and Gynecology."

It was there that I first became aware of the rich language of medicine. Some of the best words began with the letter C. Carcinoma, I read, and thought it was that aria from "Rigoletto" that mother used to sing while she washed and dried the dishes. Cerebellum. I said the word aloud, letting it drip off the end of my tongue like melted chocolate. And I read choledochojejunostomy, which later I was to learn as the name of an operation. All those syllables marching off in my mind to that terminal *y*! If that was the way surgeons talked, I thought, I would be one of them, and live forever in a state of mellifluous rapture.

I do not use these words in my writing, but I do try to use language that evokes the sounds of the body—the lub-dup, lub-dup of the garrulous heart, the gasp and wheeze of hard breathing, all the murmur and splash of anatomy and physiology. And I have tried to make use of the poetic potential in scientific language. Here, from my diary, this specimen:

> How gentle the countryside near Troy, with much farming everywhere. Farming gives a sense of health to the land. It is replenishing to watch at dusk as a herd of cattle flows like a giant amoeba toward the barn. First one cow ad-

vances. She pauses. Another pseudopodium is thrust ahead, pulling the others behind it until all of the cytoplasm, trailing milk, is inside the barn.

All along the banks of the Hudson River, oak, elm and locust trees have grown very tall. The bark of the locust is thrown into deep folds coated with lichen and moss. So old are these trees that, without the least wind, one will drop off a quite large branch as if to shed a part of its burden. This letting-fall doesn't seem to do the tree any harm. It is more an anatomical relinquishment of a part so that the whole might remain healthy. Much as a diabetic will accept amputation of a gangrenous toe in order that he might once again walk on his foot. How clever of these locust trees to require no surgeon for their trimmage, only their own corporeal wisdom.

Part I

Apprenticeship

In March 1944, a precocious fifteen-year-old student in Troy, New York, wrote a composition describing the horrors of war. His nightmarish images were drawn not from contemporary accounts of military action in Europe or the Pacific, but from a poem about World War I—"On the Wire" by Robert Service—that the boy's father often recited at home, usually bringing his two sons to tears. The beloved father, Dr. Julius Selzer, had died three years earlier.

Now Richard, the younger son, borrowed the poem's No-man's-land setting and first-person anguish while adding hallucinatory touches of his own, as well as allusions to recent readings from the high school English syllabus. His teacher, the notoriously hard-to-please Miss Buckley, may have winced at a few of the composition's florid details but obviously appreciated its imaginative intensity. She awarded the work an A+.

A quarter-century later, Richard Selzer had become a practicing surgeon. One day he felt restless, unaccountably "agitated," and on the spur of the moment he decided to rewrite the story of Jonah from a medical point of view. This experiment remained unpublished until 1985, when the manuscript was discovered by Professor Charles I. Schuster, who summarized the premise of Selzer's version: "This is a Jonah of the present, a Jonah without much history or future, and, significantly, a Jonah without God. He is an existential figure, alienated, an emotional outlaw from his own family, from himself, adrift in a world where God has no discernible presence."[1] Selzer subsequently realized that he had chosen this particular biblical tale because it offered an allegory of his own medical practice: "An operation is a reenactment of the story of Jonah and the Whale. In surgery the patient is the whale who swallows up the surgeon. . . . In an operation where the patient is restored to health, the surgeon is spewed out of the whale's body, and both he and the patient are healed."[2]

In an interview, Selzer told Professor Schuster that, when he first read his own short story, "I knew at once that I was a writer. I was in fact healed, the physician had healed himself, I was calm."[3] This new tranquility was actually the basis for furious creativity. The surgeon rose from sleep every night to write in longhand for two hours, apprenticing himself through genre fiction—particularly tales of the macabre, in which the author needed only to provoke a certain frisson. In this respect, "A Single Minute of Fear" (1970) is exemplary: The editors of *Ellery Queen's Mystery Magazine* described it as "an exceptional first story, filled with suspense and a growing sense of terror."[4]

Selzer was soon writing more ambitiously, aiming for magazines like *Antaeus*, *Harper's*, and *Esquire*. Eighteen of his early stories were collected in his first book, *Rituals of Surgery* (Harper's Magazine Press, 1974). They blend realistic details, drawn directly from medical experiences, with surreal elements made believable and haunting when seen through the eyes of the characters. The author was harnessing his naturally flamboyant style by means of subtle shifts in point of view. "Fairview," for example, begins with a lyrical and urbane love letter, only later introducing its grotesquely disabled writer. The reader is confronted with the case of an imprisoned imagination. But the imagination of the story's author has already broken free.

NOTES

1. Charles I. Schuster, "Commentary on 'Jonah and the Whale,'" *Medical Heritage* 1, no. 1 (January/February 1985), 24.
2. Richard Selzer, *Letters to a Young Doctor* (New York: Simon & Schuster, 1982), 54.
3. Charles I. Schuster, "Confessions of a Writer: The Art of Richard Selzer," *Rhetoric Review* 3, no. 1 (September 1984), 85.
4. *Ellery Queen's Mystery Bag: 25 Stories from Ellery Queen's Mystery Magazine* (New York: World Publishing, 1972), 153.

On the Wire

Richard Selzer
March 2, 1944
English III a

ON THE WIRE

It's midnight out here on the wire, and the sky is an inky pall punctuated by tiny openings, the stars, and a foolishly unreal golden disc, the moon. Last night I fell asleep for a few hours, the first in a few days, and I dreamed that the sky was a huge blanket, and the moon a hole in it. I dreamed that I floated up somehow to that hole and looked through. What I saw made my heart congeal in my breast and my throat constrict with horror. It was different from what I had expected and wanted. I wanted so much to see the angels and to speak to God. I needed him now more than ever. Yes, I looked into heaven last night, and I saw Hell. There were no angels, there was no Him, there was no beautiful, aching peace. What I saw instead was Death, dressed in a long, black robe, her hair streaming wildly in the wind, and the awful grinning skull for a face. She was standing in the middle of Heaven surrounded, as far as the eye could see, by enormous heaps of human bodies. I shrank back in horror, but the fascinating apparition drew my gaze again and again with the cling of her beady, steel-like eye. I see her now, feet spread apart, screaming with mad laughter, like one of Macbeth's witches run amok, Queen of all she surveyed—and all she surveyed was dead. A thick gray mist was clouding the air, and I caught less and less frequent glimpses of her, until finally she was obscured from my sight entirely. Down, down I fell from my ethereal perch to the reality and dirt of my foxhole.

You have no idea of what it's like here in this little hole with nobody to keep you company, and nothing to hide behind. Yes, that's the worst part. There's nothing to hide behind. You look around and all you see is inky black. But even that darkness doesn't hide you. For the eyes of the enemy are sharp, and the eyes of Death are sharper. I feel now as Rolvääg's Beret must have felt when she found herself alone on the prairie with God. I wouldn't mind the rats and the insects, the worms, the hunger and the heat so much if there were only something to hide behind.

From the foxhole just behind mine a hoarse voice whispers a command. "Over the top, over the top." At first I do not comprehend. Then I grasp the full meaning, and still I do not respond. Suddenly, I grab my gun and leap out of my grave-like hole and rush blindly forward into a hail of flashing fire and lights. The thunderous din hammers at my ears, and my temples are throbbing with the fire of battle. On, on I rush, and about me the boys I know and love are dropping one by one to the dust noiselessly, like spirits. Gone is the need for something to hide behind. Gone is all sane thought except that I must kill and run.

Look! There it is, the tangled mass of barbed wire called the "wire" immediately ahead of me. I plunge in blindly, pushing back the wire with my gun. Just one more heave—then it comes, the searing pain, a bullet tearing into my leg. I pitch forward onto the wire and lie writhing in agony, the infinity of pain wracking my body. All through the ageless night I lie thus, and then it is day again. I think, "Surely they'll come for me—they won't, they can't, leave me out here to die on the wire." I call feebly, but my voice is pathetically weak. My strength is ebbing fast and the maddening pain is driving me insane. The terrible burning heat beats down on me with all its force and my parched throat begs for death. But I know death and I'm afraid of that, too. And still I hold my horrible perch on the wire—a tangled, torn animal begging for the cheapest thing in life, life itself.

But I don't care anymore. I can take it now—that eternity on the wire. You see, I'm dead. My body is out there on the wire, but my soul, this eternal part of me, is in the heart of an American soldier who at this very moment is dying on the wire.

Jonah and the Whale

"Not bad," thought Jonah. "Not half bad."

He slipped easily off the velvety tuft of mucosa where he had been sitting, dreamily watching the ebb and flow of the great gastric pool beneath him. It was a particularly good day for fishing. The whale was enjoying a prodigious appetite today and there was a lot coming in. Jonah had seen two or three sea bass just the right size, and was waiting for them to get through their frantic period and settle down to a more catchable speed. Fishing was easy here. He waded down the sloping walls and dipped his tunic in the pool like a net. Within moments he had his catch. It was a bit sportier trying for a particular fish. For that, Jonah had to jump right in and try to corner the prey. This wasn't too hard, particularly if you waited for a day. By then the fish was pretty tired, and could be grasped with bare hands as often as not. With the fish held aloft in one hand, he would paddle through the pleasurably warm pool to the wall and climb up to his perch, stepping from tuft to tuft.

At first, only the most extreme hunger would tempt him into eating one of these fish, but he soon found that the mild digestive juices in the pool would, in a few days, soften the flesh of the fish and, in a manner of speaking, cook it. They also imparted to it a delicious flavor as of succulent marination. He had become quite a connoisseur of fish, and could taste subtle differences in flavor between the species.

He had chosen for his permanent nest, as it were, a point high on the stomach wall in a sort of bay, which doubled back toward the esophagus along the great curvature.

He discovered that this location was rarely, if ever, inundated by the ingested flood and he was safe and dry there for days at a time. It was also an excellent vantage point for surveying the gastric pool. He was quite proud of his nest which consisted of a square fence constructed from pieces of wood lashed together with strips of seaweed, all of which had been retrieved from the pool. The floor was the same spongy mucosa of the stomach which proved ideal for sleeping and walking barefoot. It had the quality of exactly fitting the contour and crevices of the body and hugging it with a slight securing suction. Because of this, walking was easy, the moist hillocks projecting between the toes to give a sure footing. Certainly it was true that the chronic low back ache which had plagued him for years was gone, and he awoke from his sleep with every muscle relaxed and fully rested.

From the beginning the climate had agreed with him: warm, humid, with occasional gusts of cold air which entered with every surfacing. The warmth and moisture suited Jonah's contemplative frame of mind and induced a wholly pleasurable laziness. The cold gusts were refreshing and prevented any monotony of climate.

"Altogether ideal weather conditions," thought Jonah.

A far cry from Nineveh which was so hot and dry that the young women shriveled quickly into old age under the relentless solar gaze. "The sun never blinks over Nineveh," the people were fond of saying ruefully, on days when the hot dust coated the tongue.

These thoughts made him squirm with delight, rubbing his bare back over the gently massaging mucosa.

And to his surprise, it was not dark, as one might have suspected. The great vault was bathed in a soft ruby glow that emanated from the walls. At first, Jonah had thought it some intrinsic quality of the lining itself, but careful observation had revealed that the pool itself was the original source of light, giving off a faint whitish luminescence which was reflected from the rosy walls as the gentle light to which he had become accustomed. The intensity of the light varied, it seemed to him, according to the contents of the gastric pool. The more opalescent the pool, the more light. When crystal clear, the great living cavern was gloomy and just a bit fetid what with those little strands of fog that hung over the pool after a particularly long period of inactivity by the whale.

Jonah lay in his nest listening idly to the muffled lub-dup, lub-dup of the heart. It was a most reassuring sound, measured, smooth—the driving force of the whole apparatus. By placing his hand on the wall near his perch, he could palpate the thrill transmitted from the heart through the body. He loved to feel it rippling through his fingers and listen to the hypnotic beat. On occasion, he would play the game of imagining words in the beat:

"Jonah-Jonah-Jonah" or, doubling, "Pomegranate-pomegranate-pomegranate."

It was only when the memory of the shipwreck returned that he grew anxious, and tossed in his nest as though to exorcise the thought by the writhing of his body. It was dreadful. The sudden darkening of the sky where low black clouds charged across it, which a moment before had been an unbroken blue. It was so sudden and shocking, from the first violent lurch of the ship to the moment when the furious sea had washed over the gunwales and flung its thunder upon the men lashed to the deck. He lay among the others clinging to the deck, the ship now out of control, and listened to the thump and crunch of the boards breaking below. Chests heaving, tangled beards flaked with salt, limbs green and glistening, already drowned and part of the sea. Terrified, Jonah had felt his grip loosening, the fingers of his hands shredding with his efforts to sink them into the planks. The ship raised upon a crest as though in deep inspiration, hung crazily for an instant, and then the agonal expiration, a long sickening fall deep, deep, deep into the green. He had felt himself bursting apart beneath the water, exploding into limpness, the sea pulling in and out of him without restraint.

What happened next was not always too clear although at times, when drifting off to sleep, the whole impossible feat came vividly into his mind. He had been flung to the surface by some internal thrust of the sea and in that moment, through a foamy crest, he saw the huge black shape sitting motionless in the sea.

"Land," he thought, "where no land had been."

Strange land it was. Sleek, shiny, mounding from the surface, but land! And Jonah began to hope only that the waves would lift him toward it. In the next instant, he felt a powerful sucking current take hold of him. Its power exceeded that of the stormy sea, and he was pulled toward the great smooth rock. At the moment of impact, his wildly rolling eyes perceived a huge opening in the rock and headlong he was carried into it. With dizzying speed he was swept into the cave, his swift excursion sucking him over a plain of white projections in neat rows. Hard they were as marble which he knew from the pain of battering against them. A great gray leathery canopy waved and curled above his head, its surface rough, abrasive. Then Jonah knew the unacceptable truth—that he had been swallowed by a whale. The blackness that now engulfed him was not only that of the great throat of the beast but the welcome loss of consciousness.

When he awoke, the world was still again. He was lying on the soft membrane which was to be his home and sustenance. The eyes he had closed to a whirlwind were now opened on a whale world.

There was pain in the memory, and Jonah abruptly sat up as if to shake from his mind the nightmare. Since then, there had been much time to think. The solitude of his new world was conducive to philosophy. Not that he was lonely. Not at all. He was always aware of the serene companionship of the whale. He had but to listen to hear its heart, but to reach out to touch it intimately without reproach or rejection. With what human had he such a union, such a mutely meaningful symbiosis, and was he not fully mindful that it was the whale who fed and housed him, shared with him the treasures of the sea and, Jonah thought, secret and joyful, took comfort from the presence of the man within him. He had come to love the whale. He hoped and dreamt that the whale loved him. Several times when he had stroked the lining gently, speaking into the caverns words of affection, had not the whale responded with a gentle rocking motion from side to side? Jonah felt that like all lovers they were beginning to find ways of reaching each other.

So the time had passed in contentment and serenity. His initial wild yearning for release, for escape, had slowly come tame. And despair grew into resignation. Resignation into peace. What was there to miss in Nineveh? The world was an unruly place. The people talked only of commerce and war—the one dull, the other stupid. Married to an acquisitive wife whose urgent voice bawled in discordant keys; sons who conspired against him and hated their heritage; daughters who patted his head and smiled at his quaintness. No, he did not long for Nineveh. It was for him a joyless waste where sincerity was found only in the pursuit of pleasure. For years he had tried hard to identify with his city, to cultivate a pride of nation, but in the end he had been alone—bored and melancholy. He had decided upon a sea voyage to get away, to regroup his thoughts, and, he hoped, to find his way again among men who strove against the sea, who were purified, washed in the waves, burnt by the sun. Perhaps he too might find a place. It was this very voyage which had culminated in his happy deglutition, and Jonah had no doubts about his preference.

His musing was interrupted by a subtle but profound sense of change. He lay still trying to assess it. There was no doubt about the fact that the whale's heart had quickened. It was racing at twice the normal rate. Jonah sat up, and in so doing became aware of a side to side motion of the beast. It was not the gentle rocking that he had come to interpret as a form of communication. Rather, it had a spasmodic jerking, tense quality. The animal seemed in a state of high excitement. The rocking became more violent, and the gastric pool was sloshing to and fro with each movement. Crouching in his nest, he became aware of sudden whipping changes of directions, as though the whale were snapping its tail in a great effort to—yes, that was it—avoid or escape something. His own sense of danger was alive now, and he lifted his head from side to side in the air like an animal holding its vibrissae stiff, alert. The turbulence of the motion increased, until Jonah was no longer able to hold to his perch, and found himself sliding into the pool whose usually unruffled surface was aboil with waves. Then, as suddenly as it had begun, the tumult was gone. There were a few last twitching movements, a long shuddering effort, then all was still.

Jonah swam to the edge of the pool and clambered out. He raced to the nest, and listened intently to the whale's heart. It was slow now, regular, the thrill comforting to feel against his hand. But all was not well. The whale was absolutely still for a long ominous moment, and then what seemed like the dissolution of the beast began to take place. As he looked out, he could see the great stomach buckling and rolling, lifting large dunes of muscular wall inward, and rolling them from below upward. The collapsing, grinding action of the walls continued always in the same direction from the dank floor up to the inlet. The cavern seemed to shrink before his eyes and to lose its capaciousness. Then the pool, which had been crowded into a narrow tunnel that was all that remained of the lumen, deepened itself to the level of his perch, and with a great grinding contraction, the entire pool was ejected from the stomach, only a small pitiful backwash falling inward at the end. The contractions paused for a moment, and then resumed building up in force, relentless, crushing the walls together. Jonah felt himself shoved and pushed by the wall which seemed to have lost its spongy softness and had become firm and muscular. With fear and a sense of loss, he was then lifted toward the gullet and forcefully expelled upward into the dark throat, past the white rows of warrior teeth. Above his head the gray canopy billowed, and he was in the sun, blind and prostrate on the sand.

The taste of salt and bile was in his mouth and he closed his eyes and lay still, giving in to the nausea which seized him. After many minutes, with great effort, he was able to raise himself on one elbow. He was on the warm sand of a beach at a safe distance from the curling tide. The land was green and dense. He could hear the chortling of birds.

He turned to look once more at the sea, and, squinting in the direct rays of the sun, thought he could see far out the tall stand of a bifurcate tail. Then it flipped, arcing into the waves, and was gone.

A Single Minute of Fear

She had sat wrenlike on the edge of an old ladder-back chair—small, thin, white-haired, with blue eyes and a startlingly youthful voice. It had struck him that if he had heard that voice without seeing her he would have expected a young girl. The voice was clear, light, with a bit of boldness in it. For an instant he had a vision of a beautiful young girl imprisoned in an old woman's body. "Yes, it is a big house, I suppose, but it's home," she was saying. "I was born here and never lived anywhere else. From up here on the hill you can see the lights on the water in the harbor. Come, I'll show you."

They walked up the curving staircase to the library. From the window the lights far below darted and zipped, like phosphorescent bugs. It was so quiet. That was what he liked best—he could study here, undisturbed. Warren was older than the other students and needed to regain the discipline of studying. Five years of solitude in the Forestry Service had depleted his drive. Passive and shy at his return to the world, he needed the isolation he saw here.

When they returned to the living room, she had said, her blue eyes pale and unswerving, "Of course, no girls in the house. And no liquor."

"May I smoke?"

"In your room."

They arranged for him to work out his rent in chores, giving her eight hours of work each week. She always took in forestry students, she said. "They understand hedges and grass. You really can't get much out of a classicist." She had made that mistake once and that year had ended up hiring a gardener.

His room was on the third floor, really more than he had hoped for. The walls were dark walnut, rather somber, but less distracting than wallpaper. There was a bathroom with ancient porcelain fixtures and a naked bulb at the end of a string. One window was darkened by the middle branches of a pine tree. The other window looked down over the steep curving drive of the private road.

He had meant to keep his distance, do his chores, and stay in his room. For a while it worked out that way, and days would go by when he wouldn't see her. Once or twice, while mowing or raking on the grounds, he had the feeling he was being watched, but when he turned to look up at the house all the windows were blank.

Then one night she met him at the door.

"Won't you have dinner with me tonight?"

"Yes, thank you, Mrs. Pierson. I can't stay long, I have so much to do, but I'd like it very much." He was downstairs at six and went to the kitchen.

"Sit down in the dining room and I'll serve in a minute."

At dinner they had talked of many things. She was an aggressive conversationalist, initiating each subject and asking questions. She seemed far more interested in his history than in recounting her own. "Not quite in character," he thought. He was pleased, nevertheless, and enjoyed telling her of his experiences in the Forestry Service.

At the end she said, "I'm glad you're here, Warren. I feel safe. These days it's not good for an old woman to live alone in a big house. There are too many burglars."

After that first dinner he found himself spending more and more time in her parlor. It became a matter of course that they would eat dinner together. Warren reluctantly admitted to himself that he enjoyed her company. Actually she knew many things and could talk intelligently on a number of subjects, from jury duty to conservation. Unlike other women he had known, she had an earnestness, an open strength of mind, that appealed to him. After the years of solitude he relished her company and, no less, the semblance of family life that she offered.

After his classes he did not adjourn to the coffee shop with the other students but went home, more and more eagerly, and always with a sense of impending comfort. There was the night she talked of her father.

"He was a hunter—not great, but certainly avid." She smiled in nostalgia. As for herself, she admitted a reluctance to shoot animals for sport. "In fact, after he died, I removed stuffed birds and beasts from every mantel and cabinet in the house, and put them in the attic. Why, there was even a great horned owl on the piano, if you please. No wonder I hated to practice, with those reproachful eyes on me. Would you like to see his gun collection?"

"I would indeed, Mrs. Pierson. I know a bit about guns myself."

"I'm sure you do. Well, after dinner I'll show them to you."

Later she unlocked a large breakfront in the library and he took one gun after another from its rack, feeling the polished barrels, the rich wood. They still had a faint odor of oil about them. She stood aside and watched him expertly cock a rifle. She seemed immensely pleased at his excitement.

"There are boxes and boxes of shells of all sizes in the drawers. See?"

She opened a drawer and he noted the carefully labeled, neatly stacked boxes.

"Have you ever shot a gun?" he asked her.

"Heavens, no! I'm not strong enough for that."

"It doesn't take much strength if you know how. Someday I'll show you."

"I'd love to watch you shoot. There's plenty of room on the back lawn."

"Good. I'll set up a target and we'll have some fun."

What had started as a game quickly assumed a more and more central focus in the time they spent together. They would meet in the library and after a brief consultation at the gun cabinet would walk together down the great staircase to the back of the house.

One day she said, "May I try?" There was timidity in her voice.

He had stood behind her. It was all so gentle. Outside, on the far end of the lawn, in front of a cluster of copper beeches, the targets he had set up stared up at them like bloodshot eyes. His left hand helped her support the weight of the rifle, his right guided her eye to the sight, her finger to the trigger.

"Now," he had whispered in her ear. The tiny body jerked once beneath his steadying grasp, but remained straight, defiant, before the recoil. She learned quickly. He felt all the pride of the trainer, the tamer of beasts, the drawer forth, the realizer of potential. She was elated at her progress, ran to examine the target, and kept her score with a scrupulousness that was almost fanatical.

At dinner they talked of guns and bullets.

"I must learn to protect myself," she said. "An old woman like me all alone. There are burglars throughout the neighborhood. They know we're helpless. Now we can fight back, can't we, Warren? Thanks to you, we can give a good account of ourselves."

She seemed then to imagine the very confrontation itself, and discovery of the intruder, the gun raised, the breathless moment of aiming, the report, the impact, the stung body's crumple and fall.

"Well, I doubt you'll ever need to use it," laughed Warren. "I suppose it doesn't hurt a bit to let them know you've been target-practicing. But it's fun."

"Yes, it is," she said, with a voice that seemed not to have finished the sentence. . . .

Warren had lived in Mrs. Pierson's house for eight months. It was November and the big house seemed darker than ever. After five o'clock in the evening there was virtually no light from the outside.

For the past few weeks he had been increasingly restless, bored. His rehabilitation at school was complete. He was tired of the old lady's company now, tired of her constant talking of guns and shooting. She was obsessed with it. He began to get home later and later in the afternoon. Often it was too late and too dark for any practice, and on those days she seemed quieter, not glum but disappointed, and he ate quickly and went upstairs to study.

There was a girl who worked as a secretary in the Forestry School, and he had begun to watch her. One day she sensed his gaze, looked up, and smiled. For Warren that smile was a land of liberation. They had talked, eaten lunch together, and he had taken her to the movies. Later he had kissed her, feeling the warm sweet-smelling body through her thin blouse. From then on he was with Paula every day.

"I won't be home for dinner tonight, Mrs. Pierson."

"Why? Is anything wrong?"

"No, I—I have some work to do in the library." Somehow he couldn't tell her about the girl. She had looked at him for one moment extra.

"We'll have coffee when you come home, then."

"I think I'll be too late tonight. Thanks, anyway."

That was the first time. In the beginning he would tell her each morning that he wouldn't be home for dinner, but when it happened every day he stopped telling her. The more he saw of Paula—and that "more" had developed into a love affair, his first—the less he saw of Mrs. Pierson.

For the past week he had merely lived there in the big dark house. They had not had occasion to speak and he tried to avoid her when possible, waiting until he heard her in the kitchen before he came quickly downstairs and ran out the front door. He felt a certain guilt in the abrupt way he had terminated their relationship, but it only bothered him when he saw her standing, tiny and silent, at the library window upstairs. The rest of the time he did not think about it.

And now tonight. He had left Paula at six o'clock. They had arranged to meet at ten for a beer. As he walked up the long steep driveway he thought he saw Mrs. Pierson at the library window. He looked again, but saw nothing.

He was stopped in his tracks by the sound of the shot and the spray of pebbles that kicked up not five feet in front of him. He was nailed to the spot. Raising his hand to shield his eyes, he peered up at the dark house. Another shot rang out, and the paved driveway bore a gouge several feet to his left.

Galvanized, he ran half crouching to the safety of the garage. Now she could not see him. He knew it was she, beyond any doubt. He unlocked the door of the garage that led to the basement and went inside. "I've got to get to her," he thought, "before she hurts herself. Crazy old bitch. I'll sneak up behind her and grab the gun. Then out I go, out of here permanently."

He noted that the house was in complete darkness, and thought, "Better not turn on any lights." He crept up the back stairs to the kitchen, flattening along the wall, then into the great hall and up the curving staircase. It was completely dark and utterly quiet. At the door to the library he stopped. The shots had come from there.

Should he run in, flick on the light, and rush her? Or creep in on the floor? He slipped off one shoe and, stepping well out of range, threw it into the library. There was a resounding crack and zing which echoed for a few moments. His skin crawled with tension.

The gun cabinet! He had to reach it and get a rifle. He had to meet her on more equal terms, so that if she were truly insane or wouldn't talk to him, if worse came to worst he could shoot, not to kill but to disarm.

The gun cabinet was at the far end of the room, near the back entrance to the library. A frontal assault was out of the question. Retreating, he slipped off the other shoe and threw it into the library. There was another shot, followed by the tinkle of shattered glass. At the same time he raced lightly and silently through a side hall to the other entrance of the library. The cabinet was now no more than three feet away.

He dropped to his haunches and inched his stockinged feet toward the cabinet. For what seemed an hour he crouched there, staring out into the blackness, then reached up to try the glass cabinet door. It was open! He had thought to quickly smash it and snatch a weapon through the broken glass. He knew which ones were already loaded. She must have forgotten, in her nervousness, to close and lock the door.

"Take one," came the youthful voice.

He froze.

"Take one. I won't shoot while you're there."

He waited. His eyes were accommodating to the darkness and he saw her as a small mound of blackness between the large windows in the far wall. He reached for a rifle and quickly slid it from the cabinet. An open box of shells stood on the lower shelf, and he took a handful and dropped to the floor. Crablike, he scuttled backward to the doorway and out of the room. No sooner had he left the library than two shots in quick succession flew across the room. He heard the glass of the gun cabinet shatter.

"Please, Mrs. Pierson, this is crazy. Can't we stop and talk about it? Someone can get hurt."

He tried to keep it light, give her a chance to quit, laugh, agree that it was only a game, and that it was now time to stop and have dinner. She answered with a shot that cracked at the other end of the dark room, spending itself in metallic echoes. Warren knelt at the turn of the hall leading out of the library.

"You need help, Mrs. Pierson. You're sick. Come on, put down the gun. Come out where I can see you. I won't shoot and I won't hurt you. I'll get you a doctor, and when you get well we'll forget the whole thing."

His voice was too loud, he knew, but it was hard to control. He was frightened.

"Mrs. Pierson," he called. "Please. Mrs. Pierson, let's stop this. Calm yourself. Why are you doing this? Why do you want to kill me? You're upset, and maybe I—I don't blame you. But surely we could talk about it."

A pause. "Can't we?" There was no answer. "Look, Mrs. Pierson." He made his tone firm, slightly menacing. "If it comes to that, you can't outshoot me. I taught you a lot but not everything." And then more gently, "I don't want to hurt you. Answer me, damn it!" he shouted. Still no answer. "O.K., that's it."

He hated her now, hated her for frightening him, threatening him. Hated her as much as she must hate him. He could feel her hatred and his own like two dark clouds filling the house, insinuating poisonous strands into each other's substance. It amazed him how immediately hatred arose, full-grown. All it took was a single minute of fear. Good lord, how he hated her now!

What had she expected? A lasting emotional attachment? Warren could not imagine the basis for her desire to possess him. All right, they had both been lonely, but that was certainly not new to her, and he had honestly enjoyed her company. At what point did reason and propriety snap? When did she announce, in silent authority, her ownership of him? It was only thwarted possession that could produce such a murderous jealousy. Even now the irony of having been the instrument of his possible destruction did not escape him.

Maybe there was time to get out of the house. He rose halfway and backed into the side hall. A shot. He ducked and fled into the library again, coming out the front entrance. Good! She had gone down the side hall, thinking he was still there. He crossed the hall and raced into a bedroom. He knelt there next to the doorway, rifle ready. At the very first sound he was going to shoot. Maybe that would scare her and make her surrender.

He stared out into the blackness; then, on the other side of the stairwell, he saw the dim shape floating toward him. He raised the gun to his shoulder, took aim at a point just behind the shape, and fired. She did not so much as start or change her speed.

"I've got to get out of here or get her." He rose to his feet, fired two shots in the direction of her shape, then plummeted down the stairs to the first floor. As he reached the bottom he heard the crack of a rifle and simultaneously felt a breathtaking pain in his left hip. There was a moment of terror, when he wanted to slump to the floor and give in to his wound; but steeling himself he plunged on, feeling his trousers grow warm and wet from the blood.

He was sweating heavily. That shot had been too close for comfort. She couldn't be that good, she couldn't. He was forced to admit that she had improved a great deal in the last weeks of their practicing. The thought crossed his mind for the first time: What if she gets me? True, he was a better shot, but she knew this house. It was like an extension of her own body. For over sixty years it had surrounded her like a carapace. Surely that would count in her favor.

"Don't be careless, Warren," he thought.

He had never wanted to kill anything so much as he wanted to kill her. The hate was like a hot branding iron in his head. He twisted and clenched to contain it, but each minute that it went unslaked was torture. He felt his brain draw itself together like an animal, grow dark and concentrated, sitting poised on the floor of his skull, ready to spring. Was he to pay for a lifetime of her spinsterhood?

"The bullet didn't hit the bone, or I couldn't run," he reasoned.

He raced across the open expanse of the living room into the solarium. This was a long narrow room with a French door at each end. It was completely windowed and full of plants. He flattened against a wall and waited for her. He knew now that he would have to shoot—to shoot to kill. And he wanted to kill her.

Then he knew she was there, in the room with him, at the other end. He could not see her but her presence was palpable. He had to kill her with the first shot or she would kill him by learning the origin of his blast. His hip was throbbing unbearably, and his right sock was sticky with blood. He had to kill her soon.

From where he crouched, Warren watched with mounting alarm as slowly, icily, the moon slid across the windows, frosting the dark leaves of the plants with a sinister shine. Here and there on the walls, tapers of its cold glare threatened to dilute the thick darkness to a vulnerable dusk. In another moment he would be revealed.

Then suddenly, absurdly, the telephone rang. His muscles jumped in fright, making his hip throb anew. It rang again and again and then again. In the middle of the fourth ring it stopped and he heard the youthful voice say, "Hello?"

Lurching forward he fired shot after shot in the direction of the telephone. It stood on a small table at the other end of the solarium. When he stopped, another shot screamed into his ear, hard, grating at first, then purifying into a single silver sound that filled his head. "My God, she's at the other phone."

From the extension in the living room he heard, or thought he heard her say, "Police—hurry. I've just killed a burglar."

Fairview

My dearest Vera,

There is such a bustle and stir at the hotel. It is as though we will be visited today by an important personage. A queen or an archangel or, wild wild hope, by you, my darling. Nothing else would do to explain the "high" that one senses here today. A dozen times have I turned from my book (although it has spice enough to mesmerize de Sade) to peer expectantly down the road. Even the lilies at the gate are bobbing and ducking to get a better view. Perhaps we should all look up, as I should not be surprised if our guest were to arrive from on high—one of your silvery astronauts carrying a tiny planet for his son, or a rug merchant from Tabriz riding smugly on his merchandise. Won't he be put down to learn this hotel doesn't take used furnishings? The swank fairly oozes from the walls. I myself shall inform the cheeky carpet beggar that even the beds are discarded each morning. We never use anything twice! Well, we shall simply have to pocket our watches (pun) and try to keep from going mad with anticipation. Be still, my heart, and all that. Perhaps a walk will help. My neighbor here is an indefatigable walker. Not heath nor steppe, not veldt nor mesa is safe from his clodhoppers. All, all he violates with his lecherous prancing. No virgin territory here. Not on your life. Old Richardson has taken care of that with his mindless laying waste. I myself am an ambler, a meanderer. I just don't like to butt into Nature's business. She knew what she was about, arranging her grass and her sand that way. It doesn't need my boot to sock it askew. No, ma'am. I'll slither through the blades like a little green snake, leaving it all arranged just as she put it, or melt away a morning on a barnacle-bearded rock in the tide waiting for a mollusk to open wide and say "Aaah." But Richardson and I are good for each other. We even look well together, I'm sure. So, of course, we would have to wear each other like apparel for the benefit of the lobby. He is big and red with white sideburns, and I—well, you know what I look like.

Oh, Vera, hurry back to me. Man cannot live forever by whimsy and caprice. And I must get back to the serious work of my life—you, my magnum opus, my unicorn. There is so much left unfinished. The two spots I have neglected to kiss, the one on your neck beneath your earlobe—luckily I have forgotten which one, and will have to do both for the sake of completeness—and the other on your left instep. I cannot have you sailing the seas uncovered by kisses lest some beetling Beelzebub find these heels of Achilles, and slay Love for me.

Your last letter should have been written in light on hummingbirds' wings. It is love perfused with air. To be loved by you is all in all.

Dr. Allain gunned his car up the winding road toward the Fairview Convalescent Hospital. There was not a jot of eagerness in him. He had not visited this one before, but knew well enough what to expect. They were of two types—one, darkly old with wrinkled antimacassars limp upon the chifforobes and samplers on the walls; the other, geometrically "decorated" in plastic and aluminum upon which no self-respecting germ would light. In general he disliked less the old converted houses with samplers that said IN GOD WE TRUST, or JESUS LOVES, or even GOD BLESS THIS PLACE. If he were to stitch one, it would say HELP, HELP right out. This type of convalescent home made no pretense. Just pack them in around the Victorian pieces and dust it all once a week.

He steered his car up the winding steep street atop which he would find the place. It had to be on top in order to justify the inclusion of the word "view" in its name. This one was Fairview. Others were Soundview, Bayview, Oceanview, Mountainview—all precursors, he mused dryly, of that ultimate convalescent home, Skyview, where the insurance never runs out.

Beyond which turn in the road would it become visible? Squat, flat-topped, with ramps like tongues sticking out of every orifice. He knew he had reached the site when he began to see them, here and there on the lawn, propped into deck chairs or standing immobile over canes like withered cornstalks. They would wait there peering through their cataracts, drooped and dripping, until attendants came, white and grim, to coax them back to Fairview. He pulled into the parking lot, driving very slowly, half expecting to find a stray strewn across the path. They seemed to have been flung about by an explosion. Getting them out of bed in the morning must be tantamount to disinterment, he thought. There it is, Fairview.

In front was a huge elm tree in the advanced stages of disease. It seemed devoid of life save for three or four courageous branches near the top, whose few leaves waggled still above the skeleton. The desiccated trunk teemed with fungi which burst through the bark like a horde of marauding goblins. It was in a state of virtual death, or technical life, depending on one's point of view.

He consulted the list of patients to be seen. Alvin Richardson was the first name: ulcer of foot.

"Where can I find Mr. Richardson?" he asked of the nurse at the desk.

"Room fifteen, doctor. I'll send someone down to assist you."

"Thank you."

He passed a long table in the lobby where a clutch of crones sat weaving colored ribbons into potholders. Others painted flowers on clay vases. The grave-smell of wet clay seemed appropriate. Perhaps they were here just to get used to it, he thought. He passed open doors on either side of the corridor, through which could be seen the still mounds of the bedridden. He heard stertorous breathing, noted the smell of feces and urine. There was a rich productive cough and the emphatic spit that followed like an exclamation point. He encouraged his step toward number fifteen. On the bed, all four extremities twisted and frozen into the shape of a pretzel, Alvin Richardson took no note of the doctor's arrival. He lay on his back staring at the tangle of his feet that hung suspended above his head like antlers. One was covered by a bandage moist with drainage from a concealed wound.

"Mr. Richardson?" He asked a tentative question. No response. He opened a package of instruments, the rubber gloves, and gauze squares, setting everything on the bedside table. He had developed an indecent curiosity about the contents of these night tables, upon which the patients piled all of their keepsakes, mementos, get-well cards, and edibles. This one was bare save for a lonely glass of faintly turbid water, one sip of which he was certain would lay him mad and frothing.

A nurse arrived and, leaning over the bed, grasped the leg to steady it while he unwrapped the soggy gauze. The odor of rot was strong and, the wound undressed, he could see the reason. A serpiginous ulcer wound along the entire side of the foot and across the sole. He donned the gloves and proceeded to attack the scab with scissors and forceps, cutting and pulling away the hidelike tissue.

"How long has this been present?" he asked the nurse, trying to keep reproach out of his tone.

"It's gone very fast, doctor. It wasn't there two weeks ago. He must have gotten himself into a bad position with his foot pressed against the railing somehow. Poor soul, but he moves now and then, you know. We find him in the weirdest tie-ups." She laughed ingratiatingly.

Bad boy, Mr. Richardson. You shouldn't move at all, he thought. You should just lie still where you're put. Now see where your rocking and wriggling have got you. A sore foot, and with bone showing at the bottom. We'll be a long time getting that in shape.

"Doctor, may I call the other girls? I want them to see this, too."

"Of course."

Alone with the patient, he bent over the dead foot, directly beyond which he could see the man's face. The eyes roved in their fissures, briefly reconnoitering the operation above, then, preoccupied with a fog of their own, moved on.

The first *pop* he did not hear, nor the second or third. It was only later that he realized them back from below the threshold of hearing. At the fourth or fifth *pop*, he began to wonder idly what was causing it. The sounds were spaced irregularly, about two to three minutes apart, and were not all of the same intensity, some being stronger than others. At the sixth *pop* he turned and with a jolt realized that there was another person in the room, a second or third, depending on how much one emphasized Mr. Richardson.

He straightened completely, still holding the scissors and forceps in his gloved hands, and faced the intruder, or had he been there all the time?

"I beg your pardon. I didn't see you. You startled me."

The man was sitting in a low wheelchair with his back to him. He did not answer.

"I mean, have you been here all the time?"

In front of the wheelchair was an ancient typewriter, and as he watched, an arm flung itself from the man's body, bending and winding as though it had more joints than it should. Arched at the wrist, rotating, flailing, it swung behind his head. Then the other arm appeared, flying up to meet its fellow, steering by the same incomprehensible stars. As they struggled in the air, the huge head tipped forward on his neck, lolling between the shoulders, and turned to face the right hand, squinting to get it in his sights. With a sudden violent jerk the hand was brought down on the typewriter and, *pop*, the index finger struck a key. His body slumped and the arms settled slowly, sinuously to his sides.

Allain caught his breath. The man was typing! He was short. This Allain could discern despite the man's sitting position. His feet, encased in the heaviest of black shoes which came to the ankles, hung freely. The shoes were far from new, but strikingly unscuffed. Worn by no walker, they were either weights or ornaments. The voluminous trousers were black and suspended from his shoulders. He wore a gray undershirt, from the orifices of which emerged two arms and a neck of whiteness so stark as to belie the presence of blood coursing beneath the surface. He had not yet seen the man's face. The right arm was again stirring, scurrying away from the torso, swinging up and out in a grandiose overshooting of the mark, falling in back of the bowed head. Again its fellow took sudden awkward flight and shot up to meet it. They tangled and turned in the air like birds. One, having spotted its prey, dipped, shuddered, then shot, finger extended, toward the key. *Pop* went the typewriter. The great head rose to eye the page and saw the doctor.

His surprisingly red lips were pulled into a grimace that might have been a smile. To Dr. Allain they had the quality of bruised fruit.

"Hello." The doctor cleared his throat.

"Aow." The voice had the same lack of control as the arms. It gave the distinct impression that unless great care were taken, it would shoot off into outer reaches of sound that would terrify both listener and speaker.

"You're typing," he said blankly, aware at once of his awkwardness. "I am Dr. Allain. I've come to treat your roommate's bad leg."

After a long pause, during which he seemed to be gathering himself together, the man began to laugh. It took a few moments for Allain to define the unrestrained scraping in the throat and the heave of the shoulders as laughter. Why was he laughing? Allain wondered. Can it be that he sees some irony here—Richardson's foot, the nurse, my being here at all? Or was he merely embarrassed at being seen?

"What's your name?"

"A-Arold."

"Harold?"

"Ayss."

Allain wished ardently that he had not started the conversation. The man had not turned back to his typewriter, and seemed to be expecting more or, at least, waiting to see if any more would be said. So he was without embarrassment. It was Allain who was ill at ease.

Pardon me for intruding, he wanted to begin. I could not help but be impressed by your ability to type. But something like intelligence sparkled in the man's eyes, and he could not say it.

"Have you been here long?"

"Ayss."

"Where are you from?"

Again there was a pause, followed by the same shaking of shoulders and scraping laugh.

"Well, I've got to finish this job. Nice talking to you, Harold."

Harold did not shift his gaze, but continued to watch him, holding him.

"What are you writing?"

"A ledder."

"How long does it take you to type a letter?"

"A mon."

"A month?"

"Ayss."

From where he was standing, he could see that the page in the typewriter was three-quarters covered with type. He had moved to within a few feet of the man, and darted a glance at the page.

"My dearest Vera," he read.

My dearest Vera! God in Heaven! He's writing to a woman, calling her "my" and "dearest"! Allain's hands shook with a fine tremor. He inched closer, knowing that he would read the letter, knowing, too, that he would be seen; caring, but feeling a compulsion to do it. Within reading distance now, he quickly scanned the page. It was almost illegible, surrealistic. There were many letters crossed out with X's (costly). Words ran together without spacing, and whole lines slanted wildly.

When he finished, he looked down to see Harold, half turned, grinning up at him wetly through his purple lips. There was no accusation in that grin, no resentment. Only, again, an ambiguity. Allain stood silently, no longer embarrassed. It was as though the letter had broken down the experience into its component parts, stripped it of pretense and formality. They seemed to have discovered each other.

He looked at the night table near Harold's bed. It was a wasteland of tissues, postcards, loose crackers, and a carafe of water. In the center stood the framed photograph of a woman, glossy, dark. She was gazing coolly over the shoulder of the viewer, no trace of a smile on her perfect features. Her black-sequined gown dipped dangerously across her white bosom. In the lower right corner was written with a flourish:

"To Harold with love," and under that, "Joan Crawford."

Allain nodded slightly at the picture.

"Vera?" he asked quietly.

"Ayss." Harold grinned.

Part II

Anatomy Lessons

Richard Selzer often said that he felt immediately at home when first entering the dissection laboratory as a medical student. For him, the lab was an intimate arena of truth and beauty, displaying the brute facts of mortality in the awe-inspiring complexity of the human form. In an essay of advice to a young surgeon, Selzer offers a compelling simile: "The cadaver toward which I have again and again urged you is like an abundant nest from which the birds have long since flown. It is a dry, uninhabited place—already dusty. It is a 'thing' that the medical student will pull apart and examine, seeking evidence, clues from which he can reconstruct the life that once flourished there. The living patient is a nest in which a setting bird huddles."[1]

This visionary mindset typifies Selzer's literary forays into the body. Early in his writing career, as he turned from fiction to nonfiction, he was guided by Gordon Lish at *Esquire*. Lish has become best known for enforcing an aesthetic of minimalism in editing such short story writers as Raymond Carver, but he encouraged Selzer's highly mannered style, one that drew on the cadences of the King James Bible and the seventeenth-century essays of Sir Thomas Browne. The result was a new kind of medical writing: comic and gruesome, meditative and digressive, lyrical and even consciously musical.[2] Selzer was trying to see the body "as if I had been in on its creation, or at the least, in the way Adam must have done his first lo-and-beholding in the Garden of Eden."[3] After publishing the essays included here on liver and bone—and comparable essays on skin, kidney stones, and the digestive system—Selzer received a 1975 National Magazine Award from the Columbia School of Journalism.

In Selzer's writing, "Nature" (often capitalized) can seem benevolent, as exemplified in the "fierce energy" of the body attempting to heal itself. But he never allows readers to forget that the natural cycle is also a spiral toward death. When he witnesses coyotes at Yellowstone attacking a mother elk and her calf, or when he examines various options (all grim) for the disposition of human remains, Selzer looks for meaning by first confronting things as they are. In "Flesh Holds the Truth, Mortality"—his introduction to a book of surgical photographs by Max Aguilera-Hellweg—he begins by asserting that "we must admit to whatever exists, deny nothing. Only then can we achieve enlightenment."

One aspect of that enlightenment is humor, and "The Corpse" ends on a note of merriment as the worst is contemplated, and then toasted. In this respect, an essay dedicated to Thomas Browne captures something of the spirit, as well as the style, of a doctor-writer whose meditation on death led to an eloquent affirmation in Chapter 5 of *Urn Burial*: "But man is a Noble Animal, splendid in ashes, and pompous in the grave, solemnizing Nativities and Deaths with equal lustre, nor omitting Ceremonies of bravery in the infamy of his nature. Life is a pure flame, and we live by an invisible Sun within us."[4]

In the 1990s, Selzer's anatomical expertise informed several lectures on painting and sculpture, conceived as lunchtime talks in the Yale Art Gallery.[5] His commentary on "Fragment of a Crucified Christ," an ivory carving by an unknown seventeenth-century artist in Portuguese Goa, shows how this aesthetic depiction of Jesus' suffering transcends the gruesome reality of crucifixion in the Roman era. Selzer's close attention to surface texture and deep structure illuminates both the craft of the carver and the majesty of the living being whose tusk became a literal *embodiment*.

In dealing with the body as represented in art, whether in the ivory crucifixion, in Aguilera-Hellweg's photographs, or in Leonardo da Vinci's anatomical drawings, Selzer's own art as a writer becomes paramount. His descriptions, with or without benefit of visual illustration, encourage the reader to see the truth—and, like the young medical student in the dissection lab, to contemplate the paradox of beauty in the midst of mortality.

NOTES

1. "Letter to a Young Surgeon—III," in *Letters to a Young Doctor*, Touchstone edition (New York: Simon & Schuster, 1982), 56.
2. In an interview with Charles Schuster, Selzer talked specifically about musicality in the opening paragraph of "Bone"—the rhythm of a heartbeat, the inversion of normal word order, the consciously archaic vocabulary—as "a way of poeticizing prose." See "Confessions of a Writer: The Art of Richard Selzer," *Rhetoric Review* 3, no. 1 (September 1984), 92.
3. Richard Selzer, preface to *Mortal Lessons: Notes on the Art of Surgery*, Touchstone edition (New York: Simon & Schuster, 1987), 9.

4. *Hydriotaphia, or Urne-Buriall* reprinted in *The Collected Works of Sir Thomas Browne*, ed. Geoffrey Keynes (Chicago: University of Chicago Press, 1964), I:169.

5. *The Whistlers' Room: Stories and Essays* (Washington, DC: Shoemaker & Hoard, 2004) includes seven of Selzer's art lectures. Of special interest is "Seeing Red: A Clinical Look at Rothko's *#3*," 236–43.

Liver

What is the size of a pumpernickel, has the shape of Diana's helmet, and crouches like a thundercloud above its bellymates, turgid with nourishment? What has the industry of an insect, the regenerative powers of a starfish, yet is turned to a mass of fatty globules by a double martini (two ounces of alcohol)? It is . . . the liver, doted upon by the French, assaulted by the Irish, disdained by the Americans, and chopped up with egg, onion, and chicken fat by the Jews.

Weighing in at three to four pounds, about one fiftieth of the total body heft, the liver is the largest of the glands. It is divided into two great lobes, the right and left, and two small lobes, the caudate and the quadrate, spitefully named to vex medical students. In the strangely beautiful dynamism of embryology, the liver appears as a tree that grows out of the virgin land of the foregut in order to increase its metabolic and digestive function. Its spreading crown of tissue continues to draw nourishment from the blood vessels of the intestine. Legion are the functions of this workhorse, the most obvious of which is the manufacture and secretion of a pint of bile a day, without which golden liquor we could not digest so much as a single raisin; and therefore, contrary to the legend that the liver is an organ given to man for him to be bilious with, in its absence we should become rather more cantankerous and grouchy than we are.

I think it altogether unjust that as yet the liver has failed to catch the imagination of modern poet and painter as has the heart and more recently the brain. The heart is purest theater, one is quick to concede, throbbing in its cage palpably as any nightingale. It quickens in response to the emotions. Let danger threaten, and the thrilling heart skips a beat or two and tightrope-walks arrhythmically before lurching back into the forceful thump of fight or flight. And all the while we feel it, hear it even—we, its stage and its audience.

One will grant the heart a modicum of history. Ancient man slew his enemy, then fell upon the corpse to cut out his heart, which he ate with gusto, for it was well understood that to devour the slain enemy's heart was to take upon oneself the strength, valor, and skill of the vanquished. It was not the livers or brains or entrails of saints that were lifted from the body in sublimest autopsy, it was the heart, thus snipped and cradled into worshipful palms, then soaked in wine and herbs and set into silver reliquaries for the veneration of the faithful. It follows quite naturally that Love should choose such an organ for its bower. In the absence of Love, the canker gnaws it; when Love blooms therein, the heart dances and *tremor cordis* is upon one.

As for the brain, it is all mystery and memory and electricity. It is enough to know of its high-topping presence, a gray cloud, substantial only in the bony box of the skull and otherwise melting into a blob of ghost-colored paste that can be wiped up with a sponge. The very idea of it, teeming with a billion unrealized thoughts, countless circuits breaking and unbreaking, flashing tiny fires of idea on and off, is too much. One bows before the brain, fearing, struck dumb. Or almost dumb, saying pretty things like "The brain is wider than the sky," or silly things like "The brain secretes thought as the stomach gastric juice, the kidneys urine." Or this: "Rest, with nothing else, corrodes the brain," which is a damnable lie.

It is time to turn aside from our misplaced meditation on the privileged brain, the aristocratic heart. Let the proletariat arise. I give you . . . the liver! Let us celebrate that great maroon snail, whose smooth back nestles in the dome of the diaphragm, beneath the lattice of the rib cage, like some blind wise slave, crouching above its colleague viscera, secret, resourceful, instinctive. No wave of emotion sweeps it. Neither music nor mathematics gives it pause in its appointed tasks. Consider first its historical role.

Medicine, as is well known, is an offshoot of religion. The predecessor of the physician as healer was the priest as exorciser. It is a quite manageable leap for me from demons to germs as the source of disease. It is equally easy to slide from incantation to prescription. Different incantations for different diseases, I gather, and no less mysterious to the ancient patients than the often mystic formulae of one's family doctor. The mystery was and is part of it. Along with the priest as exorciser was the priest as diviner, who was able to forestall illness by his access to the wishes of the gods, a theory that has since broadened into the field of preventive medicine. The most common method of divination was the inspection of the liver of a sacrificial animal, as is documented in cultures ranging from the Babylonian through the Etruscan to the Greek and Roman. Why the liver as the "organ of revelation par excellence"? Well, here it is:

In the beginning it was the liver that was regarded as the center of vitality, the source of all mental and emotional activity, nay, the seat of the soul itself. Quite naturally, the gods spoke therein. What a gloriously hepatic age! A man could know when and how best to attack his enemy, whether his amorous dallying would bring joy unencumbered with disease, whether the small would be great, the great laid low. All one had to do was to drag a sheep to the temple, flip a drachma to an acolyte, and stand by while the priests slit open the belly and read the markings of the liver, the position of the gallbladder, the arrangement of the ducts and lobes. It was all there, in red and yellow. This sort of thing went on for three thousand years and, one might ask, what other practice has enjoyed such longevity? Even so recent a personality as Julius Caesar learned of the bad vibes of the Ides of March from an old liver lover, although that fellow used a goat instead of a sheep, and a purist might well have been skeptical. Incidentally, the reason the horse was never used for divination is that it is difficult to lift onto altars, and also does not possess a gallbladder, a fact of anatomy that has embarrassed and impoverished veterinarians through the ages.

It was only with the separation of medicine from the apron strings of religion and the rise of anatomy as a study in itself that the liver was toppled from its central role and the heart was elevated to the chair of emotions and intellect. The brain is even more recently in the money, and still has not quite overcome the heart as the seat of the intellect, as witness the quaint reference to learning something "by heart." Soon the heart was added to the organs used for prophecy by the Greeks and Romans, who then threw in the lungs, and finally, with an overdeveloped sense of organic democracy, the intestines. Since the liver was no longer *the* divine organ in the animal, out it transited along with Ozymandias and other sic glorias, which decline so dispirited the hepatoscopists that soon they gave up the whole damned rite and went off to listen sulkily to Hippocrates rhapsodize, tastelessly I think, about the brain and heart. As if that were not bad enough, Plato placed the higher emotions, such as courage, squarely above the diaphragm, and situated the baser appetites below, especially in the liver, where they squat like furry beasts even today, as is indicated in the term "lily-livered," or "choleric," or worse, "bilious." The assassination was complete. Still, there are memories, and the sense of history is a power and glory to all but the most swinish of men.

Today all that is left of the practice of divination is the unofficial cult of phrenology, in which character is interpreted from the bumps of the skull, and the science of palmistry, which is a rather ticklish business to get into, and seems to me merely a vulgar attempt to transfer divination to a more accessible part of the body. Nevertheless, my palmist always places great emphasis on the length and curve of the hand marking known as the "line of the liver."

The closest thing to liver worship still in business is the reverent sorrow with which the French regard their beloved *foie*. It is at once recalcitrant child and stern paterfamilias. This national preoccupation is entirely misunderstood, and thus held in ill-deserved contempt by the rest of the world, which regards such hepatism as a form of mass hypochondria. In fact, it is wholly admirable after the shallow insouciance and hectic swilling of the Americans, for instance. The French understand the absolute fairness of life, that if you want to dance you have to pay the fiddler. Nothing in our country so binds the populace into a single suffering fraternity, any of whose members has but to raise his eyebrows and tap himself below the ribs to elicit a heartfelt *moue* of commiseration from a passing stranger. In the endless discussions of the relative merits of the various mineral waters, or whether the cure taken at Vichy or Montecatini effects a more enduring remission, class distinctions become as vague as mist. Princes of the Church, Communists at the barricade, légionnaires d'honneur, and chimney sweeps lock hearts and arms in the thrill of fellowship. Napoleon himself, wintering bitterly near Moscow in 1812, yearned not for Paris, or the Seine, or Versailles, or even for Josephine, but for Vichy and *the cure*. Obviously it is in the camaraderie of the liver and not in fragile treaties or grudging coexistence that the hope of the world lies—for ardently though one might wish to wash the brain of one's enemy, to bomb, bug, or hijack him, never would one sink to the infliction of harm upon his liver.

That these same French viciously funnel great quantities of grain into the stomachs of their geese in order to fatten the livers for pâté de foie gras, I consider simply a regrettable transference of their own hepatic anxiety onto their poultry. It is as though by bringing on such barnyard *crises de foie* they are in some way exorcised of their own. Ah, the power of insight! To gain it is to forgive and to love.

Deplorable is the constipated English view, delivered with nasal sanctimony, that the Continental liver phobia is an old wives' tale. One has but to glance at any recent map of the British Empire to know the folly of this opinion. Equally regrettable is the *que sera, sera* attitude in the United States, where the last homage to the liver was paid by the faithful users of Carter's Little Liver Pills, until the federal government invaded even that small enclave of devotion by ordering the discontinuance of the word "Liver." Now, oh, God, it's just plain Carter's Little Pills and we are the poorer.

Man's romance with alcohol had its origins in the Neolithic Age or earlier, presumably from the accidental tasting by some curious fellow of, let's say, fermented honey, or mead as it is written in *Beowulf*. The attainment of the resultant euphoria has remained a continuous striving of the human race with the exception of the perverse era of Prohibition, which presumed to tear asunder that which Nature had joined in absolute harmony. Even in the

Scriptures it is implied that Noah had a lot to drink, and Lot could not say Noah. From its first appearance on the planet, alcohol has never been absent from the scene. An early hieroglyphic of the Eighteenth Egyptian Dynasty has a woman calling out for eighteen bowls of wine. "Behold," she cries, "I love drunkenness."

The human body is perfectly suited for the ingestion of alcohol, and for its rapid utilization. In that sense we are not unlike alcohol lamps. Endless is our eagerness to devour alcohol. Witness the fact that it is absorbed not only from the intestine, as are all other foods, but directly from the stomach as well. It can be taken in by the lungs as an inhalant, and even by the rectum if given as an enema. Once incorporated into the body, it is to the liver that belongs the task of oxidizing the alcohol. But even the sturdiest liver can handle only a drop or two at a time, and the remainder swirls ceaselessly about in the bloodstream, is exhaled by the lungs, and thus provides the state police with a crackerjack method of detecting and measuring the presence and amount of alcohol ingested. Along the way it bathes the brain with happiness, lifting the inhibitory cortex off the primal swamp of the id and permitting to surface all sorts of delicious urges such as the one to walk into people's houses wearing your wife's hat. Happily enough, the brain is not organically altered by alcohol unless taken in near-lethal amounts. The brain cells are not destroyed by it in any kind of moderate drinking, and if the alcohol is withdrawn from the diet, the brain rapidly awakens and resumes its function at the usual, if not normal, level. One must reckon, nevertheless, with the hangover, which retributive phenomenon is devised to make the drinker feel guilty. In fact, it is not more than a nightmarish echo of the state of inebriation brought on by excessive fatigue and the toxic effects of congeners, the natural products of the fermentation process that give distinction to the taste of the various forms of alcohol. In *The Adventures of Huckleberry Finn*, we find Huck awakening to "an awful scream. . . . There was Pap looking wild, and skipping around every which way, and yelling about snakes. He said they was crawling up his legs; and then he would give a jump and scream, and say one had bit him on the cheek—but I couldn't see no snakes. He started and run round and round the cabin, hollering, 'Take him off. Take him off; he's biting me on the neck!' I never see a man look so wild in the eyes. Pretty soon he was all fagged out, and fell down panting; then he rolled over and over wonderful fast, kicking things every which way, and striking and grabbing at the air with his hands, and screaming, and saying there was devils a hold of him. He wore out by and by, and laid still awhile, moaning. Then he laid stiller, and didn't make a sound."

It was a French physician, quite naturally, who first described the disease known as cirrhosis of the liver, near the turn of the nineteenth century. His name, René Théophile Hyacinthe Laënnec. This fastidious gentleman was the very same whose aversion to applying his naked ear to the perfumed but unbathed bosoms of his patients inspired him to invent the stethoscope, which idea he plagiarized from a group of street urchins playing with rolled-up paper. The entire medical world continues to pay homage to Laënnec for his gift of space interpersonal. As if this were not enough, he permitted himself to be struck by the frequent appearance at autopsy of livers that were yellow, knobby, and hard. This marvel he named cirrhosis, from the Greek word for "tawny," *kirrhos*. The liver appears yellow because it is fatty, hard because it is scarred, and knobby because the regeneration of liver tissue between the scars produces little mounds or hillocks. It was suspected by Laënnec, and is known by all the rest of us today, that by far the most common cause of cirrhosis is the consumption of alcohol.

It is a matter for future anthropologists to ponder that the two favorite companions of business are Bottle and Board. More than one eminent literary agent, Wall Street broker, and vice president have died testifying affection for them. Deep drinking and intrigue are part of all the noble professions. These, combined with the studious avoidance of exercise, have conspired to produce a whole race of voluptuaries who, by twos and threes from noon till three, sit at tables in dim restaurants, picking at their sideburns and destroying the furniture with their gigantic buttocks. These same men can be seen after five years of such indiscretion transformed into "lean and slippered pantaloons," with scanty hair that is but the gray garniture of premature senescence.

In the city of New York such is the torrent of spirituous flow as to make the clinking of ice cubes and the popping of corks a major source of noise pollution. It is as though it had been purported by the Surgeon General himself that the best means of maintaining human life from infancy to extreme old age were by the copious use of the Blood of the Grape. It might with equal credibility be put forth that tobacco smoke purifies the air from infectious malignancy by its fragrance, sweetens the breath, strengthens the brain and memory, and restores admiration to the sight.

Counting every man, woman, and child in the United States, it is estimated that the average daily intake of calories is thirty-three hundred a person. In this all-inclusive group, one hundred sixty-five calories are ingested as alcohol. Pushing on, if one were to divide these Americans into I Do Drinks and I Don't Drinks, the I Do's take in five hundred calories from this same source. This alcohol is metabolized in the liver by a fiercely efficient enzyme called alcohol dehydrogenase, and transformed directly into energy, which would all be terribly nice were it not for the unjust fact that alcohol is poisonous to the liver, causing it to become loaded with fat. If enough is imbibed, and enough fat is deposited in the liver, this organ takes on the yellowish color noted by Laënnec. Still more booze, and the liver becomes heavy with fat, swelling so that it emerges from beneath the protective rib cage and bulges down into the vulnerable soft white underbelly. There it can be palpated by the examining fingers, and even seen protruding on the right side of the abdomen in some cases.

Even today, the progression from this fatty stage to the frank inflammation and scarring that are the hallmarks of cirrhosis is not well understood. Factors other than continued drinking pertain here. One of these is susceptibility. Jews, for instance, are not susceptible. One sees precious few cirrhotic Jews. It was formerly averred by somewhat chauvinistic Jewish hepatologists that Jews didn't get cirrhosis because they didn't drink much, what with their strong, dependable family ties, and their high motivation, and their absolute need to excel in order to survive. They didn't need to drink. But Jews are now among the most emancipated of drinkers and, with all the fervor of new converts, are causing such virtuosi as the Irish and the French to glance nervously over their shoulders. Still, the Jews do not get cirrhosis. This is not to say that they are not alcoholics. It has been reported by more than one visiting professor of medicine that noticeable segments of the population of Israel get and stay drunk for quite heroic periods of time. It is also reported that their livers remain enviably healthy.

Another measure of susceptibility is, brace yourselves, the absence of hair on the chest. In males, of course. Unpelted men of the sort idealized by bathing-suit and underwear manufacturers are sitting ducks for the onset of cirrhosis. All other things being equal, women, the marrying kind, would do well to turn aside from such vast expanses of naked chest skin and to cultivate a taste for the simian. It was formerly thought that cirrhotic men lost their chest hair. Not so. They never had any to begin with.

Lastly, it is said by some that climate is a factor: the closer to the equator, the more vulnerable the liver. Thus, a quantity of alcohol that scarcely ruffles the frozen current of a Norwegian's blood would scatter madness and fever into the brain of a Hindu.

There is a difference, I hasten to add, between imbibers of alcohol and alcoholics. Both develop fatty livers, true, but no one has shown conclusively that a fatty liver is the precursor of cirrhosis. One martini increases the fat content of the liver sufficiently so that it can be seen by the use of special stains under the microscope. In other words, a single martini increases the fat in a liver by one half percent of the weight of the organ, above a normal three percent. In the alcoholic this commonly reaches a death-defying twenty-five percent. But you don't have to be an alcoholic to get cirrhosis. Some quite modest drinkers get it. Nor does it matter the purity of the spirits consumed. Beer, wine, and whiskey equally offend, and he who would take comfort from the idea that he drinks only beer, or only wine, is to be treated with pity and contempt. One correlation that does hold water is the duration of time that one has been drinking. Cirrhosis is primarily a disease of the forties or fifties. Even here we cannot generalize, however, for great numbers of younger people are afflicted, and one patient within my ken was an eighteen-year-old girl whose voluminous liver could be felt abutting on her groin just eight months after she had retired to her room with a continuous supply of Thunderbird wine.

The state of nutrition is also a factor in the development of cirrhosis. It is no secret that boozers, the serious kind, stop eating, especially protein, either because they can't afford it—what with the cost of a bottle of bourbon these days—or because the sick liver just can't handle the metabolism of protein well, and the appetite is warned off.

The nitrogenous material of protein passes directly through the diseased liver and exerts a toxic effect on the brain. If one restricts protein in the diet of cirrhotics, the brain improves. A case in point is Sir Andrew Aguecheek of *Twelfth Night*, whose fervent wish to cut a dash was aborted by stupidity, cowardice, and social gaucherie. His eccentricity, emotional lability, and restricted vocabulary were almost certainly due to the organic brain syndrome of liver disease due to intolerance of nitrogen. Sir Toby Belch assesses Sir Andrew rather highly. Still, Sir Toby cannot resist the clinical judgment that "for Andrew, if he were opened, and you find so much blood in his liver as will clog the foot of a flea, I'll eat the rest of the anatomy." Such as Sir Andrew Aguecheek are thrown into mental confusion, confabulation, and even coma by no more than a single ounce of beef. Thus their medical nickname, "one meat-ballers."

In an analysis of the inhabitants of Chicago's Skid Row, it was observed that a customary diet consisted of alcohol in any form and jelly doughnuts. Yet in the cases of thirty-nine hundred such folk whose death certificates were signed out as cirrhosis, only ten percent were actually found to have the disease at autopsy. Thus it might be stated that alcoholics exceed cirrhotics by nine to one—or that only ten percent of alcoholics get cirrhosis.

What is clearly needed is a test to find out which are the ten percent that are going to get it, so that the rest of us can enjoy ourselves. At the moment I prefer to take comfort from the example of such valiant topers as Winston Churchill, who swallowed a fifth of whiskey a day all the while leading Great Britain in her finest hour, and went on to die in his nineties, still holding his fingers up like that. It is also true that if one, moved by some transcendental vision or goaded by ill-conceived guilt, abstains from further drinking, in short order all the excess fat departs from the liver and it once again regains its pristine color and size. In this way do spree drinkers inadvertently rest their livers and avoid the cirrhosis we slow but steadies risk. Thus something can be said for periodic abstinence, a wisdom one would hesitate to translate into other vices.

Before enumerating the signs and symptoms of cirrhosis, and thus running the risk of offending sensibility, it should be unequivocally affirmed that he is no gentleman, in fact a very milksop, of no bringing up, that will not drink. He is fit for no company, for it is a credit to have a strong brain and carry one's liquor well. Saith Pliny, "'Tis the greatest good of our tradesmen, their felicity, life and soul, their chiefest comfort, to be merry together in a tavern."

Envision, if you will, a house whose stones are living hexagonal tiles not unlike those forming the bathroom floors of first-class hotels. These are the hepatocytes, the cellular units of the liver. Under the microscope they have a singular uniformity, each as like unto its fellow as the antlers of a buck, and all fitted together with a lovely imprecision so as to form a maze of crooked hallways and oblong rooms. Coursing through this muralium of tissue are two arborizations of blood vessels, the one bringing food and toxins from the intestine, the other delivering oxygen from the heart and lungs. Winding in and among these networks is a system of canaliculi that puts to shame all the aqueductal glories of Greece and Rome. Through these sluice the rivers of bile, gathering strength and volume as the little ducts at the periphery meet others, going into ones of larger caliber, which in turn fuse, and so on until there are two large tubes emerging from the undersurface of the liver. Within this magic house are all the functions of the liver carried out. The food we eat is picked over, sorted out, and stored for future use in the cubicles of the granary. Starch is converted to glycogen, which is released in the form of energy as the need arises. Protein is broken down into its building blocks, the amino acids, later to be fashioned into more YOU, as old tissues die off and need to be replaced. Fats are stored until sent forth to provide warmth and comfort. Vitamins and antibodies are released into the bloodstream. Busy is the word for the liver. Deleterious substances ingested, inadvertently like DDT or intentionally like alcohol, are either changed into harmless components and excreted into the intestine, or stored in locked closets to be kept isolated from the rest of the body. Even old blood cells are pulverized and recycled. Such is the ole catfish liver snufflin' along at the bottom of the tank, sweepin', cleanin' up after the gouramis, his whiskery old face stirrin' up a cloud of rejectimenta, and takin' care of everything.

But there are limits. Along comes that thousandth literary lunch and—pow! the dreaded wrecking ball of cirrhosis is unslung. The roofs and walls of the hallways, complaining under their burden of excess fat, groan and buckle. Inflammation sets in, and whole roomfuls of liver cells implode and die, and in their place comes the scarring that twists and distorts the channels, pulling them into impossible angulation. Avalanches block the flow of bile and heavy tangles of fiber impede the absorption and secretion. This happens not just in one spot but all over, until the gigantic architecture is a mass of sores and wounds, the old ones scarring over as new ones break down.

The obstructed bile, no longer able to flow down to the gut, backs up into the bloodstream to light up the skin and eyes with the sickly lamp of jaundice. The stool turns toothpaste white in commiseration, the urine dark as wine. The belly swells with gallons of fluid that weep from the surface of the liver, no less than the tears of a loyal servant so capriciously victimized. The carnage spreads. The entire body is discommoded. The blood fails to clot, the palms of the hands turn mysteriously red, and spidery blood vessels leap and crawl on the skin of the face and neck. Male breasts enlarge, and even the proud testicles turn soft and atrophy. In a short while impotence develops, an irreversible form of impotence which may well prod the invalid into more and more drinking.

Scared? Better have a drink. You look a little pale. In any case, there is no need to be all that glum. Especially if you know something that I know. Remember Prometheus? That poor devil who was chained to a rock, and had his liver pecked out each day by a vulture? Well, he was a classical example of the regeneration of tissue, for every night his liver grew back to be ready for the dreaded diurnal feast. And so will yours grow back, regenerate, reappear, regain all of its old efficiency and know-how. All it requires is quitting the booze, now and then. The ever-grateful, forgiving liver will respond joyously with a multitude of mitoses and cell divisions that will replace the sick tissues with spanking new nodules and lobules of functioning cells. This rejuvenation is carried on with the speed and alacrity of a starfish growing a new ray from the stump of the old. New channels are opened up, old ones dredged out, walls are straightened and roofs shored up. Soon the big house is humming with activity, and all those terrible things I told you happen go away—all except that impotence thing. Well, you didn't expect to get away scot-free, did you?

And here's something to tuck away and think about whenever you want to feel good. Sixty percent of all cirrhotics who stop drinking will be alive and well five years later. How unlike the lofty brain which has no power of regeneration at all. Once a brain cell dies, you are forever one shy.

Good old liver!

Bone

Bones. Two hundred and eight of them. A whole glory turned and tooled. Lo the timbered femur all hung and strapped with beef, whose globate head nuzzles the concave underpart of the pelvis; the little carpals of the wrist faceted as jewels and as jewels named—capitate, lunate, hamate, pisiform; the phalanges, tiny kickshaws of the body, toys fantastic, worn upon the hands and feet like fans of unimagined cleverness; the porcelain pile of the vertebrae atop which rides the domed palanquin of the very brain; the vast, the slumbrous pelvis, called to wakefulness by the sweet intrusion of sex or the stirring of an impatient fetus. Out of this pelvis, endlessly rocking, drops man. I agree with those African tribes who decorate themselves with bones. It is more to my taste than diamonds, which are a cold and soulless shine. Whilst bone, ah bone, is the pit of a man after the cumbering flesh has been eaten away.

Bone is power. It is bone to which the soft parts cling, from which they are, helpless, strung and held aloft to the sun, lest man be but another slithering earth-noser. What is this tissue that has double the strength of oak? One cubic inch of which will stand a crushing force of two tons? This substance that refuses to dissolve in our body fluids, but remains intact and solid through all vicissitudes of temperature and pollution? We may be grateful for this insolubility, for it is what stands us tall. How is it that in these rigid, massive pieces is the very factory of the blood, wherein each day, one million million red blood cells are made and discharged into the circulation to course their three-score-and-one days, then die?

Stony and still though it seems, bone quickens; it flows. It is never the same at any two moments. The traverse of calcium from the blood to the bone and back again is a continuous thing, which ceaseless exchange of mineral is governed by hormonal potentates from glands afar. Fluid, too, is pressed into, then extracted from, the bone in a never-ending current, yet slow as Everglade.

In bone, as in other life, there are the givers and the takers. Twin races of cells, one the Blasts, whose function is oppositely named, for they march resolutely, all the while laying down bone, spinning out the hard stuff, each one an Atlas, born to most grittily uphold the world as he sees it. Moving steadily is the army of Clasts. These are the borers who tunnel through a bed of bone like moles through a lawn. No granitic femur is impervious to their chewings. It is not to destroy that they burrow, but to cleanse. No killers they, but peppy sweeps, clearing away old cells, all the detritus of age, the debris of ill usage. Even as they drill their winding canaliculi, scoop out their cavitations, the rival Blasts rush in to line the spaces with new bone. Thus Blast and Clast engaged in a race between growth and decay, yet all to the single purpose of renewal. Still it must be told that it is the Clast, the devourer, that is triumphant in old age, for his energies persist, while the Blast grows weary, his deposition slow. Thus does old bone grow porous, light, and brittle. Thus does it easily break, and but slowly knit.

Cartilage earns the title Mother-of-Bone. Strategically placed in the bones of the young are belts of cartilage which are the growth centers of the bone. During the first twenty years of life, this cartilage is replaced by bone at its margins even as the center remains a fiery pit of new cartilage. It must not be too hungrily replaced, before full growth is attained, or we are too short. At maturity all of the cartilage in these centers has been transformed, save for that which remains to pad the joints or, charmingly, to ornament and hold aloft the ears lest they flop like a spaniel's. In these disks of cartilage is all our stature.

Break a bone, and almost at once the blood clot between the two fragments begins to carnify. Fibrous tissue and blood vessels invade it, turn it meaty. Now, with cast or screw or metal plate, immobilize the bone so that further disruption will not take place, and the jellied mass is entered by bone-forming cells, the Blasts. Calcium salts are accepted here, and in time there is a bridge of new bone between the fragments. It is the trauma itself, the fact of fracture, that triggers the restoration. It is a cellular call to arms, a furious mobilization, an act of drive and instinct. It is the wisdom of Bone.

Remove a rib, if you must, in order to enter the chest for surgery, but leave intact the periosteum, that sheath of the bone. Strip it back, and bite away only the naked rib, and that rib will grow again, fed by the lining of the sheath, until an X-ray taken months later will reveal the marvel of the tissues. The thoracic arch has been shored up.

Bone can be grafted from one place to another to span the gap between two unhealed fragments or to fuse an unstable joint. This bone acts as a framework upon which the new bone is woven until all the pieces are joined in a single unbending whole.

No inert span this bone, but a fact of physical life each of whose parts holds a measure of electricity. Walk, and you change the electrical potential of your bones. Here it springs from positive to negative; there, from negative to positive. The strands of bone line up to follow the direction of force at any given time, seizing the position of greatest mechanical advantage, responding to each stress and shear and impact. So does it bend and relent; so does it not break; so are forgiven all the bangs and crashings of locomotion.

Like the flesh, bone is subject to defect and disease. Should the muscles attached to a bone cease to function, as in stroke or paralysis, almost half the bone served by those muscles is quickly resorbed, and disappears. Exceed the tensile strength of a bone, and it answers with the exclamation—*fracture*! Nowhere is this event more likely than in *osteogenesis imperfecta*, wherein the process of ossification is badly done. Instead of a continuing sheet of bone, there are only scanty nests of osteoblasts. An infant so afflicted may survive the trauma of birth but with half his bones broken. Merely to diaper such a child is to risk fracturing his thighs. In the aged, many small clots form in the nutrient vessels of the bone. The replenishing blood is here and there blocked, and the bone grows withered and fragile; it cracks, most often at the neck of the femur, there where the weight is borne. Such a hip fracture may be the harbinger of death for the old one forced to share his bed with Confusion and Pneumonia.

Ah, but there is more to the skull than helmet to the brain, to the sternum than shield to the heart, to the ribs than staves of the thorax. The rest of the flesh is transient, strung like laundry upon a lattice. To dwell upon bone is to contemplate the fate of man. Bone is the keepsake of the earth, all that remains of a man when the rest has long since melted and seeped and crumbled away. It endures for a million years and, if then dug up from the ground, suggests still to anthropologists the humps of meat that once it wore, and to poets the much that was from the little that remains.

What man does not ponder the whereabouts of his skeleton—the place where it will lie? Say what you will, all sanitary and pragmatic considerations aside, these jaunty saunterers that have held us upright, have stiffened us against the grate and grind of life, are dear to us. What stands closer to a man all his days than his bones?

A savage queen contrives from the skull of her young lover a wine bowl. Years later, as she lifts the kissed and polished calvarium to her lips, her old passion shudders anew, and licking an errant drop from one socket, she smiles in wild ownership. No thank you; not for me. Far better to tumble among the unnumbered treasures of the sea.

Of higher taste were the Ottawa Indians, friends of the explorer-priest Marquette. Upon learning the whereabouts of the body of their beloved visitor, the Ottawas journeyed there, to the eastern shore of Lake Michigan.

Journeyed eastward to the lakeside,
Where beloved pale-face rested.
Dug them up, the bones of Father,
Washed and dried them, Boxed in birch bark,
And the moon upon the waters
Lay a silver path to guide them.
Paddled chanting, in procession
Their canoes all draped in mourning,
To the chapel at the mission,
Neath the floorboards there they laid them.

Homage to Longfellow! One now understands why he wrote this way. Once you start, you can't stop.

I myself have confronted the hard fact of bone and have been changed by it. Listen.

A man named Barney died. He was my friend who sprawled face down upon rocks at the foot of a cliff. The impact had flattened and spread Barney, so that when I could scramble to where he crashed, he seemed to me wider, larger, than he had been. All spaltered of limb he lay, downhill, with his head lower than his feet, his arms and legs reaching out to grapple the rocks to him, the rocks that became him so. Eagerly he had leaped, and eagerly landed.

"When I die," he had said to me that morning, "take my ashes and scatter them in this woods. Add me to this place. Do it gladly or you shall be the less for it." Barney was a hard man.

A tin can such as might be expected to hold peanuts was what the undertaker gave me, after checking the name tag. In a small clearing in the forest, where the trees leaned and interlaced above, I pried off the lid, unfolded the embossed napkin, and saw . . . not silty ash drifting and banked, but chunks of white bone the size of almonds! Here was a groove where once had ridden the trunk of a nerve; there persisted an eminence, round and smooth, to which a muscle had attached. All together they had done some act for Barney. Raised his glass, perhaps. From the can rose the faint odor of scorch. I had been ready for ash; I was filled with dread by these staring bones. From the perpetuity of ash I could have departed in peace, but from these crusts and careless crumbs, I would take away no memory of the banquet of friendship, only a nausea of the soul. Nor am I alone in my terrors. Other anatomists have touched the bones of a fellow and felt their own burial cloths winding about them. Vesalius, driven by his passion and the interdictions of society to scavenge after public hangings, poked among subgibbetal offal to retrieve yet another tibia, one fibula more. And all the while, his own heart grown ossified in his breast.

But to the task. Quickly, as though to rid myself of incriminating evidence, I walked round and round the clearing, spilling Barney's bones upon the oak leaves until there were no more. Then looked down to see them strewn as by some wizard who would read Event from the pattern in which they lay. Nearby was a small park with benches and tables and tall trash cans painted green to blend with the trees. Trembling, I went there to sit alone, for it is comforting to sit beside the dead and measure the distance between them and us.

All at once, there was a noise, an *alive* sound. Less than a thump; a scrabble perhaps. I looked behind me. There was no one, nor any creature. Only the woods where, doglike, I had dropped the bones of my friend. I sat back; again I strained toward respectful elegy. Again! A whirring. I wheeled, and . . . nothing. But now I am terrified. Who's there, I called out, and the whiteness of my voice informed the forest of my vulnerability. I started to walk away, toward the road, backing off. I must not be seized from the rear. And then I heard it again, that soft thrashing. From the rim of my vision I saw a movement. A jiggling. It was a *trash can* wobbling. Once more there was the noise, and once more the jiggling of the trash can. Now I am torn by the need to run from this demonic place and the need—yes, I must—to learn what lurks and leaps within that can that is no one-pound tin but a receptacle large enough to hold a *man.* Back and forth I flopped between resolve and panic, from No-I-shall-run-away to Stay-for-I-must. I stayed. And, stalking, crept until I had circled and sidled that horrid can three times, and heard again and again the challenge of its rattle. At last, I must act or die, and rising from a crouch, I ran full tilt toward it, kicked it with my foot high up near the top, with all my strength redoubled by fear. Over it went, rolled half a turn, and lay still. And from its gape there slouched and snarled the thinnest slice of winter I have ever seen. A raccoon. Its ribs each one visible in its flanks; its tail hairless, ignoble. Slow, contemptuous, the creature walked from the barrel. Six paces, then stopped, and turned to glare at me with loaded eyes, and lips drawn back from mauve gums, from which hung yellow teeth like tines of the gates of Hell. As I watched, the raccoon tilted back its head and loosed from its throat a sound that I shall remember all of my days. A long hiss playing out into a pneumonic rattle. It was what is left of a sigh when the rue and regret is exhausted. I felt the rank whiff upon my skin. Abruptly then, the creature walked to the edge of the woods and disappeared in the direction of the clearing where I had not gladly, not reverently thrown down the bones of my friend. I was once again alone. Barney, Barney.

Ah, you say, and smile. Spooks and banshees—childish frights. An overheated brain undoes the solid mind. Come, come, you insist. Laugh with us. And I try to join. I think fiercely of politics, of theater, and all the stuff of daytime. But even now, years later, I start from my bed as I hear the hissing of those bones. And it does not matter what you say, or if you think that what I've told is true. It matters that I have been changed by it, that I am not the same as I was.

Does the haughty orthopedist swaggering by, tapping his boot with a pet ulna, does he pretend to a courage he does not own? Does he retreat by night to his closet quaking with fear, whilst all around his head the rumble of angry bones rolls and thunders? Or is it some fetish to which he is compelled, that he must see and touch again and again all those hard smooth strokables? For who could gaze hourly upon the bones of man and not shudder at the intimations of his mortality?

So, I have decided. No gourd, nor royal drinking cup, nor forest strew for me. Upon the wall of some quiet library ensconce my skull. Place oil and a wick in my brainpan. And there let me light with endless affection the pages of books for men to read.

Most commonly, bone is afflicted with that ubiquitous degeneration that is known as osteoarthritis, wherein the wear and tear of usage is expressed as the grinding down of the disks of cartilage that cap the ends of the bones like icing and that facilitate the movement of the joints. As the cartilage is worn thin, the joint undergoes inflammation, with resultant deformity and limitation of motion. Hummocks and spurs build upon the bony surfaces, pressing against the surrounding tissues to cause pain, and thus further immobilize until the joint itself is frozen, locked, its range a pitiful semicircle or less. Live long enough, and you will win a measure of this ailment which has, more than any other, come to be synonymous with the decay of aging. That it is most apparent in the spine and hips is no more than the wages we are made to pay for the sins of our forefathers.

Of all the imprudences dared by man in his brazen reach for ascendancy, the most arrogant was his decision to stand up, to eschew his all-fours, and, piling his vertebrae one atop the other, to thrust himself erect. Admittedly, there were prizes to be won by this recklessness. An apple, heretofore waggling from a branch just out of reach, could now be plucked with ease. Ledges and rocks which had, up to then, walled him in could now be overpeered. Prey could be seen advancing; enemies too, long before their arrival. And rocks could be flung farther from the new height. Most exhilarating was the discovery of front-to-front copulation, a stunning innovation that ushered in the process of selection of a mate, now euphemistically called love. Prior to his standing up, man, like the others, copulated front-to-back, nor did it matter whose front, whose back. Now, laughing himself sick at kine and behemoth, *Homo erectus* picked and chose. This one had nice furry breasts; that one was gimpy. This one was bald; that, one-eyed. Having chosen, and wishing to keep the good parts in view, bifrontal copulation seemed but the natural sequitur. Woman, in her turn, was rewarded with orgasm, a phenomenon unknown to all other species.

It all seemed like such a good idea.

But this man who thrust himself from the earth, who wore the stars of heaven in his hair, was guilty of overweening pride. An act most audacious, he had defied nothing less than the law of gravity. He was to pay dearly for such high imposture. The vertebrae, unused to their new columnar arrangement, slipped, buckled, and wore out. Next, the arches of the feet fell. The hip joints ground to a halt. Nor was payment extorted only from the skeletal system. The pooling of blood in the lower part of the body distended the fragile blood vessels beyond their limits. Thus bloomed the fruitage of hemorrhoids; thus are we varicose. Worse still, our soft underparts have given way. Under the sag of our guts, we bulge into hernia. We turn to soft lump.

Alas, was there no pithecanthropoid Jeremiah who, horrified at the vainglory of the young, would scramble to some lofty place and cry out against this swagger? Would cry out to his fellow man, "Down, you fools. Get down, before it is too late"? So we have come to our pretty pass. Better to have maintained our low profile, content to nose among the droppings of mastodons—for it is swollen, bunched, sacculent, hung down, gibbous, hummocky, knobbed, sagging, adroop, warped, tipped, and tilted, that we are made to wage life, slouching toward our infernal copulations and our eternal reward. Such is the revenge of bone.

How Proudly It Heals

In Praise of the Body Republic

At age 20, one looks in the mirror to see if he is handsome enough. (One is never fully convinced.) At age 60, one looks in the mirror to make sure that he is still there. And so it is that from the height of my beshrivelment, I am inclined to meditate upon the body's natural powers of rejuvenation. They are a little short of miraculous.

Considering the fragility of the human body, one might well think it absurd to grow too attached to it. So very many things can go wrong with so many parts. And there is much to be said for acceptance and even resignation in facing the signs and symptoms of our mortality. After all, in our very perishability lies our charm. Precisely because immortality was such a bore (ask Apollo), the ancient gods kept coming down to earth to mess around with us. It is the natural fate of mankind and all of his made things to be born, flourish, and dwindle into ruin. Only abstractions of the mind, such as music and mathematics, last forever. All that having been said, one must remain in the state of wonderment at the ability of the human body to perpetuate itself.

Contemplate the newborn baby—a perfect creature made without heed, certainly without the tight-knit brow of concentration with which a hypothesis is made, yet with no less total engagement. Look at the baby's kneecaps. Better yet, look at her nape. See how it ascends to become the head with the same grace that the trunk of the elm spreads to become the crown of the tree.

The impulse of the body is to be whole, intact. Toward that purpose, there is a fierce energy at work. Most wounds, if left to themselves, will heal without the aid of medication or physician. Most illnesses, too, have as their natural course a slow, steady progression toward cure or containment, leaving only a small localized scar—a kind of ruin, if you will—as a memento of the ravages that went before. Should any part be invaded by a foreign body—a splinter of wood or a thorn say—the inborn impulse of the tissues is to extrude the alien piece, to cast it out. Immediately after the splinter becomes imbedded in the soft flesh, the body reacts with outrage. A dense wall of angry inflammation is thrown up around the object. Because bacteria have been carried in with the penetration, pus—that mixture of bacteria and dead white blood cells—is formed, further inciting the reaction. Slowly the infection is nudged and worked for the surface, causing the skin to bulge and form a tender red boil, at last breaking through to the outside to discharge both splinter and pus. Or, barring extrusion, the impulse of the tissues is to isolate the invader from the surrounding parts and from the general circulation. Many soldiers carry throughout their lives, and without serious discomfort, fragments of missiles or hand grenades that have been incorporated and walled off. In the same way, should the invader be bacteria only, such as those inhaled to cause pneumonia or tuberculosis of the lung, the germs and the tissue they have damaged are walled off by dense scar, or even by a shell of calcium, permitting the host to live and function normally ever after. Prior to the discovery of antibiotics, most infections and wounds were healed in just this way.

My years as a surgeon only heightened my awe of the body's ability to heal itself. An incision, like a ditch or a trench, is a purposeful slice. Through it, the surgeon reaches to repair what has gone wrong with the works. No sooner has the incision been closed, the last suture taken, when what was a moment ago an incision becomes a wound—something that implies the process of healing, which begins at once. Protein-rich antibacterial fluid seeps into the space that is like a ravine in the flesh. Squadrons of white blood cells—leukocytes, macrophages, the whole of the cleanup brigade—are mustered. That area of the wound heats up to speed the process. There is a kind of fury in it. New blood vessels are laid down along the walls of the cleft; connective tissue cells weave a mesh of tendrils throughout the proteinaceous jelly. And all the while, the bits of cellular debris and old shed blood are being eaten up and carried away by the defenders of the host. At the same time, edges of the skin are proliferating; new cells are being laid down like tiles on a roof. At last the wound is sealed. It is time for the hunter-gatherers to depart. The excess fluid is reabsorbed, and any swelling subsides. Over time, the wound contracts into a narrow stripe that will gradually pale from red to violet to white. A hush settles in. Within weeks, what was once a wound has become a scar: a dead, inert, impervious wall of cells—a ruin of the body. And like all ruins, it evokes memories of the past, whether of glory or defeat. Years later, you will run your finger idly along the scar and you will remember old suffering, a passage through darkness, the rescue.

Not every part of the body has equal ability to replace itself. The skin, that protective sleeve into which the rest of us is packed and the organ most often injured, is granted the highest degree of healing. The liver, too, that massive factory of digestion and detoxification, is a miracle of regeneration. Examine the liver of even the most dedicated alcoholic and you will see, everywhere among the sores and scars, islands of brand-new cells, each capable of carrying on the task of purifying the blood and manufacturing the enzymes of digestion. Not so the brain, which has no talent for reconstituting itself. A brain cell lost is a brain cell lost, a state of frailty that is made up for by the vast numbers of brain cells we are given, many billions more than necessary to think, remember, and imagine. We are able to rest secure in the fact of the twinning of other organs. Surely we breathe easier in the knowledge that, should one lung be destroyed, the other could sustain life. So too with the kidneys, the adrenal glands, and others. Should a portion of the stomach or intestines be stricken, there is comfort in that a great portion of these parts can be dispensed with. We have much more than we need. And so it goes, with almost every organ system of the body having a built-in replacement, a standby.

There are those unphilosophical creatures who need show little interest in the lovely process of ruination I have described. The careless starfish, for example, having lost one of its rays, will simply grow another. A salamander that, through some amphibian misadventure, is minus a leg, sprouts a new one, skeleton and all, from the stump of the old. It is humbling to think of man as less gifted in this regard. Perhaps one day science will unlock the secrets of tissue regrowth in starfish and salamander and apply them to us.

Impressive as is the ability of modern medicine to intercede on behalf of the sick or wounded human, it is to Nature that we owe the greater part of our well-being and our longevity. Even the experience of pain, bleeding, and fever are gifts of Nature, a sort of early-warning system to prevent further exposure to unfriendly stimuli in the environment. Fever informs us that it is time to rest or seek relief. Far from being curses, pain and bleeding cause us to recoil from fire, excessive cold, a cutting edge. Without the ability to feel pain, no one would live beyond childhood, what with the injuries, burns, and unannounced diseases to which we are prone. There was a time when one expected to live with pain most of one's adult life; one worked around or even against the pain. With the advent of analgesics, from aspirin to opiates, and their frequent use, we have lost some of our ability to withstand pain. We have forgotten how to live with it. To that extent we are a weaker and more vulnerable race. It will always be thus that Nature, with her vast armamentarium of protective and reparative mechanisms, will either heal us, or not. The physician with his medicines and instruments is but a device that the patient takes up in order to assist Nature in the cure.

There is, for each of us, a hidden life of which we are blissfully unaware. Only on occasion does this other existence come to our attention: when, in the silence of the night, say, with an ear pressed to the pillow, we hear the lub-dup, lub-dup of the garrulous heart or the easy whisper of the lungs. Nature has thrown a veil over the inner workings of the body, whose strongest impulse is to maintain the dynamic equilibrium necessary for the whole organism to go on flourishing. To this end, there is an entire system of protective checks and balances, rather like those that maintain the equilibrium of our government. The human body is no less a republic. Should your blood pressure fall, then your pulse speeds up to ensure the delivery of enough blood to the vital parts. Should you hemorrhage, then the elaborate mechanism of clotting is set into motion to put a stop to the loss. Should a clot obstruct an artery, enzymes are released to dissolve the blockade while, in time, a network of new blood vessels grows around the obstruction to bypass it. All through life, the body is steered expertly through the narrows, between the Scylla of bleeding and the Charybdis of clotting. Nor have we the least recognition of this process. It is good that we do not hear the machinery of our marrow or feel the currents of electricity that course through the brain, lest we be distracted from the pleasure of living in the external world. That the events of the inner body are hidden from us is further proof of the kindness of Nature, which spares us the physical self-consciousness that would interfere with practical and philosophical life.

Let us be grateful that the eye cannot see itself. It is enough that Nature looks on and takes care.

A Mother's Fury

Shortly after my retirement from a career in Surgery, I received a phone call from someone who announced himself as the director of the rangers' school at Yellowstone National Park. Would I, he wanted to know, come out to teach at the school for a week?

"There must be some mistake," I told him. "I know nothing about the wilderness. My feet have rarely left pavement. I am afraid of snakes."

The man on the phone persisted. "Aren't you the doctor who wrote those books interpreting the events of the human body in literary terms?" I admitted it. "Then you're the one we want."

And so it came to pass that in June 1985 I found myself in Mammoth Hot Springs, Wyoming. Each morning I was taken into the wilderness by one of the rangers—a geologist, an ornithologist, an animal specialist. Later, in the evenings, I was to "reinterpret" the park for the students "as though it were a human body." Here follows an entry from my journal of that week:

At 8 A.M. Jim Halfpenny, a research fellow, appears at the lodge. We set out across the park. He is 38, weathered, with hooded eyes and straight, black, shiny hair that he combs forward into broad sideburns. I think he must be an Indian. No, he says, the name is English, as in ha'penny. He is no taller than I—five feet, eight inches—perhaps even shorter, but gives the appearance of stature. Reliability makes one taller. As he walks ahead of me, his compact, solid body gives off a dry odor, like that of mice. No, something wilder. This is a body that has scrambled over rocks, bushwacked, forded streams and, over its lifetime, taken on the look and smell, doubtless the feel, of rock, forest, river, animal. He seems made of bark and leaf and oiled fur.

Today we will study tracks and scat. "Fox," says Jim as he points to prints in the earth. "Four toes with nails. The palm pad a single lobe. A loper." We walk on.

"Bear. No space between the toes. They're all cramped in. Hind foot looks human. A heel slows you down. Got to go up and down on it." He demonstrates.

"A rabbit. Indistinct. Hoppers are light on their feet. He's running away from something." Just so does Jim Halfpenny gather evidence, populating the empty wilderness with invisible creatures, divining presences. Each time we pause at a mound of stool, he makes a diagnosis.

"Rabbit. It's dry and round."

"Porcupine . . . a long pellet with a hook at the end."

"White in it? The bear's been eating bone."

"Blue? He's been at the berries." He bends to sniff. "Smells nice and sweet."

"Cat covers it up. Coyote wants you to see it." About feces, Jim is as clinical as a gastroenterologist.

"The diameter of scat is controlled by the circumference of the anus." He says this without the least irony, then kneels to pick something up.

"Lady-slipper," he says, and holds up a yellow flower.

We have been trekking for several hours when, by a hand held out, palm directed backward, one finger shushing, I am commanded to halt and be still. Jim points to a gentle slope of grassland from which we are separated by a body of water. The wooden marker names it "Floating Island Lake." A misnomer, as there is no island, floating or anchored, and the "lake" is no more than 50 yards across and a like number in length. I should think it more a pond than a lake. The countryside of Yellowstone is anything but modest.

Directly across the water, arranged in classic pose: an elk, her calf, and three coyotes; two with black-tipped tails, black again across the shoulders. The tail of the third coyote has been stripped so that it is little more than bone and ligament, no fur. For a long time, the animals stand immobile as though waiting to begin the performance of a play. All at once, they are touched into motion. One of the coyotes makes a low slink toward the calf. The elk dashes to drive it off. As she does, the coyote with the stripped tail lunges, upending the calf. We see four small hooves waving, an impossibly twisted neck, then nothing but a rumpled brown blanket on the grass. The elk charges the killer. Too late. And stands guard over the body of the calf.

For the next two hours, she will careen back and forth, first in one direction, then in another, as the coyotes feint and dodge. They are low and silver; I can see through them. Only their jaws are substantial. They give her no rest, take turns inviting her gallop, swerving out of reach of her hooves just in time. All this while, the calf shows not the least sign of life. From time to time, the elk bends to sniff the carcass, even gives it a healing lick. But then she must return to fend them off. Clearly, the calf is dead. But she will not let them have it. Again and again, she interposes herself between fangs and calf, rearing, prancing.

But now her mouth is open, her tongue hangs out, light flakes from her heaving flanks. She is afire. Her eyes, too, burn with a preternatural glare, like those of a war horse in the clamor of battle. She tires. But she will not let them have it! Now and then, in the very heat of the fight, she bends to rip a mouthful of grass and chew, so strong is the habit of grazing. That is, after all, her work. But the body of the calf is her passion. Has she not yet accepted the fact of death? Or does she act out of some maternal frenzy? Whatever, the coyotes are of equal resolve. They will have that calf. And their effort is shared; they are three. The battle is fought in absolute silence. None of them cry out, growl; nothing, only the thudding of her pistons on the ground. The tawny coat of the elk is repeated in the golden grass that bends and straightens in the wind as though the earth itself were panting. In the foothills, the sagebrush, frothing. At our feet, the cool unblinking heartless gaze of the lake.

Now the battle enters a second phase. Somehow the coyotes know she has reached her limit. Twice, the skinny-tailed one holds a thigh in his jaw. Twice the elk repels, dislodges. As though a bugle has sounded, one of the tricksters darts toward the calf, asking for pursuit. The elk obliges, and as she does, the other two seize the carcass and drag it to within a few feet of a solitary aspen tree in the center of the clearing. There they relinquish it. But now there are four against her: the three coyotes and the tree, about which she cannot circle and turn with their agility. Round and round the aspen, first in one direction, then the other, she runs, flailing.

"Look at that," says Jim. "Ring-around-the-rosy." The sound of human speech is shocking.

The coyotes grow bolder; there are whole moments when one has its snout buried in the crumpled brown thing. A great red rip appears in the flank of the carcass. One by one, the coyotes dip their muzzles in it, lifting them like Russian flags. And still the mother tries. One coyote turns to nip at her heels, but she is fearless and fights on. A pair of ravens, like black rags, shakes into the low branches of the aspen and settles there, lengthening the odds against her. But this elk says, "NO!" And, all but spent, continues to pound the air, the ground, with all her might, wheeling into the saliva that hangs from her lip. Once more she achieves the body of the calf, gives it an exploratory nudge, bends to nuzzle with the ferocity of resuscitation. I wish for her arms, fists, talons. Oh, I think, had she fists and talons, she would keep them from it. I want her to keep them from it. It is not any longer the matter of a calf, which I understand is dead. It is she. I am caught up in her mad purpose.

Then, all at once, as if a signal has been given, a handkerchief thrown, she knows. And, high, nude, sleek, she steps away to the edge of the clearing. The coyotes barge in. In a moment they are deep imbrued in gore. Their tails twitch, their soft growls of pleasure come across the water. From where she stands apart, the elk turns to cast a single lingering backward glance, then slips into the forest. The last of her is her bright rump, like a small sun. In the tree, the ravens wait their turn. Jim is silent, satisfied. He turns to see that I am full of her defeat.

"You're wrong," he says. "It was beautiful. All energy and grace. To choose sides would be to stop all nature in its tracks. A calf dies, three coyotes live another day. There is no good, no bad."

"Yes," I say. "I see." But I do not see. Is pity a less natural emotion than lust? Or hunger? Save us all from the "mercy" of the disinterested, the fair, to whom it is all the same—elk or coyote. The heart knows better.

It is the next day, and I return alone to Floating Island Lake. It is calm and quiet. Two scaup sit up to their gunwales in the water. A coot preens his wingpits with a white bill. Then, well-scratched, he quivers once and flat-foots from a reed jam into the water with the softest, wettest noise. On the opposite bank, where only yesterday gods did battle, it is convalescent, empty. Or more than empty; a vacancy hovers there, crowded with ghosts. Look! A lone elk and three transparent coyotes, one with his tail unsleeved, circling, darting in. Now the others turn. Each move begets a responding move. See that fellow hanging fast to the carcass until he is almost beneath her hooves. How she slathers. In the lake, the scaup rattle their wings, a bullfrog booms, and the yellow-headed blackbird shrieks his personal complaint.

Reading this memoir now, I think back, not to that time but to a time before that, when I sat with a woman in the solarium of a pediatric intensive care unit trying to tell her that her child had just died. I remember how, wide-eyed and perfectly still, she took the struck blow—her disbelief; then, her spasms of rage. How I fought to withstand them. At last, there came the caving in, the crumpling.

Leonardo's Drawings

Before the close of the fifteenth century the human body was seen in static terms, a piece of movable sculpture. Veiled as much by the taboo against dissection as by the integument which encased it, the interior of the body was terra incognita, an occult, untraveled place that lay hushed, keeping its mystery. But in the year 1487 Leonardo da Vinci began the first of the thirty anatomical dissections he was to perform during his lifetime. Let us visit his prosectorium:

The bodies are lean. He insists upon it. Fat obscures the organs, prevents the fine definition of the fascicles of a muscle. Then, too, there is the problem of liquefaction in the Florentine heat. And so he must choose carefully, sort. In this, he is not unlike the surgeon, who, faced with the obesity of his patient, must delve doubly, shoveling aside the yellow meadows in which the arteries and nerves have taken cover like frightened lizards. No, they must be lean. In leanness, too, there is that implication of strength that is a reminder of the much that was from the little that remains.

But gaze long enough within these peeled and cored cadavers and slowly, all but imperceptibly, the organs take upon themselves a faint suffusion of ruddiness, suggested only, yet unmistakably there. He would try for that with light and dark shading, varying the density of brown ink, heightening with white chalk. Gaze longer, and the tissues begin to swell. Another stroke of the pen, and they throb! All at once, the whole of the body seems invested with a kind of energy. The dissector is coming to it: that for which he is searching with all of his heart—the soul that resides in a muscle, a column of vertebrae, a spray of nerves. And, which to find, he must fend off his repugnance for the task, the handling, the smells. Worse still is the terror that comes over him during these long candle-lit nights spent in the company of flayed and shredded corpses.

Just see the huge bearded man hunched over the long table to which he himself has lifted his prize. (How had he secured it? Was money paid to the next of kin? Had there been clandestine exhumation?) He takes up his knife and forceps, pauses, then sets them down. For once again he has glanced up and seen that terrible head still cowled, the face relented in the opaque detachment of death. Quickly he draws this face at the top of the page; it is a kind of homage to the newly dead who has offered his body for this enterprise.

Now to the work. Everything must be done with exactitude. No symbols; only the facts themselves. It is a machine, after all. He must discover how it works. To do this, he would apply all the principles of the physical world. Mechanics and mathematics first. Later, there would be plenty of time for art. For these dissections, make no mistake, are to be done in the service of art as well as science. Only through mechanics and mathematics would he come to understand gesture and attitude, the body in action and perspective.

Soon Leonardo is totally engaged. The back of a forearm has been slit, the outer layers peeled back. With thumb and forefinger he rummages among the sinews, elevating one into the incision he has made. Now he plucks it as though to extract music from it. As he does, the little finger lifts in a gesture of immense delicacy. He lets go of the cord and watches the little finger fall to its neutral position. This he does again and again until he is certain that this is the tendon into which all of the contractile power of the muscle to the fifth finger is shot. Quickly the dissector makes another incision, this time on the back of the arm, and fishes, tugging first one, then another of the tendons there until he sees the little finger furl itself into the palm. He has found the right string. Grasping both, one in each hand, he tugs them each in turn and sees how the little finger opens and clenches, opens and clenches. Pull at the back, it opens; pull at the front, it clenches; pull them both at the same time and with equal force, and the finger is held rigid in the middle position. Just so does the marionette finger act in accordance with the will of its new master. Now the heart of Leonardo da Vinci is glad, for he has found both the extensor and the flexor digiti quinti. It is time to draw. Releasing the arm, he takes up his pen once more and begins. Within moments, an arm organizes out of the ghostly shape of a man's body shown from the rear. The arm is held rigid and a little apart from the curve of the hip. The muscles of the arm bulge in contraction. The wrist is gently dorsiflexed, the fifth finger elevated and pointing slightly away. The attitude is one of controlled power. More, it has grandeur.

Nor is any part of the body left inviolate from Leonardo's bare-fingered probing. Here, a scalped head wears its musculature as though it were a fan of feathers pendant at the nape. The eyes of this cadaver examine the ropes of his own axilla. He too seems caught up in the absorption of discovery. Here, the thoracic and abdominal organs of a pig are shown suspended from the bronchial tree like a Tiffany lamp. And here, above lines of mirror-writing, three distended urinary bladders, two of which wear the stalked ears of their kidneys. Upon another page a man stands, legs widely apart, all of his viscera—heart, lungs, great vessels, stomach—visible through a great ventral window. Upon his feet he wears the thonged sandals of his arteries. One hand presents dorsally; the other is palm up in supplication. The face wears the expression of one who has tolerated, one who has endured, and who now offers up his entrails as though it is the best he can do under the circumstances. Look further and see a quartet of arms in various stages of dissection performing a weighty dance. Even, we are shown the figures of a man and a woman in the act of coition. They are hemisected, the better to reveal the secret placement of the penis at the mouth of the womb. It is the moment of ejaculation and the semen is leaving the man to ascend into the woman's body. Her face is unrealized as though she has already departed into her orgasm. The face of the man is distant, preoccupied. All the strength of the drawing is concentrated in the great pelvic event, the two figures having been summoned back from death for this "little death" performed in the service of art and science. Nearby, an erect penis, its corpora cavernosa distended with blood, points at the buttocks of a similarly hemisected man. These are graffiti that would one day grace the walls of a castle.

All right, all right. He did not always get it quite right. But righter by far than anyone before his time. Thirty-four years later Vesalius would come along and found the science of anatomy. Still, there is a meaning beyond exactness that is more likely to be found in art than in science. These anatomical drawings of Leonardo da Vinci teach us that God is just as much present in beauty as he is in truth.

Flesh Holds the Truth, Mortality

"'Tis so appalling—it exhilarates—" wrote Emily Dickinson. Here is the terrifying truth that we have all along striven to hide from view—with clothing, makeup, beards—at last exposed. Like the surgeon, the photographer slashes open the body of his fellow man, removes his eyes, empties his abdomen of organs, hangs him up on a hook, holding up to the light all the body's palpitating treasures, sending a burst of light into its remotest depths. Like the surgeon, the photographer seeks to reveal a truth. We gaze at these chilling pictures and we are led into contemplation of the fragility and the toughness of the human body.

I have some hesitation in introducing these photographs to an innocent laity. Perhaps these things should remain the secrets of the priesthood of surgery. Perhaps it is a violation of a taboo to show them. It is not the beautiful or the sublime that is celebrated here; it is the forbidden, the truth incarnate before which even a physician's heart may quail. Anton Chekhov, doctor and writer, cried out in despair during the dissection of a cadaver: "Where is the soul in all of this?" But we must admit to whatever exists, deny nothing. Only then can we achieve enlightenment. Leonardo da Vinci, scientist, artist, vegetarian, also dissected the bodies of the newly dead—forty of them, in the heat of Florence, Italy. Each time, he located beauty and truth and reported it back to the world in his great anatomical drawings.

With the click of his shutter, the photographer hopes to transform his subject—be it a normal heart, a liver, or some hideous, pathological distortion—into a sacred icon. His will be a transforming vision, like that of a prophet. The photographer would restore the mythic to modern surgery. But surgery is devoid of the sacred. It has to be, or so the surgeons insist.

These photographs tell us what is in danger of being lost, that man sets great store by myths. We live by them. Through myth we can bypass the intellect, and free up the imagination, that bane of the technologist. In myth lies intuition and instinct. The artist who would lay open the events of the body for our interpretation is tracking down the pre-logical. He is the enemy of science, a pagan. Let us look together at some of these works.

Among them is a woman or a girl, I think, whose eyelids have been sewn shut. There is something about the brow, the eyebrows, that makes me think so. Or is it the chador of towelage she is wearing. The lids are stitched so as to protect the eyes during facial reconstruction. It is a prudent measure. Perhaps, too, there is some protection for the surgeon as well, lest he see in those eyes something that will give pause—her terror or reproach?

The heart has only just been harvested for transplantation. Harvest. Transplantation. Soft words of husbandry and the soil implying fruition, growth. Our sensibilities would be offended by the more precise term—evisceration. The heart seems smaller than imagined and all but embedded in fat. Only a few islands of red muscle show, and the cut ends of the great vessels above. The harvested heart still beats, the way the heart of a dogfish, removed and dropped into a beaker of saline, will go on beating for up to eight hours. Is it alive? Or only technically so and giving but the appearance of life? Or is it in a state of virtual death? These are questions for the philosopher, the ethicist, not the surgeon. The freshly taken liver, too, lies in the palms of the surgeon, vulnerable but with all its powers of cleansing and manufacturing intact. Soon these organs will fill with new blood and pulsate. See how the incision through which the heart has been removed has not been repaired cosmetically, as by a plastic surgeon, but is reefed up just to get the cavity closed.

The girl, we are told, has a parasite in her brain. It is cysticercosis. She has eaten partially cooked pork and become infested. The parasite has wriggled all the way to her brain. She is young, but what with her crooked teeth and poor complexion and the crown of stainless steel she is wearing, she does not look her best. Never mind, there is no place for embarrassment in the operating theater. Ten thousand years ago, a tribesfellow would have come upon her unconscious body. He would have taken one of his sharpest stones, a fleam, and bored a hole in her skull at the place where the shaman had told him the invader lay. No vise such as holds this girl's head, but the strong hands of another man to steady her. When the hole had been made, the ancient surgeon would have packed it with boar fat to lure the parasite so that he might grasp and pull it out. But now there is a stereotactic crown screwed into the skull. A CT scan has been done to plot longitude and latitude and so locate it. Same thing, almost. Wouldn't you say?

Pectus excavatum it is called. Sunken chest. The piracy took place before he was born. His ribs and sternum developed unequally so as to form a concavity in the front of his thorax, deep enough in some to press against the heart and great vessels. It is a curse handed down from father to son to grandson. This boy's chest is a maelstrom whirling down toward his most vital parts. We do not need his face to tell us how he feels. All of his anguish is expressed by the torso. Let the nipples be his eyes; let the surgical wound be a mouth open as if to howl. It is often so, that pain, rage, sorrow, will be transferred from the face to another part of the body, there to be portrayed all the more powerfully.

Look here! A man is hanging from the ceiling by a C-clamp attached to his skull. It is his spinal canal they are after. The vertebrae have enlarged to encroach upon the spinal cord. There is numbness, weakness, evidence of incipient paralysis. He, too, is wearing the uniform of his regiment—a headdress of towelage, something like Saran Wrap to cover his skin, a tube in the windpipe, and that stainless-steel crown. But there, on the back of his neck, at the place where he will he cut, are those creases, like hieroglyphs, written in a rare ink that has just been made visible by odd chemicals. A message from patient to doctor: *Primum non mihi nocere*. First, do not harm me. And here, in the next picture, through the incision, we see that the vertebrae have been chipped away, the spinal cord made comfortable in its canal. And here is an abdomen from which the liver, spleen, pancreas, and kidneys have been harvested. It is a room emptied of furniture and swept with a broom.

The outrage of birth! This boy delivered by cesarean section, "untimely ripped" from his mother's womb, as Shakespeare said of Macduff. It seems an expulsion from Eden, what with the cool air abrading tender skin unprotected by amniotic fluid and vernix caseosa, the maternal smear. No rock-a-bye baby in the treetops for him. If he cries now, it is for his placental pillow. In time, he will cry for his blanket. It is what we have all endured, then repressed—the trauma of birth. Once again the photographer awakens our deepest anxieties.

And now, an eyeball is removed for its precious cornea. It is held out like something on the end of a stalk. Just behind, in the shadow, fringed by damp lashes, the empty socket. We do not gaze into this eye; we gaze upon it. In that change of prepositions there is revealed one of our most primitive fears—that of blindness. This enucleated eyeball reminds us of the punishment of Samson by the Philistines and the blinding of Oedipus by his own hand, and now at last we cannot keep from shuddering. There is irony in this as the whole purpose of the harvest is that someone who cannot, will see.

I have tried to hold up the lamp of language to these powerful photographs. They do not need elucidation. Words cannot come near the beauty and truth they convey. Like all fine art, they speak for themselves.

The Corpse

Shall I tell you once more how it happens? Even though you know, don't you?

You were born with the horror stamped upon you, like a fingerprint. All these years you have lived you have known. I but remind your memory, confirm the fear that has always been prime. Yet the facts have a force of their insolent own.

Wine is best made in a cellar, on a stone floor. Crush grapes in a barrel such that each grape is burst. When the barrel is three-quarters full, cover it with a fine-mesh cloth, and wait. In three days, an ear placed low over the mash will detect a faint crackling, which murmur, in two more days, rises to a continuous giggle. Only the rendering of fat or a forest fire far away makes such a sound. It is the song of fermentation! Remove the cloth and examine closely. The eye is startled by a bubble on the surface. Was it there and had it gone unnoticed? Or is it newly come?

But soon enough more beads gather in little colonies, winking and lining up at the brim. Stagnant fluid forms. It begins to turn. Slow currents carry bits of stem and grape meat on voyages of an inch or so. The pace quickens. The level rises. On the sixth day, the barrel is almost full. The teem must be poked down with a stick. The air of the cellar is dizzy with fruit flies and droplets of smell. On the seventh day, the fluid is racked into the second barrel for aging. It is wine.

Thus is the fruit of the earth taken, its flesh torn. Thus is it given over to standing, toward rot. It is the principle of corruption, the death of what is, the birth of what is to be. You are wine.

SHE: Is he dead, then?

HE: I am sorry.

SHE: Oh, God.

HE: I should like to ask . . . because of the circumstances of your husband's death, it would be very helpful . . . to do . . . an autopsy.

SHE: Autopsy? No, no, not that. I don't want him cut up.

Better to have agreed, madam. We use the trocar on all, autopsied or merely embalmed. You have not heard of the suction trocar? Permit me to introduce you to the instrument.

A hollow steel rod some two feet in length, one end, the tip, sharp, pointed; to the other end there attaches rubber tubing, which tubing leads to the sink; near this end the handle, sculpted, the better to grip with; just inside the tip, holes, a circle of them, each opening large enough to admit the little finger or to let a raisin pass. This is the trocar.

A man stands by the table upon which you lie. He opens the faucet in the sink, steps forward, raises the trocar. It is a ritual spear, a gleaming emblem. Two inches to the left and two inches above your navel is the place of entry. (Feel it on yourself.) The technician raises this thing and aims for the spot. He must be strong, and his cheeks shake with the thrust. He grunts.

Wound most horrible! It is a goring.

The head of the trocar disappears beneath the skin. Deeper and deeper until the body wall is penetrated. Another thrust, and he turns the head north. First achieved is the stomach, whose stringy contents, food just eaten, are sucked into the holes. A three-inch glass connector interrupts the rubber tubing. Here one is spectator as the yield rushes by. Can you identify particular foods? Beets are easy, and licorice. The rest is merely . . . gray.

Look how the poker rides—high and swift and lubricious. Several passes, and then the trocar is drawn expertly back until the snout is barely hidden beneath the skin. The man takes aim again, this time for the point of the chin, he says. Then he dives through the mass of the liver, across the leaf of the diaphragm, and into the right chambers of the heart. Black blood fills the tubing. Thrust and pull, thrust and pull, thunking against the spine, the staves of the ribs, shivering the timbers, the brute bucking as it rides the magnificent forearm of the Licensed Embalmer in high rodeo.

The heart is empty. The technician turns the tool downward, into the abdomen once more. Now are the intestines pierced, coil upon coil, collapsing their gas and their juice to the sink. It is brown in the glass connector. Thunk, thunk, the rod smites the pelvis from within. The dark and muffled work is done: the scrotum is skewered, the testicles mashed, ablaze with their billion whiptail jots. All, all into the sink—and then to the sewer. This is the ultimate suck.

The technician disconnects the tubing from the sink, joins the tubing to a pump. He fires the motor; preservative fluid boils up, streams into the trocar, thence to thorax and abdomen.

The trocar is doubly clever.

HE: Urea combines with the phenol to make plastic. We, in effect, plasticize the body.

SHE: I do not want him plastic.

HE: It's only a word.

SHE: Jesus, words.

HE: There is the problem of the mouth.

SHE: Jesus, problems.

HE: It is all words, all problems. Trust me; I see. I . . . am . . . a physician. I really know, don't you see?

SHE: All right, then. The mouth. Tell me.

Our technician forces the mouth shut, holds it there, assessing. Buckteeth are a problem, he says. Sometimes you have to yank them to get the mouth closed. He removes his hand, and the mandible drops again. Now he takes a large flat needle. It is S-shaped, for ease of grasping. A length of white string hangs through the eye of this needle. He draws back the bottom lip with thumb and forefinger. He passes the needle into the lower gum. Needle and string are pulled through and out, and the lip allowed to rest. Next, the upper lip is held away, and the needle is passed up into the groove at the crest of the upper gum, thence to the left nostril, through the nasal septum into the right nostril, finally plunging back into that groove and once again to the mouth. This stitchery will not be seen. Pledgets of cotton are inserted to fill out a sag here, a droop there, lest the absence of teeth or turgor be noticed.

What? No penny enslotted here for Charon? No bite of honey cake for mad Cerberus?

No. Only cotton.

About this invented fullness the jaws are drawn to as the string is tied. One square knot is followed by two grannies. Prevents slippage, Death's tailor says. Gone is all toothy defiance. In its place, there is only the stuffed pout of anything filled too much. Now the plastic caps are inserted beneath the eyelids—pop, pop. And here—hold still—we are ready for cosmetics.

The case is opened importantly. It is of alligator hide, imitation of this. Within are shelves for the jars, slots for the brushes, as many as the vanity Death's whore requires. The technician selects three jars. Red, yellow, blue: daubs a bit of each on the palette; mixes, turns, and wipes—until the color of your skin is matched. More blue for Negroes, says he; less yellow and more blue for them. He has said something unarguable—and is now quiet. Many a sidelong glance later, he is ready. He steps to the head of the table and applies the paint, massages the color into the skin of face and hands. This is what shows, he says. And one must do, but not overdo, he says. At last our fellow approves. How lovely the morning, pockless glow! It is a wholesome look—a touch of evening blue in the hollows of the lids. Oh, yes, art is truly bottled sunshine.

Who, but a moment ago, was huffing rider of the belly artist, configuring Death, shaping it. He has rebuilt a ravaged chin, replaced an absent nose, he says. Give him enough plaster and a bit of paint and he can make a man, he says. I wait for him to lean over and blow into these nostrils. He can make anything except life, he says.

Thus combed and shaved (lemon-scented Colgate is nice) and powdered, the corpse gleams, a marquis upon ruched velvet, banked with fierce forced blossoms.

SHE: Embalming belittles death.

HE: On the contrary, art dignifies. It is the last passion. For both fellows, don't you know?

SHE: But there must be some other way. As for myself, mind you, I prefer to be of use. I have made arrangements that my body be given to a medical school for dissection. I carry this little card that so states. In case of accident.

HE: A gesture in the grand style. You join a gallant band. So many are concerned with the appearance of the flesh, leaving ill-considered its significance. Well . . . its usefulness.

Forty feet long, four wide, and seven deep is THE TANK. It is set into the ground at the very bottom of the medical school. If Anatomy be the firstborn of Medicine, then the tank is its sunken womb. Here at the very center of stench it lies; here is the bite of embalming fluid sharpest. Tears overwhelm the eyes. The tank demands weeping of this kind. It is lidded, covered by domed metal, handle at apex, like a casserole of chow mein.

Let me remove this lid. Behold! How beautiful they are, the bodies. With what grace and pomp each waits his turn. Above the fluid, a center rod, like a closet rod, suspends them in a perfect row; forty soldiers standing in the bath, snug as pharaohs, only heads showing, all facing, obediently, the same way.

Come, walk the length of the tank. We review these warriors who, by their bearing, salute us. Arteries have been pumped full of fluid. It helps the flesh to sink, lest feet float to the top in embarrassing disarray. Thus weighted, the bodies swim readily to erect posture. Upon each head, worn with a certain nonchalance, are the tongs, the headdress of this terrible tribe. The hooks of the tongs are inserted one into each ear, then sunk home by pulling on the handle. Each set of tongs is then hung from the center rod by a pulley. In this way the bodies can be skimmed back and forth during the process of selection or to make room for another.

We end skin overcoats on a rack.

A slow current catches the brine and your body sways ever so slightly, keeping time. This movement stirs the slick about your shoulders. Iridescent colors appear, and little chunks of melt, shaken off in annoyance, it seems, bob up and down.

Does some flame far below, at the center of the earth, thus bring this tank to lazy boil? Or is it the heat from hell? Look. A dead fly floats, one wing raised in permanent effort at extrication. A fly? Well, of course. There is food here.

It is wine.

SHE: I want nothing done. Let him be put in the ground as he is.

HE: You are distraught. Perspective. What you need is perspective. Listen. Outside the rain is falling, soft as hair. [A pause] No toilette, then?

Dead, the body is somehow more solid, more massive. The shrink of dying is past. It is as though only moments before a wind had kept it aloft, and now, settled, it is only what it is—a mass, declaring itself, an ugly emphasis. Almost at once the skin changes color, from pink-highlighted yellow to gray-tinted blue. The eyes are open and lackluster; something, a bright dust, had been blown away, leaving the globes smoky. And there is an absolute limpness. Hours later, the neck and limbs are drawn up into a semiflexion, in the attitude of one who has just received a blow to the solar plexus.

One has.

Even the skin is in rigor, is covered with goose bumps. Semen is forced from the penis by the contraction of muscle. The sphincters relax, and the air is poisonous with loosed sewage. Colder and colder grows the flesh, as the last bit of warmth disperses. Now you are meat, meat at room temperature.

Examine once more the eyes. How dull the cornea, this globe bereft of tension. Notice how the eyeball pits at the pressure of my fingernail. Whereas the front of your body is now drained of color, the back, upon which you rest, is found to be deeply violet. Even here, even now, gravity works upon the blood. In twenty-four hours, your untended body resumes its flaccidity, resigned to this everlasting posture.

You stay thus.

You do not die all at once. Some tissues live on for minutes, even hours, giving still their little cellular shrieks, molecular echoes of the agony of the whole corpus. Here and there a spray of nerves dances on. True, the heart stops; the blood no longer courses; the electricity of the brain sputters, then shuts down. Death is now *pronounceable*. But there are outposts where clusters of cells yet shine, besieged, little lights blinking in the advancing darkness. Doomed soldiers, they battle on. Until Death has secured the premises all to itself.

The silence, the darkness, is not for long. That which was for a moment dead leaps most sumptuously to life. There is a busyness gathering. It grows fierce.

There is to be a feast. The rich table has been set. The board groans. The guests have already arrived, numberless bacteria that had, in life, dwelt in saprophytic harmony with their host. Their turn now! Charged, they press against the membrane barriers, break through the new softness, sweep across plains of tissue, devouring, belching gas—a gas that puffs eyelids, cheeks, abdomen into bladders of murderous vapor. The slimmest man takes on the bloat of corpulence. Your swollen belly bursts with a ripping sound, followed by a long mean hiss.

And they are at large! Blisters appear upon the skin, enlarge, coalesce, blast, leaving brownish puddles in the declivities. You are becoming gravy. Arriving for the banquet late, of course, and all the more ravenous for it, are the twin sisters Calliphora and raucous Lucilia, the omnipresent greenbottle flies, their costumes metallic sequins. Their thousands of eggs are laid upon the meat, and soon the mass is wavy with the humped creamy backs of maggots nosing, crowding, hungrily absorbed. Gray sprays of fungus sprout in the resulting marinade, and there lacks only a mushroom growing from the nose.

At last—at last the bones appear, clean and white and dry. Reek and mangle abate; diminuendo the buzz and crawl. All, all is eaten. All is done. Hard endlessness is here even as the revelers abandon the skeleton.

You are alone, yet again.

HE: Come, come, we are running out of time. How, at last, would you dispose of your husband? You must make a decision.

SHE: Why must I?

HE: Because you are the owner of the body. It is your possession.

SHE: Oh, cremation, dammit. I'm sick of this business.

HE: Brava! Man is pompous in the grave, splendid in ashes.

SHE: A smaller package to mail.

HE: You are doing the right thing, I assure you. The physiognomy does not endure in the grave. There is no identity. Cremation is tidy. I can see that you abhor the slough of putrefaction. Who wouldn't?

To the prettiness again. . . .

The good fellow slides you into the oven, and ignites the fire. If you are burned in your casket, an exhaust fan sucks away the wood ash, until there is only your body. He observes through a peephole at the back of the oven. Now he turns off the exhaust, and lets the flames attack the body. Three hours later, at two thousand degrees Fahrenheit, it is done. The oven is turned off, is let cool overnight. The next day a rear door is opened, and the ashes are examined. Intact pieces of bone are pulverized with a mallet. With a little broom the residue is whisked into an urn. The operator is fastidious, down to smallest bits of dust.

The modern urn is no garnished ossuary, but a tin can indistinguishable from that which holds coffee by the pound. It is unadorned. Pry open the lid and see the expensive white doily, of the best embossed paper, creased like a priest's napkin. Unfold it, and gaze upon the contents. Shocking! They are not ashes but chunks of bone, and recognizable as such. Some as big as your thumbnail, chalky, charred. A tin of cinders. Coals and calx—with the odor of smoke and the semen-smell of cooked bone.

SHE: How do I know that it is my husband's ashes that you give me? That they are not his but some other's—an old woman's, a dog's?

HE: A vile and baseless suspicion. Now, in the matter of the cremains . . .

SHE: The what?

HE: Your husband's cremains.

SHE: His ashes?

HE: Yes. Many bereaved find it a soothing term, less harsh than . . . you know . . .

But you are right to question.

Who knows the fate of his bones? His ashes? To what purpose tamp them into sad sepulchral pitchers? I have seen the cremation of two, even three, together. Later, the ashes were shoveled into cans in equal amounts, and labeled. Why not? Great religions have flourished on more spurious assumptions. The idea is not new. Were not the ashes of Achilles mingled with those of his lover Patroclus? Ah, you say, it is one thing to burn lovers, then fondly stir their ashes together; quite another to have one's urn-fellows selected at random. Yet are not all our greatest intimacies merest chance?

HE: Have you considered the disposition of the ashes?

SHE: The toilet?

HE: I am afraid, madam, that we have reached an impasse. You prefer neither cremation nor embalming. You are repelled alike by anatomical dissection and the moist relentment of putrefaction. Why don't you admit that you are ashamed of death? You think it is a disgrace to be dead.

SHE: That's it. Yes. A disgrace. That's it exactly.

HE: Exactly, yes.

SHE: If you know everything, then what is your choice? For yourself?

HE: That is not the point.

Ah, but it is the point. Listen. On the banks of the Hudson, midway between Manhattan and Montreal, squats the lizard town of Troy. In the back room of Moriarity's Saloon, the November meeting of the Druids of Eld is taking place. Harry Bascomb rises to deliver the invocation:

"From insomnia as from bad dreams, from lack of love, from waiting so long you forget why, from enlargement of the prostate, from running out of coal, from constipation, from a sniveling son and a daughter who flunks Deportment, from the pox and from the gout, from a grave full of worms—in Moriarity's, in the woes of day and the throes of night, O Lord, deliver us."

This is followed by the ineffably sad sound of men trying to laugh together.

"The subject for tonight is what to do with your mortal remains. You first, Georgie."

Georgie assumes a leprechaun stoop and a high Irish voice. "I want me heart cut out and placed in a little silver box," he says, "with napkins and red candle wax all around. The rest ye can cast on terra damnata, and piss on it."

"You're next, Doc. Surely you've learned from the dying whispers of your fellow men?"

"Nothing. Nothing."

"What? A physician? Sawbones? Nothing? We can endure your hideous facts."

The doctor shivers despite the warmth of the saloon, and hugs his chest with his arms. He is fresh from debate with next of kin, weary, weary. There is a stain on his vest more terrible than the Ancient Mariner's eye.

"I want," he begins, "to be buried—unembalmed and unboxed—at the foot of a tree. Soon I melt and seep into the ground, to be drawn up by the roots. Straight to the top, strung in the crown, answering the air. There would be the singing of birds, the applause of wings."

"Fed to a tree? All right, then. But a cow would do the tree more good."

Then all sing:

O what shall be done with our dead, old boys?
We'll run out of ground very soon.
Why, pack 'em in straw for a bed, old boys,
And freight 'em straight off to the moon.

O what shall we do with our dead, old boys?
It seems a shame to waste 'em.
So after your tears are shed, old boys,
Why, spit 'em and roast 'em and taste 'em.

Then all drink their wine.

Wine?

The Ivory Crucifixion

From time immemorial, ivory has been used for carving. Extremely smooth and without the granular character of marble, ivory has the paradoxical property of being both sensuous and pure. The tusk of an elephant is a highly developed upper incisor tooth, mostly dentine with a thin cap of enamel. In the Middle Ages, the chief market for ivory carvings consisted of the Church and the royal households. There was always a shortage of the raw material until Marco Polo opened up the trade routes that passed through Baghdad and Damascus. When banditry made these roads impassible, the ivory trade dwindled until the early sixteenth century, when the Portuguese Empire included Goa (an enclave on the western coast of India), parts of China, and Macao.

In 1541 no less a personage than St. Francis Xavier went to Goa to convert the heathen, with mixed results, although by 1570 three-fourths of the city was said to be Christian. This might have been due as much to ethnic cleansing as to missionary success. Today the city of Goa is in great disrepair. The only buildings of note are the churches, one of which houses the skeletal remains of St. Francis Xavier. With the comparative availability of ivory in the sixteenth and seventeenth centuries, carvings became largely secular—combs, pommels, dice, buckles, buttons, and chessmen.

The ivory crucifixion was acquired by the Yale Art Gallery in 1967 from a dealer in Dublin. It is thirteen inches long and weighs three and a half pounds.

It happens invariably that when I have left the presence of the figure, it seems so much larger than it really is. Out of sight, it is in the mind's eye many times its real size, evidence that suffering magnifies the sufferer. The tusk in its original state is calculated to have been one yard long. It was carved in the late sixteenth or early seventeenth century in Goa. In all prob-

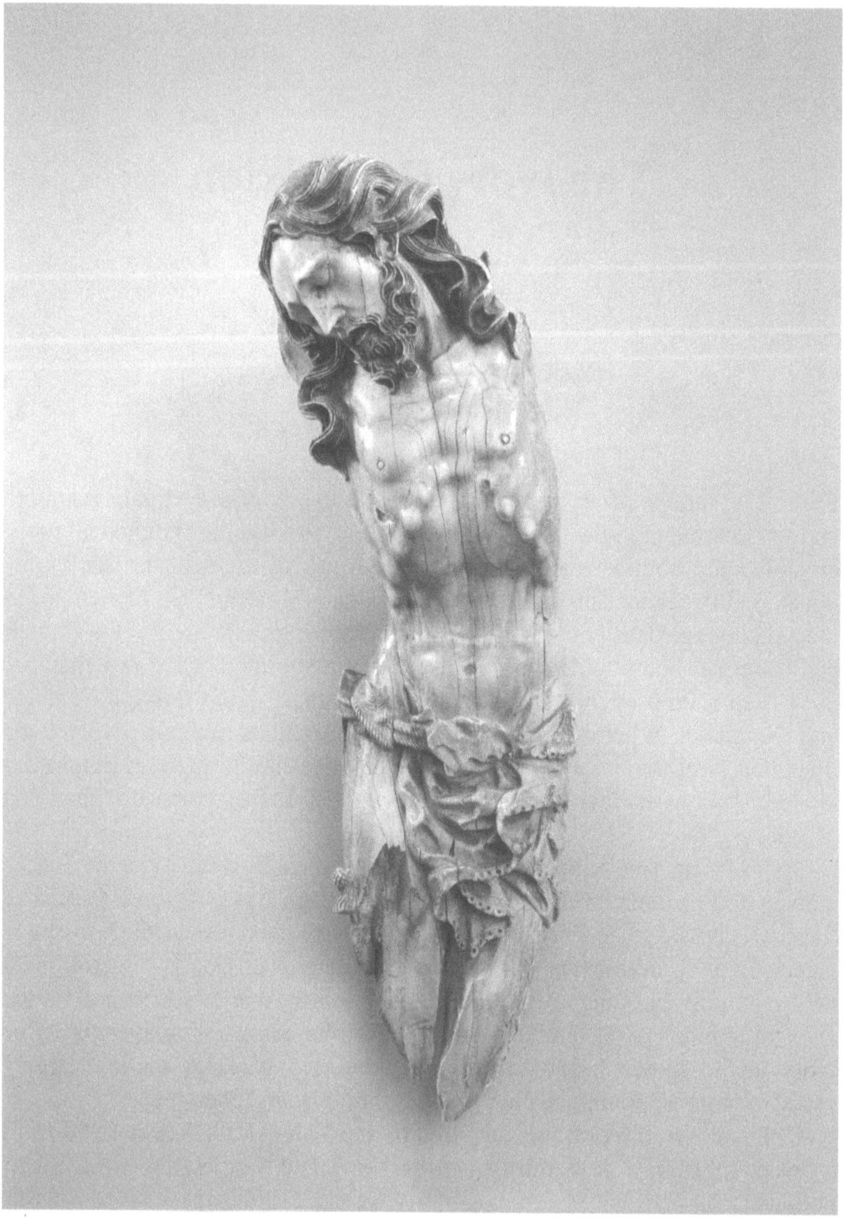

"Fragment of a Crucified Christ." Courtesy of the Yale University Art Gallery, New Haven, Connecticut (Director's Purchase Fund).

ability the sculptor was a native convert or someone in the employ of the missionaries. The bulk of Goan ivory carving has been deemed of little artistic merit. I don't know about that. The usual subject was Jesus as the Good Shepherd sitting among his lambs and ewes, with the repentant Mary Magdalene lying about. In another Goan carving, the Virgin Mary is shown wearing a sari. She has distinctly Asian features, including long black hair in a simplified style. The Yale Christ is, beyond doubt, the masterpiece of the genre. Gazing at this ivory Christ, one cannot help but think of its anonymous sculptor, think of him applying his knife, chisel, and mallet to the raw tusk; think of the months and even years spent in creating the statue; think of the way he must have held the tusk with one hand, cut and scraped with the other, pausing to blow away the ivory dust, realizing the essential crucifixion that lay hidden in the mass of dentine; think of him smoothing and polishing the surface. Had he pumice with which to rub it? Or did he use a paste of crushed seashells, ashes of bone, coarse fish skin? Had he tiny drills? Spoonbits? Did he soak the tusk in wine or vinegar or a solution of phosphoric acid to soften it for the knife and chisel? All these tools and techniques were used: matters of craft and handiwork that would appeal to the curiosity of a surgeon.

Now see him, our unknown artist, crouching at his workbench, darkening the tusk with the shadow of his own body, letting his breath play on it. These things are important—how else infuse the inert mass with his own aura? How else incorporate his personality and temperament? I like to think that piety was the engine that drove him in this enterprise, that his was a worshipful knife, but we know very well that it is not always good heart that makes good art. Cezanne did not attend his mother's funeral because he didn't want to lose two hours of good light. And Giotto, shortly after he painted St. Francis of Assisi taking Lady Poverty for his mistress, rented looms to the impoverished women of Florence at a return of one hundred and twenty percent. So far as I know, no one has ever claimed that Robert Frost was a man of generous heart toward his fellow artists.

Gazing further, one thinks of the great lumbering beast that had dumbly, and unbeknownst to its handlers, carried glory in one of its tusks. The Yale Christ is of a soft shade of brown, with highlights suggestive of the candlelight in which it was doubtless most often seen. The ivory is seamed, cracked, pitted, and weathered. This is a tusk that has labored and endured, perhaps suffered its own form of crucifixion. An altogether fitting undifferentiated substance, a mesenchyme, for the depiction of an event that has enthralled much of Western Civilization for two thousand years.

This statue is an ideal convergence of beauty and pain. He is closer to the lissome, androgynous Christ of the Italian Renaissance than He is to the sixteenth-century Isenheim altarpiece by Matthias Grunewald, in which there is no trace of transfiguration—no Savior, only a martyr. There, the wounds are detailed. Broken bits of wood still stick in the flesh. Blood drips. The hands are convulsively cramped, the feet deformed. The parched yellow skin is turning grayish green. It is festering and bruised. There is exhaustion in the drooping face, with its scraggly beard and open bluish lips. The tortured brow is rent by thorns. All in all, the Grunewald altarpiece exudes a dreadful splendor. But this Yale Christ shows none of the fleshly torment. In the accepted style of the period, Christ's suffering is placed at an aesthetic distance, so that it becomes less human than universal.

The arms are not present. Surely the girth of the tusk would not permit them. They would have to have been carved separately and then fixed into sockets at the shoulders. One imagines arms outstretched upon a crosspiece. The legs, too, are absent, brutally amputated, truncated, and fractured at mid-thigh. The deformity gives a mute eloquence to the figure. Why, one wonders, had the artist not begun to carve a few inches higher up on the tusk? There would have been room for the legs. Because, the sculptor is likely to reply, *here* was the Christ, only here and nowhere else. That is the way artists talk.

It is noteworthy that the position of the body makes use of the natural curve of the tusk, not unlike the prehistoric cave paintings, whose artists made use of the mounding and declivities of the cavern walls to suggest movement and to give perspective. The knees, had they been present, would have been drawn forward and upward as if to ward off a blow to the midsection. Precisely because of the absence of arms and lower legs, the figure is all the more expressive. It is often so; an absence makes a declaration that a presence cannot, much as a silence can be more evocative than a shout.

John Keats instructed us that "heard melodies are sweet, but those unheard are sweeter." Similarly, the German poet Rainer Maria Rilke gazed at a headless torso of Apollo and found that the vision of the God had transferred itself from the absent eyes to the torso, which "glowed like a chandelier, his gaze, only turned down, not dead, persists and burns." Rilke offers proof of this: If not, how could the surge of the breast blind the viewer? And what of the "smile that passes and returns in the thighs"? In the end, Rilke's "Antique Torso of Apollo" is looking at the viewer. The roles are reversed. "There is no part that does not see you." And then comes the command from the poet through the torso: "You must change your life." A meditation that might apply equally to this Yale Ivory Christ.

No less than Rilke's "Antique Torso of Apollo," this figure is imbued by the artist with the property of unearthly persuasion. Apollo's is a proud and godly sermon that evokes remorse and self-examination, while Christ uses His wounded body to arouse compassion and pity. The face is not the only doorway to the spirit. I have seen sorrow more fully realized in a buttocks eaten away by bedsores, vulnerability in a kyphoscoliotic spine, supplication in an arthritic hand, fear in the arching of a child's neck, despair in the blind numb placement of a diabetic foot on the ground. Not long ago I was informed by a man's kneecaps that he was going to die. Turning blue, they notified me that he was running out of oxygen. As soon as I got their cyanotic message, I summoned the family for a last visit.

Before some works of art, we are humbled, stunned. They seem to exist apart from and beyond the human; they speak, if only "murmuringly heard." Such mysteries are not meant to be solved; they are meant to be deepened. This Christ is not supernatural or magical. It is our imagination that makes it seem so. Some objects realize their full potential only in our vision of them, and whether one is Christian or not, this derelict Yale Christ, without arms or legs, speaks powerfully to the emotions.

Where the ivory figure triumphs is in the uncanny achievement of both serenity and anguish in Christ's face. Viewed from the left and below, the expression is one of suffering, pain; viewed from the right and below, there is the countenance of everlasting peace. What we have, then, is a Christ suspended between two worlds, the world of the body (not yet entirely abandoned) and the world of the spirit (not yet entirely attained). It is the moment of transition, the interface between the human and the divine. While the pain is almost over, the sculptor has held back the repose of death that would have extinguished all character from the face, that would have caused it to descend into bland insensibility. Even at rest, there must be character. Here, repose and agony—call it Passion, if you will—are locked in mutual opposition. The contrast is dramatic, the expression unstable. Nor is there any sign of what is called the Hippocratic facies, the classic mask of the dying described by the Father of Medicine, and characterized by pinched nostrils, pointed nose, sunken eyes, hollow cheeks, and leaden skin.

The anonymous sculptor shows an instinctive knowledge of facial anatomy. See how he has shut the eyes gently, as if in sleep. He understands that it is only the upper eyelid that moves in closing. The lower lid has no muscle that would help it to meet halfway. He has placed the whole burden of the agony on one or two skin folds, making precise use of that portion of the frontalis muscle called the corrugator supercilii—the knitter of the brow. This muscle is composed of transverse fibers that are attached at one end to the frontal bone at the inner end of the orbital socket, where nose and eye meet. The other end is attached, not to the bone as is usual, but to the dermis, the deepest layer of the skin itself. Even without benefit of gazing into the eyes, we are entirely absorbed in His condition, which is one of utter self-absorption. He is alone, isolated in his Passion and aglow with His suffering.

As for the expression of the body of Christ, it is exerted entirely by the tension of the torso, which both writhes and sags limply. The exaggerated rib cage and the engorged neck veins serve to convey the straining of the body as it strives to exhale against the inertia of the diaphragm. Each rib ends in a bony knob that is riveted to the sternum as to a battleship. The posture of the body combines with the dramatic fall of the head to the right shoulder. There is the wealth of His hair, grown past the shoulders and spreading like a dark star from the crown of His head. Missing, too, is the crown of thorns, although a faint trace of red at the hairline may be evidence that it had once been there. There is also a bit of red at the mouth and at the side wound. The head fallen thus is reminiscent of the passage of *The Aeneid* in which Virgil describes the death of one of his heroes, Euryalus:

> . . . And on the shoulder
> the neck droops over, as a bright-colored flower
> Droops when the ploughshare bends it, or as poppies
> Sink under the weight of heavy summer rainfall.

The idealized posture of Virgil's dead hero, who was also one of the good guys, is typical of heroic death, such as that of Leander or St. Sebastian. It is characteristic of the death of a hero or a righteous man. Notice that there is not the natural equipoise of the sleeper, whose muscles and joints are relaxed. Nor does it have the heaviness of a corpse. There is tension in every part of His body.

The drapery that conceals Christ's nakedness is tied to the body by rope that weaves in and out. The folds are dramatically accentuated by being sharply incised and by a rather sophisticated use of light and dark. If there is anything in Christian art more hypocritical than Christ's loincloth, I don't know what it could be. The blame is not the artist's; he is, after all, a child of his time. It was thought pious to protect the modesty of Christ, and he made no distinction between nakedness and nudity. The nude in art is most often an erotic figure designed to arouse carnal thoughts. The naked human form, on the other hand, is far from erotic. It is piteous, vulnerable, supplicant, and ashamed. The nude is not ashamed, but joyous and proud of the fact. To be naked is to be devoid of physical pride, defenseless. It should come as no surprise that, to a doctor, the human body, whether naked or nude, is the greatest subject for art.

Covering up Christ with a loincloth at all, even a plain diaper, is a trivialization of the Incarnation. In the same way, it is far more diagnostic for a doctor to watch a man remove his soiled underwear to show his wounded body than it is to read a yard of data from the computer. And here on this Ivory Christ we have the Imperial Diaper itself, an obi right out of kabuki theatre. Festooned and draped, it produces the ironic effect of riveting the imagination on the genitalia cowering way beneath. If one is asked to believe that what existed at the very beginning entered the atmosphere of His creation in human form, then one must accept that, while in human form, He engaged in human activities and that he had the complete anatomy of a man. It is not only hypocritical to carve or paint for Christ a loincloth, it is artistically dishonest. It is a far cry from the phallic religions and fertility cults that antedated or were coeval with Christianity, and that celebrated the sexual and the procreative. In stripping off the loincloth in his rendition of the Crucifixion, Michelangelo was not trying to *épater le bourgeoisie*; he was restoring dignity to the Incarnation.

The artist who would prettify or soften the Crucifixion is missing the point. The aim was to kill horribly and to subject the victim to the utmost humiliation. It involved a preliminary whipping with the dreaded Roman *flagrum*—a leather whip with three tails. At the tip of each tail there was a small dumbbell-shaped weight of iron or bone or wood. With each lash of the whip, the three bits dug into the flesh. The victim was tied or chained to a post, and two centurions stood on either side. The wounds extended around to the chest and abdomen. Profuse bleeding ensued. Then the man was beaten on the head with reeds so that his face was bruised, his nose broken. In the case of Jesus, in order to further deride him and to mock his appellation as King of the Jews, a crown of thorns was placed on his brow and temples.

At one point a Roman soldier hurled the spear that opened the wound in His side. Jesus, weakened by a night of fasting and prayer, as by the flogging and blood loss, was not able to carry his own cross to the place of execution as the punishment required. Simon of Cyrene did it for Him. Then His hands were nailed to the crosspiece, and the whole apparatus was raised and set into a groove on the upright part. The height was approximately seven and a half feet. To add to the suffering, Jesus was assailed by extreme thirst, as is usual in instances of severe blood loss and dehydration. On one occasion, a disciple was able to reach up and give Him a drink through a hollow straw. To ensure maximum humiliation, the cross was set up in a public place, along a main highway or at a crossroads or on an elevation of land such as the hill of Calvary. Death resulted from shock, both traumatic and hypovolemic, and from respiratory failure due to the difficulty of expelling air from the lungs in the upright and suspended position, in which the diaphragm does not rise easily. It is altogether understandable that Jesus, the night before, said to God: "If at all possible, let this cup pass from my lips."

Crucifixion was practiced not only by the Romans, but by all of the peoples of that time, including—rarely—the Jews. After the slave uprisings led by Spartacus in Rome in 71 B.C., six thousand insurrectionists were crucified at one time. In A.D. 70, in Judaea, five hundred Jews were similarly executed each day. In the late 1970s, a burial mound outside the city of Jerusalem was excavated and the skeleton of a young man unearthed. A spike had been driven through both heel bones and was still in place. Ordinarily the iron spikes were withdrawn after death and reused many times. In this instance, the spike had become bent during the driving and could not be retrieved.

A sculpture such as the *Ivory Crucifixion* exists all by itself; it has no companions, no background or surroundings to describe or to reflect upon. The entire artistic burden is carried by the figure affixed to a plain brown piece of cloth and hung inside a glass case. Alone, it retains its purity. Christ is portrayed apart from all *situation*, unmolested by any intrusion. And yet, full of the vitality and the allure produced by the coalescence of body and spirit. I mean no disparagement, but at the Yale museum this beautiful Christ hangs on the wall immediately adjacent to a sacrilegious elevator. It is rather like giving a little girl a doll, then nailing it up on a wall out of her reach. Out of harm's way, you tell her, but she is not consoled. She had wanted to take care of it, to hug and kiss it. But that is a shortcoming of The Museum, and no, Art is not Life, we are told. Surely a more congenial place might be found? A niche, say, lit by candles to encourage the possibility that, at any moment, He might relent into the uncarved tusk from which he had been wrested. In much the same way, hanging a Titian in an apse makes the dark shadows of a church work for him.

I deplore the practice of covering paintings with glass. The reflection is always wrong, so that you can't see for the glare. And if the painting is dark, a Murillo say, or a Zurbaran, all you can see is yourself. Not long ago, at the Cleveland Art Museum, I watched a woman putting on lipstick in front of a *Temptation of St. Anthony*!

Confronted by the Yale Christ, with its missing parts, the cracks and darkening of the ivory, it is only natural that one's thoughts turn to ruins. In the matter of ruination, I am all on the side of the ravages of time. It is not destruction but gentle evidence that everything created and those who created it will one day return to that state of shapeless quiescence from which might spring a new art or even a new species. Could this have been on the mind of John Keats when he addressed the sky children? "For on our heels a fresh perfection treads." I'm opposed to the restoration of old paintings. Such cleaning, scraping, and touching up are futile attempts to deny the finitude of things, rather like embalming a corpse. In the end, it is all the same. The restored painting has little resemblance to the lovely "ruin" it had become. The new product is apt to be garish and vulgar as well as counterfeit. Surely it has been robbed of its dignity, and looks for all the world like someone elderly who has been got at by a swarm of plastic surgeons. When will art historians learn that Time adds its own slow strokes to every work of art? A scab of lint, soot, dead bugs, and cobwebs gives a kind of fourth dimension to a painting, just the right hallucinative touch to an *Annunciation. A Deposition from the Cross*, seen through a film of mildew and flyspeck, is suitably darkened, the sorrow of the Virgin magnified. As in the ruin and decline of the living human body, Time is the gentle nurse that eases a work of art into the irretrievable past. As far as I'm concerned, she can have her way with me, too.

I'm not at all sure that a museum is the best place to encounter this figure. You aren't allowed to touch it, to palpate it, as a doctor would examine a patient—arguably no less sacred a personage. You can't brandish it *en militaire* and then go off on a Crusade to the Holy Land to rescue Jerusalem from the likes of me. Nor can you pick the statue up and march in procession behind braziers of incense to the angelic blare of trumpets. It is not, after all, a trophy, something won on the field of battle or in a contest. No, all you can do is peer at it through glass, which is all right for an icon that carries with it the implication of being on high and at a respectful distance. Icons are meant to be prayed to, knelt before. They're nowhere near as useful as amulets, charms, or the welter of *bondieuserie*—scapulars, rosaries, medallions—that are on sale outside shrines. An amulet can be palmed, worn about the neck, kept in a pocket or, if no one is looking, kissed. An amulet gets you safely through the day. An amulet asks of you no worship, piety, or confession. It simply offers all the ancient power of superstition, and in the absence of faith, I have found that superstition does very nicely.

Still, the Yale *Ivory Crucifixion* teaches the essential holiness of the body. Just as every elephant contains within its tusk such a possibility, so is every body pregnant with the sacred, the unspeakable, the beautiful. The clearest evidence of this is in the body wounded, of which the crucified Christ is the literary, religious, and artistic exemplar.

There is a book called *The Bestiary* that was hand-copied by monks in the twelfth century. In one chapter, we learn that an elephant, having fallen down, cannot get up again. Therefore, when an elephant wants to sleep, it leans against a tree in order to do so. A hunter, wishing to kill the beast and harvest its tusks, saws partially through the tree so that, when the elephant leans, the tree and, with it, the elephant will tumble. The fallen elephant cries out for help. The largest elephant in the herd comes running, but is unable to raise him up. Together they trumpet for help, and the other twelve elephants arrive, but they cannot raise their fallen comrade either. All fourteen elephants call out together, whereupon a runt of an elephant, the smallest and most insignificant in the tribe, appears. He pushes his proboscis and his tusks under the fallen one and lifts him easily to his feet. According to *The Bestiary*, the runt is Jesus Christ who, although He was the greatest, was made insignificant and obedient even unto death in order that He might raise up men. To the readers of the twelfth century, this was a wonderful story. It gave them real pleasure to think of Christ as an insignificant elephant. Just as eight hundred years later, it gives us pleasure to know that one elephant, the Yale elephant, carried within its tusk a powerful image of that same Jesus Christ. It is a dramatic closure that is utterly satisfying.

Part III

Being a Doctor

Richard Selzer's memoir *Down from Troy* (1992) is subtitled *A Doctor Comes of Age*. While the book details the author's lifelong education in medicine, it focuses most sharply on lessons learned by observing and accompanying his father, Julius Louis Selzer, a general practitioner in Troy, New York. In all of Richard Selzer's writing, Julius emerges as a loving father and an ideal physician—brave, intelligent, and genuinely caring: "He was a compassionate man who loved his patients as they loved him, and that is probably most essential in the practice of medicine."[1] When his father died suddenly of a heart attack in 1941, Richard's vocation became clear. In "Reflections on Doctoring" he explains: "If I could no longer find him in the flesh, I would find my father through the work that he did."

While working as a medical resident at Yale in 1955, Selzer was drafted into the Army and sent to Korea. At twenty-six, he became commander of a rudimentary medical company in a small village, where he insisted on treating Korean civilians as well as American servicemen. His duties were unlimited: "Surgery, obstetrics, purifying the water, general medicine, dermatology, treating all the diseases—it was everything."[2] Selzer also kept a journal and later fictionalized his experiences in a manuscript called *The Bronze Gong*. Fifty years later, this manuscript, revised as *Knife Song Korea: A Novel*, was published by State University of New York Press and was honored with an Independent Publishers Book Award.

The chapter from *Knife Song Korea* reprinted here dramatizes the harsh physical challenges of performing basic emergency medicine under primitive conditions. But Selzer's writing has more often dramatized ethical challenges. His short story "Mercy," for example, is just one of several narratives dealing with euthanasia. In other stories and essays, Selzer has explored conflicts about abortion, patient privacy, the mechanization of medicine, and the AIDS epidemic.

Selzer's reportage about AIDS in Haiti, "A Mask on the Face of Death," appeared in *Life* magazine, and then was selected by Annie Dillard for inclusion in *The Best American Essays: 1988* (Houghton Mifflin). An earlier example of his reportage, "The Scalpels of Arequipa," appeared in *Vanity Fair*, an edited version of which became the title essay in Selzer's 1986 book, *Taking the World in for Repairs*. Both essays make effective use of the present tense to convey the immediacy of medical encounters, as well as the interior monologues of a restless mind in a foreign setting. Selzer's occasional work as a medical missionary also led to "Imelda"—a tale so densely layered that even some sophisticated readers have assumed that it is another example of brilliant nonfiction.[3] In fact, "Imelda" is simply one of Richard Selzer's greatest short stories.

Two previously unpublished lectures, one light and one meditative, ask what it means to be a good doctor, and both circle back to Julius Selzer as a model of medicine as vocation. "Three Doctors" was a witty address to members of the New Haven Sherlock Holmes Society. "Reflections on Doctoring," a brief talk to Yale medical students, concluded with vignettes drawn from three of Selzer's published essays, each capturing a sudden compassionate insight. These haunting epiphanies also anticipate the sacramental moments detailed in this book's next section, "Illuminations."

NOTES

1. Richard Selzer, *Mortal Lessons: Notes on the Art of Surgery*, Touchstone edition (New York: Simon & Schuster, 1987), 178.
2. Peter Josyph, ed., *What One Man Said to Another: Talks with Richard Selzer* (East Lansing: Michigan State University Press, 1994), 34.
3. The story was anthologized, for instance, in *The Touchstone Anthology of Contemporary Creative Nonfiction*, ed. Lex Williford and Michael Martone (New York: Simon & Schuster, 2007).

A Hero in a Rowboat (from Chapter 2 of *Down from Troy: A Doctor Comes of Age*)

When the flood came, no one thought of moving to higher ground. That was not our way. And so we stayed and watched the river licking bricks out of the walls, stones out of the street. For days on end the rain came down in sheets. From the kitchen window, the empty lot and King Street were a single lake. One time, through a scrim of rain I saw the figure of Christ walking on the water just as he had done at Galilee. I ran to get Billy.

"Look!" I cried, pointing to the apparition. "It's Jesus!"

Billy peered through the curtain of rain. "That," he announced in a voice dripping with disgust, "is no such thing. It's Old Man Sheridan standing on the roof of his Chevrolet."

"Don't tell anyone," I pleaded.

"I might and I might not," he offered, by which I guessed he would not.

Later I watched from the bay window as Father set out from the front porch to make a house call in a rowboat.

"Where are you going?" I shouted.

"Down to Washington Park," he called back.

"Can I come? Oh, please wait for me!" But, sitting in the boat, wearing his fedora and long overcoat and with a Lucky Strike clamped between his teeth, the bravest man in all Troy set out alone into the raging current that had been Fifth Avenue. Almost at once he seemed to be having trouble with the oars. At the corner of Fifth and Federal the two marauding streams turned incompatible and threw themselves into one another. With mounting horror I saw the little boat go tipsy and begin to circle in the maelstrom.

"I surely do hope it is not an emergency down there at Washington Park," said Mother. Then, as an afterthought, "He doesn't know how to swim."

Occupying the other seat in the rowboat was Father's black bag with its rows of pill bottles and jars of salve, each neatly labeled in his baroque handwriting: nitroglycerine; digitalis leaf; phenobarbital, half- and quarter-grain; tincture of opium; rhubarb and soda; glycerine and rosewater. As for the salves, there was unguentine for burns, ammoniated mercury for impetigo and a black ointment called Ichthyol that brought boils to a head. And Father's own creation—Will's Foot Balm, named for my brother Billy. It was a specific for athlete's foot, the active ingredient being coal tar and a desquamating agent. It operated on the premise that since athlete's foot was skin disease, you had to get rid of the skin. There was Beef, Iron and Wine for anemia. And a supply of mustard and turpentine for making plasters and stoups. Potassium permanganate for painting an ailing part purple. (I can think of no other reason.) Potassium chloride helped raise phlegm and, in a town full of tuberculosis, was in great demand. A compartment at the bottom of the bag held rolls of plaster of Paris, gauze and adhesive tape, a scalpel, scissors, forceps, metal probe, needle and thread, a rubber catheter, a few glass syringes, a test tube of boiled twine for tying off the umbilical cord and an alcohol lamp and a silver spoon for preparing injections of morphine.

With such an armamentarium, what couldn't he cure? But mostly it was himself just stepping into a sickroom that effected the cure. He had that *je ne sais quoi* of all great shamans, an aura that informed his patients that their doctor was in touch with the secret powers of healing.

The people of Troy thought he could bring back the dead.

("Is it true?" I asked him once.

"Not yet," he said modestly. "I specialize in the half dead." And so he did, with injections of bee venom and jolts of electricity from his diathermy machine, a large black apparatus on wheels with wires, electrodes and a dashboard of many knobs.

"Someday he is going to electrocute someone with that thing," said Mother on more than one occasion.)

When, hours later, the little boat heaved back into view, it contained, in addition to one exhausted general practitioner and his black bag, a blood-stained parcel in newspaper.

"Another damned chicken!" said Mother from the bay window. And so it was, freshly slaughtered: Father's fee for setting a broken wrist, applying the cast and suturing a laceration of the forehead. An old man, it seems, had fallen down a flight of stairs.

The day after the flood the sun came out. It was precisely then that Troy turned beautiful. Gone was all the sooty grayness; the peeling lackluster buildings wore the rich patina of antiquity; the whole town and everything in it took on a kind of mineral splendor. It shimmered as though having risen from the pavement on a hot day. The men and women all wore halos. I mentioned it to Mother.

"Not only that," said Billy, "he saw Jesus on King Street."

"I thought so," said Mother. "We'll have your eyes tested." Two weeks later, with my new eyeglasses pinching the bridge of my nose, Troy was once again Troy and the dazzling uncertainty had vanished. It was the reverse of a glory. A happy conjunction of myopia and astigmatism had given the city that mirage-y look. O the cruelty of twenty-twenty vision that sees too much that exists on the surface and nothing of the *real* real that lies just beneath! As soon as I was out of the house, I took off the hated glasses and—presto! Troy was once again Ilium. Bare-eyed and squinting, I decided, was the only way to look at Troy.

Father's hero was Ambroise Paré, a sixteenth-century barber-surgeon. Barber-surgeons were distinguished from real doctors by "another stupidity of the church," the law that forbade physicians from shedding blood. After three or four years spent dressing wounds at a hospital in Paris, Paré spent the next thirty years as a military surgeon attached to the armies of France. These armies were not equipped with medical services. Each great noble was accompanied by his private physician. The common soldiers doctored themselves or used the barber-surgeons and quacks who followed the campaigns as adventurers. Like all the surgeons who came after him, Paré learned to treat wounds not from books but by trial and error. Year in and year out, he fished for bullets in the bodies of the wounded, amputated ruined arms and legs, splinted fractures and dressed wounds, often under a hail of bullets on the field of battle. Nor did he refuse the enemy his ministrations but treated them with equal care. It must be so, said Father, for a doctor's allegiance is to his Hippocratic oath instead of to his king and fatherland.

Paré received no regular payment save what the soldiers gave him: food, an article of clothing, wine, a horse and, once, a diamond straight from the finger of a duchess for saving the life of a nobleman.

"That's like you," I said to Father, "when the patients give you a chicken or some fish or apples."

"Yes," he said, immensely pleased, "like me."

Paré was a modest man. He refused to take credit for his astonishing success at saving lives. "I dressed him and God healed him," was his constant refrain. He was the most tender-hearted of doctors, again like Father, who told me of the time that the French army, after a long and bitter siege, entered a city, passing over the dead bodies and some not yet dead. Hearing them cry out under the horses' hooves made Paré's heart ache. After a while, he found a barn where he thought to stable his horse. Inside, he found four dead soldiers and three more still alive propped against the wall, their faces contorted with pain, their clothes still smoldering where the gunpowder had burned them. As Paré gazed at them with pity, an old soldier came up and asked whether there was any way to cure them. Paré shook his head sadly. Whereupon the old soldier went up to the wounded men and cut their throats "gently, efficiently and without ill will." Horrified at what he thought a great cruelty, Paré cried out to the executioner that he was a villain.

"No," said the man. "I pray God that if ever I come to be in that condition, someone will do the same for me."

"What else about Paré?" I wanted to know.

"Well," said Father. "Paré observed that because of their pain and terror and the noise of the battle, the wounded men could not sleep. So he induced sleep by making artificial rain. Everybody knows you can't stay awake with the sound of rain on the roof. He did it by causing water to be poured from a high place into a metal caldron so that the men might hear the sound of falling water and go to sleep."

"Like the freight trains?"

"Yes, like the freight trains."

Emergency Medicine (Chapter 12 of *Knife Song Korea: A Novel*)

After three months he had seen nothing of the war. Now and then on a hillside he would find vestiges of it—a scatter of craters or the carcass of a tank twisted and rusting like a plated dinosaur—and he would wonder at their antiquity, wonder what warriors had left them. Then one morning Sloane awoke to the presence of battle. He knew it from the first tentative sniffing of the air, a mixture of oil, blood, sulphur, and a richer smell like that of flesh liquefying into the ground. Gears were grinding, men shouted, and a wild blare rolled back and forth across the air. Bombs, shells, machine-gun fire, zing and bunk-bunk ratta-tatta—boom! They never saw the enemy. With no corpus against which to marshal one's energy, one could listen only and heard too late the sexless whine of his own missile and suddenly there are flames in the tangled willows. Compared to this, hand-to-hand combat must have been a kind of lovemaking.

Then the first three casualties appeared at the dispensary. They were like biblical visitors presenting their wounds as though they were jewels, rich bursts of red flesh gingerly held out by their bearers.

Sloane stood amid the stretchers, dazzled at their costliness.

Beneath one blanket a spike of bone pointed through torn muscles. The boy's face was moon-white, his leg flailed helplessly as he was lifted to a cot, and through his open shirtfront the narrow neck was ridged by an Adam's apple bobbing slowly up and down.

The second man was holding something on his stomach with both hands as though it were a cat that might leap off. Sloane loosened the bandage and peered between the cupped hands. A floral pattern of intestine wound sinuously between the fingers. From beneath an eyepatch festoons of clotted black blood looped the cheek of the third man.

"Soak it off with peroxide," Sloane ordered, and the loosened patch gave suddenly with a sucking sound. Still stuck to it came the torn and empty globule that was the eye.

*

Sloane pointed to the boy with the abdominal wound.

"That one first. Send ahead that we *cannot* handle *any* more majors for six hours. It'll take that long for these three. Six hours. At *least.* Tell them to send *everyone* they can on to Ui Jong Bu *if possible.* Otherwise, we'll take them, but *only* the minors. They *must* give us six hours."

The boy with the belly wound was lifted to the high wooden table. Sloane punched open a can of ether and started dripping it into a cone over his face.

"Breathe deeply. Blow it away. Don't fret. You're safe now. I'm not going to let *anything* happen to you. When you wake up you'll be fine, just fine. *Trust that.*"

He dripped the ether until the hands holding the intestines fell softly away to the sides.

"Here, Jang. Drip this. *Slowly.* One drop every three seconds. One drop, three seconds. No more, no less. You get it? *One* drop every *three.*"

Jang nodded eagerly and began to pour the ether. Sloane watched him for a moment.

"Not so fast. Too fast, no good. You be careful or I'll get someone else." As though there *were* someone else.

"Pour that alcohol. Hands and my arms. There—that's enough."

He rubbed his hands together fiercely, cleaning under nails with other nails. He was thinking about the inside of the abdomen and what he would find there when he entered.

"Now more."

He splashed the alcohol over his arms and let it drip off his elbows. "Again. All right, now the instruments."

At each order the men jolted into action. He saw how clumsy they were, naïve, driven into automaticity by their awe of that limp and crawling loop of bowel, their own nearness to it. He scrubbed the abdominal wall around the wound with soapy water and outlined a rectangle of skin with towels. Inserting his index finger into the wound alongside the intestine, he drew the scalpel down across the abdomen. A bloody stripe appeared. He stroked again with the blade. The yellow fat lay parted at the base. Again, then again until the stray loop was joined by its fellows. He inserted the retractors.

"Hold these just like this."

Yoon took them.

"Pull harder."

Yoon pulled.

"Now don't move until I tell you. Good. Bring the other light over. *Come on*—bring it *over*."

He was barehanded as usual. Long since, he had run out of rubber gloves. He grasped the bowel and began to withdraw it. He would have to examine every inch of it, making sure there was no perforation. Let there be no leakage of feces, no hole in the gut please. Otherwise he'd have to resect the pieces, stitch the severed ends together. When the pile of intestines outside the body had grown to a large mound hanging from the incision, he could feel his assistants watching him in horror. Slowly he surveyed the surface of the bowel, running it between the thumb and fingers of one hand, turning it to examine the under-surface. No odor of feces, no hole. His hand dipped into the clef, feeling for any interruption in the smooth contour of the organs. Spleen. Left kidney. Colon. Bladder. Then around to the right kidney, his hand now immersed in the abdomen almost up to the elbow. Liver. Stomach. Now to replace the bowel.

"Lift high and hard. Almost up to the ceiling."

The bowel began to slip wetly out of sight.

"Look out, he's waking up. Pour, dammit—*faster*."

The muscles of the abdominal wall tightened and the bowel threw itself up and out of the wound. He leaned on it with his hand, trying to hold it in. A large coil escaped between his fingers and fell across the back of his arm.

"Pour. Pour faster. Get him *down*, he's going to *vomit*. Turn his head to the side. Hold it, keep it down. *Don't* let him *choke*. Now pour, *please*, pour goddamnitall. Never mind the mess."

He felt the boy's body loosening again, sliding into unconsciousness, the edges of the wound relaxing.

"Keep going."

With infinite care he replaced loop after loop.

"Lift harder."

It was all in.

When it was done, he said, "You are good good boys. Number one. Put him to bed. Wash the table. Get the next."

*

He pointed to the eye wound. The youth's uncovered eye followed his movements, swinging from his hands to his face.

"Peroxide. Pour it slowly on the gauze."

He gently irrigated the eye socket, wiping away clots, picking out loose stringy ends of tissue, bits of vegetation that had been driven in. There was bleeding at the base, too much to let alone. This is going to hurt.

"Hold his arms and his legs. Grab his head, too. Tight. Hold it tighter. *Tighter*. He mustn't move."

He leaned down and breathed into the boy's ear, close enough for his lips to touch.

"Okay now, it's going to hurt. Try to keep still. Really try. I'll be quick."

He prepared the sutures, threading the black thread through the eye of a curved needle, then fitting it into the jaws of the hemostat.

"Now. *All* of you. *Hold* him. Tight. Understand? *No movement.* Tied down tight."

He mopped the bloody pool out, pressing vigorously, no longer tender. The body stiffened, became rigid but did not struggle. When he had the spurter in view he sank the needle into the tissues around it, pulled it through, then sank it again in a figure of eight. The other eye was shut now, turned in upon a screaming brain, shutting out the world, utterly absorbed in the private agony. He tied the first knot. That's got it. Then the second and the third.

"Now pour again."

It was washed clean. There was no fresh bleeding.

"Ointment."

He emptied the tube of aureomycin into the socket, filling it to the brim, packing gauze squares on top of it for pressure.

"Put a bandage over it, round and round the head. Leave his ear *out.* Would *you* like to have an ear *squashed* like that? Put him to bed. Clean up, get the next one ready."

He stepped out of the Quonset hut and headed for the outhouse, the demands of foreign amoebae tunneling into his bowel. The night was full of bellowing and bumping. Strange that he had heard nothing inside. He had a period of weakness as the diarrhea took him. The cramps, the odor, the sweating all over, the bruised and burning hemorrhoids, the sight and the thought of where he was. Living or dying or even fighting in a place is not the same as being sick there. Dysentery and malaria had combined to establish a kinship of disease between the Koreans and himself. It drove them together. Perhaps therein lay the solution to the struggle of ideologies, he thought. Give both sides amoebiasis, give them malaria, give them a common ground of suffering with neither the time nor the energy for war.

He bent forward and put his head between his knees until it passed. At least it waited until now. At least no one else came to join him. Often he had to suffer with a man on each side of him. When all three were sick, the place was unbreathable. With his eyes closed he started to dream a little but then he roused himself to finish. How he would have loved to drop down deeper. "Surgeons are not for sleeping," he was told during his residency. There's a boy out there who is waiting for his leg. In a much better world they would both dream deeply without this duet. As he walked down the hill he had to stop and ask whether that was an aftercramp or whether he needed the three-holer again. The answer turned him around and back up the hill. "It just doesn't end, does it?" he said aloud. Such merciless rejection when the body doesn't want something in it. Not most of it out—*all of it.* It was something he couldn't bluff, something he couldn't argue with, not even if Eisenhower were down there wounded and waiting.

*

For two hours he cleansed and washed the wound of the third patient, cutting away all the devitalized and contused tissue, chipping at the blackened spicules of bone for a semblance of cleanliness.

"Hold him under the arms and pull. Yoon. Take the foot and pull as hard as you can. We must try to straighten it out. Harder. Now *keep* it that way. Plaster rolls. Bucket of water."

He dipped the rolls one by one and wrapped them snugly about the leg from toes to groin while the Koreans, standing opposite each other, pulled as hard as they could. Over the wound he left a window in the cast to change the dressing.

"A few minutes more till it hardens, then to bed."

There was a new arrival, a young man lying on a stretcher. He had raised himself up on his elbows and was staring down at his crotch with silent fascination. A dark stain covered the entire front of his pants, expanding down the legs. It spread slowly even as he watched. Later Sloane would have to tell him he had lost his testicles.

Mercy

It is October at the Villa Serbelloni, where I have come for a month to write. On the window ledges the cluster flies are dying. The climate is full of uncertainty. Should it cool down? Or warm up? Each day it overshoots the mark, veering from frost to steam. The flies have no uncertainty. They understand that their time has come.

What a lot of energy it takes to die! The frenzy of it. Long after they have collapsed and stayed motionless, the flies are capable of suddenly spinning so rapidly that they cannot be seen. Or seen only as a blurred glitter. They are like dervishes who whirl, then stop, and lay as quiet as before, only now and then waving a leg or two feebly, in a stuporous reenactment of locomotion. Until the very moment of death, the awful buzzing as though to swarm again.

Every morning I scoop up three dozen or so corpses with a dustpan and brush. Into the wastebasket they go, and I sit to begin the day's writing. All at once, from the wastebasket, the frantic knocking of resurrection. Here, death has not yet secured the premises. No matter the numbers slaughtered, no matter that the windows be kept shut all day, each evening the flies gather on the ledges to die, as they have lived, *ensemble.* It must be companionable to die so, matching spin for spin, knock for knock, and buzz for buzz with one's fellows. We humans have no such fraternity, but each of us must buzz and spin and knock alone.

I think of a man in New Haven! He has been my patient for seven years, ever since the day I explored his abdomen in the operating room and found the surprise lurking there—a cancer of the pancreas. He was forty-two years old then. For this man, these have been seven years of famine. For his wife and his mother as well. Until three days ago his suffering was marked by slowly increasing pain, vomiting, and fatigue. Still, it was endurable. With morphine. Three days ago the pain rollicked out of control, and he entered that elect band whose suffering cannot be relieved by any means short of death. In his bed at home he seemed an eighty-pound concentrate of pain from which all other pain must be made by serial dilution. He twisted under the last of it. An ambulance arrived. At the hospital nothing was to be done to prolong his life. Only the administration of large doses of narcotics.

"Please," he begs me. In his open mouth, upon his teeth, a brown paste of saliva. All night long he has thrashed, as though to hollow out a grave in the bed.

"I won't let you suffer," I tell him. In his struggle the sheet is thrust aside. I see the old abandoned incision, the belly stuffed with tumor. His penis, even, is skinny. One foot with five blue toes is exposed. In my cupped hand, they are cold. I think of the twenty bones of that foot laced together with tendon, each ray accompanied by its own nerve and artery. Now, this foot seems a beautiful dead animal that had once been trained to transmit the command of a man's brain to the earth.

"I'll get rid of the pain," I tell his wife.

But there is no way to kill the pain without killing the man who owns it. Morphine to lethal dose . . . and still he miaows and bays and makes other sounds, like a boat breaking up in a heavy sea. I think his pain will live on long after he dies.

"Please," begs his wife, "we cannot go on like this."

"Do it," says the old woman, his mother. "Do it now."

"To give him any more would kill him," I tell her.

"Then do it," she says. The face of the old woman is hoof-beaten with intersecting curves of loose skin. Her hair is donkey brown, donkey gray.

They wait with him while I go to the nurses' station to prepare the syringes. It is a thing that I cannot ask anyone to do for me. When I return to the room, there are three loaded syringes in my hand, a rubber tourniquet, and an alcohol sponge. Alcohol sponge! To prevent infection? The old woman is standing on a small stool and leaning over the side rail of the bed. Her bosom is just above his upturned face, as though she were weaning him with sorrow and gentleness from her still-full breasts. All at once she says severely, the way she must have said it to him years ago:

"Go home, son. Go home now."

I wait just inside the doorway. The only sound is a flapping, a rustling, as in a room to which a small animal, a bat perhaps, has retreated to die. The women turn to leave. There is neither gratitude nor reproach in their gaze. I should be hooded.

At last we are alone. I stand at the bedside.

"Listen," I say, "I can get rid of the pain." The man's eyes regain their focus. His gaze is like a wound that radiates its pain outward so that all upon whom it fell would know the need of relief.

"With these." I hold up the syringes.

"Yes," he gasps. "Yes." And while the rest of his body stirs in answer to the pain, he holds his left, his acquiescent arm, still for the tourniquet. An even dew of sweat covers his body. I wipe the skin with the alcohol sponge, and tap the arm smartly to bring out the veins. There is one that is still patent; the others have long since clotted and broken down. I go to insert the needle, but the tourniquet has come unknotted; the vein has collapsed. Damn! Again I tie the tourniquet. Slowly the vein fills with blood. This time it stays distended.

He reacts not at all to the puncture. In a wild sea what is one tiny wave? I press the barrel and deposit the load, detach the syringe from the needle and replace it with the second syringe. I send this home, and go on to the third. When they are all given, I pull out the needle. A drop of blood blooms on his forearm. I blot it with the alcohol sponge. It is done. In less than a minute, it is done.

"Go home," I say, repeating the words of the old woman. I turn off the light. In the darkness the contents of the bed are theoretical. No! I must watch. I turn the light back on. How reduced he is, a folded parcel, something chipped-away until only its shape and a little breath are left. His impatient bones gleam as though to burst through the papery skin. I am impatient too. I want to get it over with, then step out into the corridor where the women are waiting. His death is like a jewel to them.

My fingers at his pulse. The same rhythm as mine! As though there were one pulse that beat throughout all of nature, and every creature's heart throbbed precisely.

"You can go home now," I say. The familiar emaciated body un-tenses. The respirations slow down. Eight per minute . . . six . . . It won't be long. The pulse wavers in and out of touch. It won't be long.

"Is that better?" I ask him. His gaze is distant, opaque, preoccupied. Minutes go by. Outside, in the corridor, the murmuring of women's voices.

But this man will not die! The skeleton rouses from its stupor. The snout twitches as if to fend off a fly. What is it that shakes him like a gourd full of beans? The pulse returns, melts away, comes back again, and stays. The respirations are twelve, then fourteen. I have not done it. I did not murder him. I am innocent!

I shall walk out of the room into the corridor. They will look at me, holding their breath, expectant. I lift the sheet to cover him. All at once, there is a sharp sting in my thumb. The same needle with which I meant to kill him has pricked *me.* A drop of blood appears. I press it with the alcohol sponge. My fresh blood deepens the stain of his on the gauze. Never mind. The man in the bed swallows. His Adam's apple bobs slowly. It would be so easy to do it. Three minutes of pressure on the larynx. He is still not conscious, wouldn't feel it, wouldn't know. My thumb and fingertips hover, land on his windpipe. My pulse beating in his neck, his in mine. I look back over my shoulder. No one. Two bare IV poles in a corner, their looped metal eyes witnessing. Do it! Fingers press. Again he swallows. Look back again. How closed the door is. And . . . my hand wilts. I cannot. It is not in me to do it. Not that way. The man's head swivels like an upturned fish. The squadron of ribs battles on.

I back away from the bed, turn and flee toward the doorway. In the mirror, a glimpse of my face. It is the face of someone who has been resuscitated after a long period of cardiac arrest. There is no spot of color in the cheeks, as though this person were in shock at what he had just seen on the yonder side of the grave.

In the corridor the women lean against the wall, against each other. They are like a band of angels dispatched here to take possession of his body. It is the only thing that will satisfy them.

"He didn't die," I say. "He won't . . . or can't." They are silent.

"He isn't ready yet," I say.

"He *is* ready," the old woman says. "*You* ain't."

Taking the World in for Repairs

INTERPLAST. It stands for International Plastic Surgeons, Incorporated. The organization was conceived in 1969 by Donald Laub to bring plastic and reconstructive surgery to indigent people of the Third World, to train the native surgeons in operative techniques and to forge professional relationships that would endure, would outlast any political differences between countries. Twenty-five years ago I was chief resident in surgery at Yale. Don was one of my interns. Now he practices plastic surgery in Palo Alto, California. Since it began, INTERPLAST has performed more than ten thousand operations on many dozens of expeditions to those parts of the world termed "undeveloped"—Mexico, Honduras, Ecuador, the Philippines, Jamaica, and Peru. Sometimes a single person is sent out; sometimes, a team of twenty. All are volunteers. The length of this expedition to Peru will be two weeks. The doctors, nurses, and technicians will come from five universities—Yale, Stanford, Johns Hopkins, Emory, and the University of West Virginia—and from seven of the United States—Nevada, Kentucky, California, Connecticut, Georgia, West Virginia, and Maryland.

*

The trip from North to South America is hardly Xenophon's march from Babylon to the Bosporus; still, it is in the heroic mold. Twenty people, all unused to and resisting regimentation, each with that certain "sweet arrogance" that belongs to men and women trained to a fare-thee-well in their life's work—it is not easy. In Miami, a surgeon wanders away; in Lima, a nurse stops listening and misses a vital connection. Yet in the end we have been coaxed and prodded on and off the succession of planes, buses, and cars that have carried us to Peru. Seventy crates and cartons of equipment have been ushered through customs. INTERPLAST uses none of the precious resources of the host country. We have brought our own—sterile gauze, hemostats, scalpels, all.

We are assembled in the lobby of the Hotel Crillon in Lima. The next morning we fly to Arequipa in the southern highlands. We shall work there in a government provincial hospital named Honorio Delgado. In the evening an exuberance possesses us, a kind of glee at the prospect of shared labor and adventure. Friendships which had been initiated in airports along the way are cemented. Absent is the wariness of new acquaintances inching toward intimacy. There is no taking of measure, no hesitation. The team is being forged. A MASH mentality prevails. Veterans of previous expeditions regale novices with tales of surgical derring-do. The initiates sigh and fidget. Later I fall asleep dreaming of Peru. Of condors and gold, of llamas and emerald mountains, of cruel Pizarro and his conquistadores.

The flight from Lima to the mountain city of Arequipa takes little more than an hour, but I think the direction must be straight up. Soon we are flying among the white peaks. What a harsh rudimentary land! It is at once epic and mysterious. Even the sky seems studded with hieroglyphs. Abruptly, Peru vanishes and we are engulfed in fog. Peaks and crags dodge our wings and miss, but barely. The plane flutters, banks, rolls all but over, and we are on the ground. It is less a descent and landing than a careful insertion into Arequipa. Half of us are to be housed in Peruvian homes, the rest are wedged, three to a tiny room, at Turistas, a pink and green hotel made of volcanic rock. We do not stop to unpack but rush to the hospital to begin our work. The great clinic we are told, is already in session. CONSULTORIO CHIRUGIA PLASTICA DE INTERPLAST reads the sign on the wall. Black crayon on yellow paper. Within minutes we are fully engaged in the examination and selection of patients for the days of surgery ahead.

The hospital of Honorio Delgado is slowly, imperceptibly settling into a state of splendid ruination. One day it will be the twentieth century's medical Machu Picchu. The floor bears great gouges where tile and stone have crumbled. The ceiling is a constellation of cracks. Should something break, it stays broken. There is no such thing as restoration or replacement. Again and again Honorio Delgado has run out of catgut, scrub suits, dressings. Rubber gloves are mended and reused the next day and the day after that. Each scrap of gauze is retrieved from a bucket, washed and folded, and made ready to blot another patient's blood. The scalpels of Arequipa enjoy longevity. If these knives could speak, they would each spin tales of their dozens of incisions. At Yale or Stanford, a knife has a lifetime of a single operation. Each procedure here is dictated by the cost of the material needed to do it. The staff is paid, but poorly. Before an emergency appendectomy, the patient must buy the suture material, gauze, and knife blade to be used upon him. If there is no money, as is usual, the residents themselves must buy the material, paying for the right to heal their patients. While INTERPLAST, ah INTERPLAST, has come to Peru, its cartons bursting with throwaway knives, suture material of every caliber and variety—catgut, nylon, vicryl, silk; and tanks of anesthetic gas, intravenous fluids and an array of clever instruments—dermatomes, staples, retractors, endotracheal tubes. We are both proud of and embarrassed by our plenty. Under the awed gazes of our hosts we squirm. Always, we are the rich gringos.

Clinic is held in two tiny examining rooms in which there are never fewer than a dozen people. Four examinations are being conducted simultaneously. In one corner Iris Figueroa, a beautiful fourteen-year-old girl, glows among our white coats. Her mother holds up the girl's right hand for us to see. It has but one finger, the index, which protrudes like a talon. The rest are absent save for a cluster of soft nubbins bunched at the knuckles.

Leo is our hand surgeon. "What is your name?" he asks her.

"Iris," she says and lowers her gaze.

"Wiggle your thumb," says Leo. His English is translated into Spanish by a nurse. But what can he mean? There is no thumb. He means only to see if she moves the bone at the base of what should have been her thumb, the one hidden in the featureless pad of tissue in which all five metacarpals exist uselessly. Iris tries to wiggle it; she tries very hard to do what the doctor has asked her to, even shakes her head at the effort. There is no movement to be seen. Still, palpating, Leo feels *something* at work within that pad of flesh.

"We can separate this ray out," he thinks aloud. "Make a web space, deepen it all the way to the wrist. Then she will be able to pinch." The girl's mother lifts Iris's other hand and we see that this one too is blank, blind, dumb. And fingerless. For a moment we are still. Then:

"Is she right- or left-handed?" The interpreter is busy.

"Right," she says at last. And we smile as though we have just received the best news. And we have. All this while, the girl has been eating our faces with her eyes.

"Put her on the schedule," says Leo. "I'll do her tomorrow."

"There's no more room on the schedule tomorrow," says Fran. She has charge of making out the operative list. "In fact, you're all booked up for the whole two weeks." Leo says nothing, only looks down at the small unfinished hand, paw really, that he still holds in his own.

"It's just the way it is," says Fran. "We can't do them all."

"You tell her, then," says Leo. There is a short volley of Spanish. Something pale and vague flits from the face of the girl. I think it must be hope. Her head drops down and away. She is trying not to show what is churning inside. But courage has its limits, in Peru as everywhere else, and there are tears. With her single finger she reaches up to wipe them away.

"No room?" Leo asks again. He cannot seem to understand.

"No room," says Fran.

"Give her a high priority slip for next year. We'll be back next year," he says to Iris. "I'll fix it then." Fran writes out a slip of paper, marks it "priority" and hands it to the mother of the girl.

Paper is shuffled, the door is let open a bit, and a woman leads a seven-year-old boy into the room. He climbs upon the table that Iris has just left. Where his lip should be is a nude rubbery insect from which a single tooth projects.

"What's your name?" asks Don. In California, he is famous for his large series of sex-change operations.

"Miguel."

Don laughs as though the name itself were funny. "Say '*el gato*,' Miguel," he says. "Say 'Coca-Cola.'" The boy looks at his mother. She nods.

"*El gato*," says Miguel. "Coca-Cola." But it is only an approximation. The vowels leak out of his nose; the consonants are blunted, furry.

"Unilateral cleft lip and cleft palate," says Don. "We ought to get it fixed now. Later, there will be less chance for speech improvement. He's at the right age."

"Now," says Fran. "You know there's no space for it. Why do you make me say it again and again?" She tells the mother it cannot be done, tells her to bring him back next year. She gives her a slip of paper. They rise to leave.

"Good-bye, Miguelito," said Don. "*Adios, amigo*." It is the boy's turn to smile.

Just at noon the sun comes out for the first time. In its rays the hospital of Honorio Delgado blanches. Through the tiny window of the examining room we turn to see the huge snowy cone of Misti, one of the three volcanoes that ring the city of Arequipa. It is dead, they say, burnt out. But I don't know about that. There is just the whiff of temper in that bit of cloud the peak has snagged. With volcanoes as with people, I suspect eruptions are a matter of anger or spite. If the gift of prophecy has not deserted me, we can expect a rush of hot lava when the "No!" index in this clinic reaches a critical point. What mountain could hold its peace in the face of so much heartbreak? Once, I arrived in Paris some hours later than I had planned only to find that the hotel had given away my room reservation. "*Complet*" announced the desk clerk, dismissing me with her back. Very Parisian, I was to learn, after dragging my reluctant luggage into a dozen other lobbies in search of shelter only to be met each time with another "*Complet*." It is a small thing to sit up all night in a foreign city waiting for the dawn. I know that. "No room" in Peru is worse than "*complet*" in Paris. Still, as I watch the disappointed children leave the clinic, I think of that cold and tired night.

"Look at this, will you?" says Aida, one of the nurses. She is registering the patients, carrying out triage.

"Look at what?" I say. And see the balled-up hand of the young man. Fifteen years ago he had grabbed something hot, something which stuck to his palm. When the burn had healed, his fist was permanently clenched.

Mano embalito it is called here.

"Needs excision of the cicatrix and full-thickness skin graft. Or a pedicle."

I look over at Fran. "Don't," I say. Later Fran will admit that it took her four years and six expeditions to be able to say no without crying. Fran is a specialist in international medicine. She is pretty and petite. She is fluent in Spanish. She gets things done.

The door opens. Three young women enter. They are sisters, each with the fused fingers of syndactyly on their left hands. Once again, Fran wrings out the operative schedule and a single operating space is found.

"You must decide," she says to the sisters. They whisper to themselves for a moment, then two point to the third.

"Why that one?" I want to know.

"She is getting married. Without the operation, she cannot wear her wedding ring."

I step out into the waiting room from which the throng spills to the out-of-doors where there is a topiary garden—shrubs in the shape of a llama, a condor, an ocelot, an angel, each one carved precisely as if by a surgeon of INTERPLAST. From this garden I spy on the patients. How beautiful they are. Tiny. Even the tallest of them is shorter than the least of us. Every shade of brown and gold is represented in their skin. Their hair is full and black. All their sexuality seems to reside in their hair. Again and again the children are scooped up and pressed into their mothers. The children eye each other's deformities with quiet solemnity. The mothers too cast quick glances. It is said that the Incas were all exterminated during the Spanish conquest, that their race is extinct. But I don't believe it. The genes of the Incas are here in this courtyard full of *serranos*. Now and then I see a perfect pre-Columbian face, and then I am sure.

Here, in this waiting room, one would think deformity the natural state of mankind. No child but with his cleft lip, burn scar, webbed hand. The marred and the scarred far outnumber the others. The children are quiet, reserved. There is no restlessness in them. Only, they wait. The longing in their faces is all for a clever scalpel, a tiny row of meticulously placed sutures that will redeem their lives. See how the examining room opens again. Something billows forth from the crowd. Yet no one moves. It is only their breath that has surged. The lucky name is called out: "Fabian Platera Choquehuanca." A woman carries a fully swathed infant into the examining room. The rest inhale, exhale, and settle back into waiting. Many have come on foot from great distances, from villages high in the Andes. Still, they are not disgruntled. Nor are there predatory lawyers circling at the periphery. There is only the eternal eloquence of the wound. All at once, from the examining room, another "no room" followed by a hush in which I think I hear the volcano rumbling. I go back to duty. The door bangs open and a young boy of eight runs in and hugs Fran. They cling to each other, laughing. There is a barrage of Spanish. Fran explains:

"He had a double cleft lip. We fixed it last year. He and his mother have come all the way from Puno to show us. Look. You can't even tell." She turns to the boy.

"You are handsome," she says. He laughs and races out of the room.

It is a long walk from Turistas to the hospital. At eye level, the swarm and buzz of Calle Jerusalén. Glance upward and there, pale with snow and cloud, the great Andean ghosts—Misti, Chachani, Pichu Pichu. Somber and outsize, they are inert in a way that the Alps or the Rockies never are. And how much older they seem. Arequipa is white, every building made of the gleaming lava stone called *sillar.* It is porous, with many natural gouges. Plastered and whitewashed, it makes an irresistible writing surface for the slogan-crazed Peruvians. Straight through the center of the city charges the river Chili, from a distance a veritable whitewater shaking its mane over the banks. Come closer, and it is brown, feculent, stinking. Upon its banks, you stay mum. You had better. A single drop of spray upon your lip would lay you mad and frothing.

Another day. Another ten cleft lips and palates. We are pushing to get them all done, all that we have promised before we leave. Among the Indians it is believed that a congenitally deformed child is a reproof to the mother for excessive passion or aberrant desire, whatever they are. If this were so, these legions of lips and palates would accuse all of Peru.

A short lesson in embryology: Mesenchyme is that all-purpose undifferentiated tissue of which we are largely comprised early in fetal life. Mesenchyme is not stationary, but flows, folding upon itself, rising into ridges, incorporating within itself little sacs and hollows. Within the first trimester of pregnancy it happens sometimes, far oftener in Peru than in America, it seems, that the mesenchyme destined to form the upper jaw, the lip, and the palate fails either to fuse in the midline of the face, or even to migrate to the midline of the face. And so there is a cleft where there should have been an uninterrupted smooth and attractive joining. Such an intrauterine mishap runs in families. Should a mother or a sibling have a cleft lip, then the odds turn grimmer for the unborn. Inbreeding, it is said, plays a part, the grouping and concentration of negative influences. And malnutrition. And multiparity in which an eleventh or twelfth child is born to a woman in her forties or later.

The Indians of Peru live in just such a state of genetic vulnerability. INTERPLAST has come here to repair and reconstruct, to correct the inborn errors to which society and culture have made these people susceptible. So we tell ourselves and others. So we believe. But that is not the only reason we have come. Honesty insists that each of us is here for our own entirely other reasons. The surgical residents have come for the experience of operating on great numbers of these deformities. Within two weeks they will have performed more of these operations than most surgeons will do in a lifetime. For some, it is the opportunity for virtue that we are seeking. Such opportunities are not without the element of self-aggrandizement. For still others it is the exhilaration of the exotic that beckons, or the lovely sense of camaraderie that is to be found in working together for a purpose we think high. Last, there is the need for human beings to challenge themselves. In surgery it is best done by tackling the most difficult of clinical situations and prevailing. Next to the control of the birth rate, the correction of malnutrition, genetic counseling and the teaching of simple hygiene, all our surgery is nothing. Still, that we have come to do it is enough for us.

In the great central hall as in the courtyards outside the hospital, endless lines of Indians, many exhausted and malnourished, wait for a turn at the *farmacia*, the *sala de radiografia.* There is almost no noise, no movement. Only now and then a small enigmatic cry, a whisper, a cough. The faces of the people are patient, blank. A visit here takes an entire day, at the end of which half will not have been seen and must return the next day. The *sala de operaciones* is on the fourth floor. One climbs, of course. From the head of the stairwell to the doors of the operating theater, the corridor is jammed with the relatives of those inside and undergoing surgery. Some member of the family will remain with the patient throughout his hospital stay. Food will be brought in and fed to the patient.

Now that the days of our great clinics are over, physical examinations take place in every nook and cranny of the hospital—in the middle of a hallway, on the stairs. Indians arrive at any time, unannounced, and ask to be seen. No one is turned away by INTERPLAST. Most are given slips to return the next year. One or two lucky ones are taken then and there into the operating room and added to the day's schedule. Somehow, a woman with a paralyzed arm has made her way through the operating-room doors and into the surgeons' dressing room. She stands against a row of metal lockers hoping to be examined. Nearby a Peruvian doctor is undressing for his work. I ask the woman to remove her shirt. It is a long-sleeved pullover which she cannot manage unassisted. I help her. Now she is naked from the waist up. One year ago, she tells me, a surgeon in Cuzco removed a tumor from her armpit. Ever since, her arm has been dead. She cannot care for her children. Now the woman and the Peruvian surgeon are equally naked, each taking no notice of the other. A brachial plexus injury, I think. From the surgery. There is nothing to be done. I help her to put on the shirt.

In the operating room the ancient pedagogy of surgery goes on, but here as in Babel. The doctors and nurses of Arequipa speak no English; we, no Spanish. Still, hand guides hand within a sleeping patient. Voices murmur.

"*Paciencia, paciencia. Despacio, por favor.*" And after a difficult technique newly mastered: "*Felicitaciones, amigo.*"

As usual, the surgeons are confident; the anesthesiologists nervous. It is the role of the anesthesiologist to rein the surgeon in, restrain him, lest, in his enthusiasm, the surgeon endanger life. These surrogates are the conscience of the operating room. They, the statesmen. We, the warriors.

"*Milagro*!" It is Iris who is the patient on the operating table. A last-minute cancellation. An infant with too low a blood count, crackles in his lungs. An anesthesiologist has said no. The infant's misfortune is Iris's good luck. Now we are in the middle of the surgery. The skin flaps have been cut. A full-thickness skin graft has been taken from the girl's groin. There is still much to do.

Anesthetist: "How much longer will you be at it?"

Surgeon: "Another hour and a half or so. Why?"

Anesthetist: "The trouble is . . . we are almost out of oxygen. The tank is on EMPTY."

Surgeon: "No."

Anesthetist: "Yes."

Surgeon (angrily): "How could you let that happen?" Then, "We'll have to find a good place to stop."

Anesthetist: "That would be *right now.* I'm going to have to wake her up."

Surgeon: "Can you wait one minute?"

Anesthetist: "No."

Just then, the door to the operating room opens and a huge headless tank is rolled, wobbled, carried even, into the room. Two tiny Peruvian nurses are supplying the brawn. They are dwarfed by the giant tank. Still, they use their breasts and their breath to propel it forward. A monkey wrench is found and the tubing is switched from the dead tank to this new one. A knob is turned. All eyes are on the gauge. No one knows how much, if any, oxygen the tank holds. The needle pops to the halfway mark. It is enough. The surgeon and the anesthetist breathe heavily as though it were they who had run out of air.

Surgeon: "Now can we get on with it?"

Anesthetist: "Trouble is, now there's no oxygen in the recovery room. This is their tank. The only one."

Surgeon: "Suture!"

I am invited to the operating room of a Peruvian surgeon to observe and comment. The room and everything in it sparkle. The walls, ceiling, linen—all white. The surgeon is a flamboyant older man with a gray moustache. He speaks no English but explains each step of the procedure at a shout; I might be deaf. I shout back at him in rudimentary Spanish.

"*Bisturi*!" he calls out to the scrub nurse at his elbow. And, making a quick small Sign of the Cross over the woman's belly with the scalpel, he makes a huge deep incision in the upper-right abdomen. None of the bleeders is clamped. Unaccountably, they stop after a minute or so. The Sign of the Cross?

"*Gorda*," growls the surgeon. Her fat annoys him. He looks up at me and shakes his head, asking commiseration from a colleague. I shake my head in return.

"*Muchissima gorda*," I say and cluck my tongue hard. His two assistants speak only when spoken to. Nor do they perform any single step of the operation but stand holding what he tells them to hold with an obedience that is as remarkable as it is absolute. I think of the backtalk I get in New Haven, where I am lucky to be let into the operating room at all, and then must painstakingly attend to each intern and resident according to his level of experience. They would settle for nothing less. Nor would I, actually. It is the American way. Youth is stroked and cosseted. But here in Peru it is age, petulant, cantankerous age, that commands. I rather like the idea.

"*Calculo in choledochus*!" the surgeon shouts at me.

"*Si! Si!*" I shout back. He opens the common bile duct, scoops out several spoonsful of sludge and gravel, then tries to pass a dilator down through it into the duodenum. It will not go.

"*Otro calculo*?" I suggest.

"*No*!" he thunders. "*Espasmo*!" It is the anesthetist's fault somehow. The surgeon informs the hapless anesthetist that in America he is quite certain that the anesthetist is helpful to the surgeon, that he does not become part of the problem. Abashed, the anesthetist checks the patient's blood pressure and injects something into the intravenous tubing. More passes with the dilator. At last it goes through the narrows into the intestine.

"*Muchas gracias*," I tell him. "A beautiful job."

"I do another one tomorrow," he hollers in Spanish. "You must come and watch me."

In the central corridor of the operating suite, next to a wall, stands a small gaudy altar, no more than a crucifix on a tablecloth strewn with artificial flowers. No one pays it the slightest attention. But it is there. In the same tiny storeroom that is stuffed with the cartons of our equipment, the men and women of INTERPLAST dress and undress together. We have not the modesty of the Peruvians who seem shocked by our shamelessness. Here too, between operations, we chew away at the slabs of tough fried meat and buns that are handed out by a beautiful young woman who is always dressed to the nines for the occasion—flowered silk dress and high heels. What could she possibly be thinking? Someone takes the roll of toilet paper from the table and disappears. Already, for our sins, the diarrhea rages.

Emergencia! One of the palates done yesterday is bleeding. A nurse wheels the rattletrap gurney through the doors of the *sala de operaciones.* The boy, Juan, is eleven years old. A gauze has been stuffed into his mouth. The end protrudes and is draped over his chin. It is blood-soaked and more blood drips from it to his bare chest. With one finger, as he has been instructed, he presses the wad against the roof of his mouth. He is utterly calm in his martyrdom. We place him on his side on the operating table. He will be put to sleep in that position, tilted forward, in order to prevent blood from running into his windpipe. A mask is held over his face. Above it, dark slanted eyes gaze at something far beyond the swirl of doctors, nurses, and equipment in which he is engulfed. Only once does he raise one hand to point to the angle of his jaw where the anesthetist is pressing too tightly.

"Your finger is hurting him," someone says.

"Sorry," the anesthetist says to the boy. "How do you say 'I'm sorry' in Spanish?"

"Never mind. He speaks only Quechua, anyway. He's from a village far up. Not even Pizarro got to it." Only when the boy is asleep and the tube is secure in his airway is he turned on his back. The packing is removed from his mouth. It is chased by a red froth, then pure blood.

"I see it," says the anesthetist. We peer into the open mouth of the boy and we too see the torn artery at the front of the incision in his palate. Two four-by-four-inch gauze pads have been unfolded and packed in the throat to prevent aspiration. A metal mouth gag is inserted behind the front teeth and screwed open. Now the site of hemorrhage can be seen with ease. Tick, tick, ticking away. With each beat of the pulse another expensive red jet. A single stitch of 4-0 vicryl in a figure-of-eight, and we are dry. We are safe. The anesthetist holds out his hand which is completely painted with blood.

"Can someone wash me off?"

A nurse or a doctor, like an artist, must have an illiberal human heart, the kind that is unmoved by news of a far-off massacre, in Cambodia, say, but breaks each time at the death of Juliet. Juan is wheeled to the recovery room, his mouth still stuffed with gauze packing. The lump is in *my* throat.

I am scheduled to remove an Indian woman's gallbladder at 8:00 A.M. All night my own abdominal griping has spiraled to truly marvelous heights, my bowels vibrating like a harp. An operation performed under such intestinal duress is likely to become a photo-finish race. How I envy the antibodies of the roomful of Peruvian doctors and students who have gathered to assist and observe. And how I curse my insipid Connecticut colon. In the room where I work no one speaks English. We shall see. The patient is a short chunk of a woman somewhere between thirty and fifty years of age.

"*Donde le duele*?" I ask her. "Where does it hurt?" She points to her gallbladder. I press the area firmly. She winces. "O.K.," I say eloquently.

The anesthetic is peridural; she is to be awake. Still, she has descended into a mysterious condition of apartness from the world. She is elsewhere. My assistants and I scrub in silence. Masked, gowned, gloved, we are no longer able to use the sign language that has sufficed for conversation heretofore. The abdomen has been prepared.

"*Bisturi*!" I say, holding my hand for the scalpel. There is a sudden quick slice. But it takes place somewhere within my own belly. The diarrhea. A wave of faintness is fought down. There is to be none of that, I tell myself. And we start. Dense adhesions obliterate the gallbladder as completely as the fog on that first day hid the airport of Arequipa. There is more bleeding than I like.

"Jesus," I say in English. "She is bleeding all over South America." I say it again, this time, for some reason, in French. Then it is that Maria, the scrub nurse, who has up to now been silent, says, all but inaudibly, "*Je parle francais*."

Her very words are hemostatic for the patient, anti-diarrhetic for me. From then on I speak to her in French which she translates into Spanish for the others.

"*Il y a beaucoup de calculs, calculs grands et petits, dans le cholecyste, mais rien dans le choledochus*." I listen to her repeating these things in Spanish.

"*Je prefere deux ligatures de colon pour le canal cystique*." Again, she interprets.

"*Les jeunes filles de Peru sont tres charmantes*," I drone on. Maria gives a tiny giggle and says nothing.

"*Mais, traduisez, s'il vous plait.*" With obvious reluctance, she does. The men in the room laugh appreciatively.

"*Et Maria est mon ange gardien. Traduisez.*" This last with all the sadism of a conquistador. With a sweet blend of pleasure and pain, she does. The surgeon rules here, remember? More laughter, after which Maria and the men have at each other in high spirits. I see that she is more than a match for the whole lot. Whatever nerves I had before are now settled. The gallbladder is quickly and neatly removed. Without untoward event, as we say in surgery.

"*Felicitaciones. Muchas gracias. Perfecto.*"

I peel off my gown and gloves and race to the toilet.

The Indians chew coca leaves wrapped about a small piece of limestone. The wad is held in the groove between the cheek and the gum. It is the slow activation of the cocaine by the stone and saliva that serves to disconnect, just a bit, the chewer from his hardships. Such usage does not make him happy, nor is it meant to. Only to alleviate. Very sensible, we decide. At the hospital, in the long waiting lines, the eyes of the coca eaters are withdrawn, unfocused. It does seem true that in every culture there is some national elixir to which the people turn for their dreams and for relief. In the spirit of experimentation, shall we say, we pay a little money to a man outside Turistas. Within minutes there are pebbles, there are leaves. In the evening, self-consciously, we try to feel what it is that they feel. *Nada.* Only, we cannot sleep. And so we go to Pena, the native cabaret. Bottles of pisco on the tables. The nurses and doctors with whom, hours earlier, we had shared disappointment and triumph in the operating rooms teach us to dance. German Munoz, a specialist in the treatment of burns; Luis and Alfredo who dream of going abroad to finish their surgical training—Luis, to the States, Alfredo, to Brazil. And the nurses, Maria, Eleana, and the rest, clapping their hands to the beat, now and then uttering tiny birdlike cries, their eyes gone muzzy with longing. We watch them court each other, the men all gallantry, the women a blend of eagerness and coquetry. Here at Pena, it is INTERPLAST that is shy, awkward, encased in a Puritan cuirass that holds stiff our hips and shoulders and necks. We marvel at the oiled hinges of our counterparts. At last midnight, and with it, lubrication. Then we too come ashake and aswivel. The music is made with wooden flutes, reed pipes, guitars, and drums. It is immensely erotic, feral. The flutes and pipes cry, shriek, moan. The guitars shuffle chords this way and that. But it is the great drum that governs. Like a cardiac muscle it drives our blood. When, abruptly, the beat changes, we suffer arrhythmia.

Don is assisting a local surgeon, Alfredo Montes, in the repair of a cleft lip. Alfredo is the single most important man here for it is he, if anyone, who will inherit the mantle. In a few days INTERPLAST will have departed. Alfredo will be left to carry on. He is immensely Peruvian—short, beefy, brown, with a wealth of black hair which he has had "styled." There are gold chains around his neck.

"*Tinte*," says Alfredo to the scrub nurse, and with a sharp stylet dipped in ink he marks out the flaps on the mound of chaotic flesh.

"No, no," says Don. "Make it longer laterally. Look. Here is the vermilion border. That's the Cupid's bow. Yeah, now you've got it. *Bravissimo*!" An hour later, Alfredo is suturing the two halves of the orbicularis oris muscle, the one used in pouting, sucking, sipping, kissing, all of that. With each suture he restores a new function to that mouth. Minutes later, the flattened nostril rises in a lovely curve to match that of the other side. The defect narrows, is closed. Over the head of the child, the American and Peruvian shake gloved hands. This, then, from Don: "Give a man a fish and he will eat one meal. Teach him how to fish and he will not be hungry the rest of his life. And he will feed others." He is given to adages.

"Old sawbones," I say.

Next to the hospital is a kind of Indian funeral parlor. It is a canny choice of location. We are walking past when a man emerges carrying a flat limp bundle wrapped in a blue alpaca blanket. He is followed by a woman with a more than usually solemn face. She has the inevitable protruding abdomen and wide pelvis of the Indian female. These women are masterpieces of fecundity. Many go decades without menstruating once, proceeding directly from lactation to pregnancy. Aida says it is one way of saving on sanitary napkins. The woman is wearing a stiff short skirt of many colors. It has the shape of an elongated tutu. But the shape only. Beneath, wide-set skinny rachitic legs. An ancient battered car is waiting. The man tries to insert the bundle into the backseat, but cannot. The bundle is too long. After a few clumsy attempts, he gives it up, opens the trunk of the car and lays the bundle inside. Just before he closes the lid, we see five small dark toes emerging from the blanket. The sound of the trunk closing is the most utterly serious sound in the world. The man and woman get into the car and are driven away. We stare at the trunk of the car until it is out of sight. A few steps from where the car had stood, the topiary garden of Honorio Delgado Hospital needs clipping badly. The once crisp green creatures have quite gone to seed. The little llama is whiskered; the angel, shaggy. My own melancholy is a foot thick.

I am walking in the city with Don.

"Clean, isn't it?" he says. "No discarded paper or plastic in the streets. No dog shit." And it is true. Not Paris, but Arequipa is the city of light. If blue skies, herds of mountains, sprays of stars and clean streets are proof of divine approval, then God surely loves Arequipa. Praise how you will the city that boasts the Cathedral of Notre Dame; if to walk there with unsoiled shoes you have to keep your eyes on the pavement and practice a kind of broken-field running, it just isn't worth it. In Arequipa the dogs are confined to rooftops and courtyards. In Arequipa in the evening, you can walk and look up at the stars.

Sunday, Carlos Galda, the chief of surgery, has arranged an outing for us at a restored Inca grain mill. After weeks of surgery, clinics and rounds, we are eager for leisure. We are a caravan of four cars each holding five *interplasticos.* There is much hilarity. At El Molino there will be a feast; octopus marinated in lime juice, slices of charcoal-broiled beef heart, pisco, and beer. And dancing without which a party is not a party in Peru. Peruvians cannot imagine a party where people sit around and converse. What fun is that? they ask. Not much, we admit. The mill is about twenty miles from Arequipa, in the country. I am in the backseat of the last car. Near the halfway mark we cross a narrow bridge that spans a deep gorge at the bottom of which is a swiftly running river. Immediately having crossed, we find that the road ascends sharply, then curves out of sight. The leading cars have already disappeared from view. It is in mid-ascent of that incline that Fate casts upon INTERPLAST its most ironic smile. The car stalls. Before the hand brake can be applied, we have rolled backward a few feet and struck a small car filled with people. It is an ancient blue Volkswagen. The driver of that Volkswagen leaps from the car, neglecting, in his ardor for battle, to close the door. Now he and our driver are fully engaged in a passionate discussion which promises to be interminable. I get out of the car to assess the damages. None to our car, I see; a dent, only, in the front bumper of the other. Never mind, I say. I'll give him money. Let's get going. Just then, thinking to disengage us from the Volkswagen, our driver releases the hand brake prior to starting the motor. It is a lapse. The hand brake is reapplied but not before we have once again nudged the Volkswagen. This time, it begins to roll backward down the hill toward the bridge. I chase after it, thinking, I suppose, to reach in and pull up the hand brake. But I cannot catch the car. Faster and faster it rolls. Through the windshield I see the faces of the passengers. Indians. Their eyes are wide with terror. Their mouths are open for shrieking. Just before the bridge, the little blue car takes a small sickening turn to the left, achieves the rim of the chasm, tips up at the front and plunges backward into the ravine. All this I watch from a few feet away. And hear the crash far below. For a moment I pause at the edge, then leap. The sides of the gorge are not quite straight. There are stunted shrubs to grab, rocks to brace a foot against. It is an utterly graceless scramble downward, at least half of which is made on skidding buttocks, heels. A series of bounces, really, until that final plummet into the river. A mouthful of raw sewage.

I am twenty feet from the rock ledge where the car has come to rest on its side. From the wreck, whimpering. They are alive! I see three old men. They are covered with blood. The river beneath the ledge is red with it. I try to pull one of the men through a window, but he is wedged. Now I am joined by Bill and Michael. They are both young and strong. I am merely old and reckless. We shout to each other above the noise of the river. Our voices echo against the walls of the chasm. The air is stagnant, palpable. Michael climbs on top of the car and tries to open the door. It will not open. He pounds it with his fist, a rock. At last it gives, and we hand the three old men out to each other. They are Franciscan monks. They wear long brown habits and rosaries. Somehow, this makes it worse. From the bridge, people throw ponchos in which the injured will be carried up to the road. Other men have come down to help. One of the monks has sustained an avulsion of his forehead and scalp. Blood from the great wound films his face. He is blinded by it. I wipe the wound with my hand, find the artery that is spurting at the base of the gouge, pinch it between thumbnail and fingernail. The bleeding slows, virtually stops. We lay him on a poncho and begin to climb. He is immensely heavy and I must use one hand to pinch the artery. The other is the tiredest hand of my life. No mountaineer ever looked more longingly at the summit of Everest than I at the bridge high above. Crampons! I cry, like a surgeon calling for his favorite scalpel. What I want more than anything in the world is to lie down too, and, lapped in alpaca, be carried up the cliff. But there is that damned artery. And I its hemostat. Is it not, I ask myself . . . is it not the calling of a surgeon to be an instrument that the patient takes up in order to heal himself?

There are no level places, no footholds. Only slanting slippery rocks. Nor can we see the placement of our feet. Has human foot ever stepped here? I wonder. Will it ever again?

"Let's stop for a minute," says Bill. "Set him down." I could weep with relief. Twice we stop to rest, panting. Each time, we turn to look down. Beneath our feet the terrific cliff sinks in awful steepness to the river fifty . . . a hundred feet below. Who cares if it is fifty? Or a hundred? Or five hundred? The insolence of mere numbers. At last we reach the top; I unpinch my fingers from the blood vessel. The bleeding has stopped. It does not resume. The three wounded men are placed in the back of a truck and taken to Honorio Delgado. The next day we will visit them on rounds. Rows of cotton sutures will crisscross their smiles. From swollen purple mouths they will cast blessings upon us. There will be no single word of reproach. All the same we will be filled with guilt. We who came to repair and have ended by damaging. Conquistadores!

But now, still standing at a cowardly distance from the edge of the ravine, I piece together the fragments of my body, which is not that of your fit and fly-soled athlete come to Peru to scale the *cordillera blanca* but that of a middle-aged padder of pavement. No, I am not one of those macho surgeons who give themselves airs over muscular prowess. Great aprons of beef do not hang from my diminutive skeleton. Ah well, Carlos and the others have come back to find us. He insists that we go on to El Molino. Shattered, and so malleable, we do. You do not refuse a Peruvian's hospitality, no matter what.

The stairways and corridors of El Molino have been decorated with paper lanterns. Just outside, a herd of alpaca graze by a peaceful stream. There is kindly massage, tumblers of pisco. And dancing. In two hours we are tipsy. Later, on the way back to Arequipa, we stop at the bridge and go to stand again at the edge of the precipice. A rank air hisses up from the depths. Like ones who have emerged from the mouth of Hell, we are returned to a state of childhood horror. You are making too much of it, we say to one another. And know that we are making far too little. We pick up stones and toss them over the side. The one I throw takes hours to strike the bottom. It has a muffled sound like the impact of flesh. A noise like that could kill you. I would not go down there again for Saint Francis himself.

A last visit to Honorio Delgado. What a far cry it is from my sleek and spanking hospital in New Haven—all glass and prestressed concrete. And yet, so like. A hospital is only a building until you hear the slate hooves of dreams galloping upon its roof. You listen then and know that here is no mere pile of stone and precisely cut timber but an inner space full of pain and relief. Such a place invites mankind to heroism. For us, Honorio Delgado has become an instrument with which to confront life, a rock that stands firm against the incessant lapping of fate. Even at Pena, at the mill, at the bottom of the ravine, this hospital clung to us like a she-wolf. We could smell her maternal odors penetrating to our hearts. Tomorrow we leave Peru carrying with us the pathetic belief that the way to heal the world is to take it in for repairs. One on one. One at a time.

Imelda

I heard the other day that Hugh Franciscus had died. I knew him once. He was the Chief of Plastic Surgery when I was a medical student at Albany Medical College. Dr. Franciscus was the archetype of the professor of surgery—tall, vigorous, muscular, as precise in his technique as he was impeccable in his dress. Each day a clean lab coat, monkishly starched, that sort of thing. I doubt that he ever read books. One book only, that of the human body, took the place of all others. He never raised his eyes from it. He read it like a printed page as though he knew that in the calligraphy there just beneath the skin were all the secrets of the world. Long before it became visible to anyone else, he could detect the first sign of granulation at the base of a wound, the first blue line of new epithelium at the periphery that would tell him that a wound would heal, or the barest hint of necrosis that presaged failure. This gave him the appearance of a prophet. "This skin graft will take," he would say, and you must believe beyond all cyanosis, exudation, and inflammation that it would.

He had enemies, of course, who said he was arrogant, that he exalted activity for its own sake. Perhaps. But perhaps it was no more than the honesty of one who knows his own worth. Just look at a scalpel, after all. What a feeling of sovereignty, megalomania even, when you know that it is you and you alone who will make certain use of it. It was said, too, that he was a ladies' man. I don't know about that. It was all rumor. Besides, I think he had other things in mind than mere living. Hugh Franciscus was a zealous hunter. Every fall during the season he drove upstate to hunt deer. There was a glass-front case in his office where he showed his guns. How could he shoot a deer? we asked. But he knew better. To us medical students he was someone heroic, someone made up of several gods, beheld at a distance, and always from a lesser height. If he had grown accustomed to his miracles, we had not. He had no close friends on the staff. There was something a little sad in that. As though once long ago he had been flayed by friendship and now the slightest breeze would hurt. Confidences resulted in dishonor. Perhaps the person in whom one confided would scorn him, betray. Even though he spent his days among those less fortunate, weaker than he—the sick, after all—Franciscus seemed aware of an air of personal harshness in his environment to which he reacted by keeping his own counsel, by a certain remoteness. It was what gave him the appearance of being haughty. With the patients he was forthright. All the facts laid out, every question anticipated and answered with specific information. He delivered good news and bad with the same dispassion.

I was a third-year student, just turned onto the wards for the first time, and clerking on Surgery. Everything—the operating room, the morgue, the emergency room, the patients, professors, even the nurses—was terrifying. One picked one's way among the mines and booby traps of the hospital, hoping only to avoid the hemorrhage and perforation of disgrace. The opportunity for humiliation was everywhere.

It all began on ward rounds. Dr. Franciscus was demonstrating a cross-leg flap graft he had constructed to cover a large fleshy defect in the leg of a merchant seaman who had injured himself in a fall. The man was from Spain and spoke no English. There had been a comminuted fracture of the femur, much soft-tissue damage, necrosis. After weeks of debridement and dressings, the wound had been made ready for grafting. Now the patient was in his fifth postoperative day. What we saw was a thick web of pale blue flesh arising from the man's left thigh, and which had been sutured to the open wound on the right thigh. When the surgeon pressed the pedicle with his finger, it blanched; when he let up, there was a slow return of the violaceous color.

"The circulation is good," Franciscus announced. "It will get better." In several weeks, we were told, he would divide the tube of flesh at its site of origin, and tailor it to fit the defect to which, by then, it would have grown more solidly. All at once, the webbed man in the bed reached out, and gripping Franciscus by the arm, began to speak rapidly, pointing to his groin and hip. Franciscus stepped back at once to disengage his arm from the patient's grasp.

"Anyone here know Spanish? I didn't get a word of that."

"The cast is digging into him up above," I said. "The edges of the plaster are rough. When he moves, they hurt."

Without acknowledging my assistance, Dr. Franciscus took a plaster shears from the dressing can and with several large snips cut away the rough edges of the cast.

"*Gracias, gracias.*" The man in the bed smiled. But Franciscus had already moved on to the next bed. He seemed to me a man of immense strength and ability, yet without affection for the patients. He did not want to be touched by them. It was less kindness that he showed them than a reassurance that he would never give up, that he would bend every effort. If anyone could, he would solve the problems of their flesh.

Ward rounds had disbanded and I was halfway down the corridor when I heard Dr. Franciscus's voice behind me.

"You speak Spanish." It seemed a command.

"I lived in Spain for two years," I told him.

"I'm taking a surgical team to Honduras next week to operate on the natives down there. I do it every year for three weeks, somewhere. This year, Honduras. I can arrange the time away from your duties here if you'd like to come along. You will act as interpreter. I'll show you how to use the clinical camera. What you'd see would make it worthwhile."

So it was that, a week later, the envy of my classmates, I joined the mobile surgical unit—surgeons, anesthetists, nurses, and equipment—aboard a Military Air Transport plane to spend three weeks performing plastic surgery on people who had been previously selected by an advance team. Honduras. I don't suppose I shall ever see it again. Nor do I especially want to. From the plane it seemed a country made of clay—burnt umber, raw sienna, dry. It had a dead-weight quality, as though the ground had no buoyancy, no air sacs through which a breeze might wander. Our destination was Comayagua, a town in the Central Highlands. The town itself was situated on the edge of one of the flatlands that were linked in a network between the granite mountains. Above, all was brown, with only an occasional Spanish cedar tree; below, patches of luxuriant tropical growth. It was a day's bus ride from the airport. For hours, the town kept appearing and disappearing with the convolutions of the road. At last, there it lay before us, panting and exhausted at the bottom of the mountain.

That was all I was to see of the countryside. From then on, there was only the derelict hospital of Comayagua, with the smell of spoiling bananas and the accumulated odors of everyone who had been sick there for the last hundred years. Of the two, I much preferred the frank smell of the sick. The heat of the place was incendiary. So hot that, as we stepped from the bus, our own words did not carry through the air, but hung limply at our lips and chins. Just in front of the hospital was a thirsty courtyard where mobs of waiting people squatted or lay in the meager shade, and where, on dry days, a fine dust rose through which untethered goats shouldered. Against the walls of this courtyard, gaunt, dejected men stood, their faces, like their country, preternaturally solemn, leaden. Here no one looked up at the sky. Every head was bent beneath a wide-brimmed straw hat. In the days that followed, from the doorway of the dispensary I would watch the brown mountains sliding about, drinking the hospital into their shadow as the afternoon grew later and later, flattening us by their very altitude.

The people were mestizos, of mixed Spanish and Indian blood. They had flat, broad, dumb museum feet. At first they seemed to me indistinguishable the one from the other, without animation. All the vitality, the hidden sexuality, was in their black hair. Soon I was to know them by the fissures with which each face was graven. But, even so, compared to us, they were masked, shut away. My job was to follow Dr. Franciscus around, photograph the patients before and after surgery, interpret and generally act as aide-de-camp. It was exhilarating. Within days I had decided that I was not just useful, but essential. Despite that we spent all day in each other's company, there were no overtures of friendship from Dr. Franciscus. He knew my place, and I knew it, too. In the afternoon he examined the patients scheduled for the next day's surgery. I would call out a name from the doorway to the examining room. In the courtyard, someone would rise. I would usher the patient in, and nudge him to the examining table where Franciscus stood, always, I thought, on the verge of irritability. I would read aloud the case history, then wait while he carried out his examination. While I took the "before" photographs, Dr. Franciscus would dictate into a tape recorder:

"Ulcerating basal-cell carcinoma of the right orbit—six by eight centimeters—involving the right eye and extending into the floor of the orbit. Operative plan: wide excision with enucleation of the eye. Later, bone and skin grafting." The next morning we would be in the operating room where the procedure would be carried out.

We were more than two weeks into our tour of duty—a few days to go—when it happened. Earlier in the day I had caught sight of her through the window of the dispensary. A thin, dark Indian girl about fourteen years old. A figurine, orange-brown, terra-cotta, and still attached to the unshaped clay from which she had been carved. An older, sun-weathered woman stood behind and somewhat to the left of the girl. The mother was short and dumpy. She wore a broad-brimmed hat with a high crown, and a shapeless dress like a cassock. The girl had long, loose black hair. There were tiny gold hoops in her ears. The dress she wore could have been her mother's. Far too big, it hung from her thin shoulders at some risk of slipping down her arms. Even with her in it, the dress was empty, something hanging on the back of a door. Her breasts made only the smallest imprint in the cloth, her hips none at all. All the while, she pressed to her mouth a filthy, pink, balled-up rag as though to stanch a flow or buttress against pain. I knew that what she had come to show us, what we were there to see, was hidden beneath that pink cloth. As I watched, the woman handed down to her a gourd from which the girl drank, lapping like a dog. She was the last patient of the day. They had been waiting in the courtyard for hours.

"Imelda Valdez," I called out. Slowly she rose to her feet, the cloth never leaving her mouth, and followed her mother to the examining-room door. I shooed them in.

"You sit up there on the table," I told her. "Mother, you stand over there, please." I read from the chart:

"This is a fourteen-year-old girl with a complete, unilateral, left-sided cleft lip and cleft palate. No other diseases or congenital defects. Laboratory tests, chest X-ray—negative."

"Tell her to take the rag away," said Dr. Franciscus. I did, and the girl shrank back, pressing the cloth all the more firmly.

"Listen, this is silly," said Franciscus. "Tell her I've got to see it. Either she behaves, or send her away."

"Please give me the cloth," I said to the girl as gently as possible. She did not. She could not. Just then, Franciscus reached up and, taking the hand that held the rag, pulled it away with a hard jerk. For an instant the girl's head followed the cloth as it left her face, one arm still upflung against showing. Against all hope, she would hide herself. A moment later, she relaxed and sat still. She seemed to me then like an animal that looks outward at the infinite, at death, without fear, with recognition only.

Set as it was in the center of the girl's face, the defect was utterly hideous—a nude rubbery insect that had fastened there. The upper lip was widely split all the way to the nose. One white tooth perched upon the protruding upper jaw projected through the hole. Some of the bone seemed to have been gnawed away as well. Above the thing, clear almond eyes and long black hair reflected the light. Below, a slender neck where the pulse trilled visibly. Under our gaze the girl's eyes fell to her lap where her hands lay palms upward, half open. She was a beautiful bird with a crushed beak. And tense with the expectation of more shame.

"Open your mouth," said the surgeon. I translated. She did so, and the surgeon tipped back her head to see inside.

"The palate, too. Complete," he said. There was a long silence. At last he spoke.

"What is your name?" The margins of the wound melted until she herself was being sucked into it.

"Imelda." The syllables leaked through the hole with a slosh and a whistle.

"Tomorrow," said the surgeon, "I will fix your lip. *Mañana.*"

It seemed to me that Hugh Franciscus, in spite of his years of experience, in spite of all the dreadful things he had seen, must have been awed by the sight of this girl. I could see it flit across his face for an instant. Perhaps it was her small act of concealment, that he had had to demand that she show him the lip, that he had had to force her to show it to him. Perhaps it was her resistance that intensified the disfigurement. Had she brought her mouth to him willingly, without shame, she would have been for him neither more nor less than any other patient.

He measured the defect with calipers, studied it from different angles, turning her head with a finger at her chin.

"How can it ever be put back together?" I asked.

"Take her picture," he said. And to her, "Look straight ahead." Through the eye of the camera she seemed more pitiful than ever, her humiliation more complete.

"Wait!" The surgeon stopped me. I lowered the camera. A strand of her hair had fallen across her face and found its way to her mouth, becoming stuck there by saliva. He removed the hair and secured it behind her ear.

"Go ahead," he ordered. There was the click of the camera. The girl winced.

"Take three more, just in case."

When the girl and her mother had left, he took paper and pen and with a few lines drew a remarkable likeness of the girl's face.

"Look," he said. "If this dot is *A*, and this one *B*, this, *C* and this, *D*, the incisions are made *A* to *B*, then *C* to *D*. *CD* must equal *AB*. It is all equilateral triangles." All well and good, but then came *X* and *Y* and rotation flaps and the rest.

"Do you see?" he asked.

"It is confusing," I told him.

"It is simply a matter of dropping the upper lip into a normal position, then crossing the gap with two triangular flaps. It is geometry," he said.

"Yes," I said. "Geometry." And relinquished all hope of becoming a plastic surgeon.

*

In the operating room the next morning the anesthesia had already been administered when we arrived from ward rounds. The tube emerging from the girl's mouth was pressed against her lower lip to be kept out of the field of surgery. Already, a nurse was scrubbing the face which swam in a reddish-brown lather. The tiny gold earrings were included in the scrub. Now and then, one of them gave a brave flash. The face was washed for the last time, and dried. Green towels were placed over the face to hide everything but the mouth and nose. The drapes were applied.

"Calipers!" The surgeon measured, locating the peak of the distorted Cupid's bow.

"Marking pen!" He placed the first blue dot at the apex of the bow. The nasal sills were dotted; next, the inferior philtral dimple, the vermilion line. The *A* flap and the *B* flap were outlined. On he worked, peppering the lip and nose, making sense out of chaos, realizing the lip that lay waiting in that deep essential pink, that only he could see. The last dot and line were placed. He was ready.

"Scalpel!" He held the knife above the girl's mouth.

"Okay to go ahead?" he asked the anesthetist.

"Yes."

He lowered the knife.

"No! Wait!" The anesthetist's voice was tense, staccato. "Hold it!"

The surgeon's hand was motionless.

"What's the matter?"

"Something's wrong. I'm not sure. God, she's hot as a pistol. Blood pressure is way up. Pulse one-eighty. Get a rectal temperature." A nurse fumbled beneath the drapes. We waited. The nurse retrieved the thermometer.

"One hundred seven . . . no . . . eight." There was disbelief in her voice.

"Malignant hyperthermia," said the anesthetist. "Ice! Ice! Get lots of ice!" I raced out the door, accosted the first nurse I saw.

"Ice!" I shouted. "*Hielo!* Quickly! *Hielo!*" The woman's expression was blank. I ran to another. "*Hielo! Hielo!* For the love of God, ice!"

"*Hielo*?" She shrugged. "*Nada*." I ran back to the operating room.

"There isn't any ice," I reported. Dr. Franciscus had ripped off his rubber gloves and was feeling the skin of the girl's abdomen. Above the mask his eyes were the eyes of a horse in battle.

"The EKG is wild . . ."

"I can't get a pulse . . ."

"What the hell . . ."

The surgeon reached for the girl's groin. No femoral pulse.

"EKG flat. My God! She's dead!"

"She can't be."

"She is."

The surgeon's fingers pressed the groin where there was no pulse to be felt, only his own pulse hammering at the girl's flesh to be let in.

*

It was noon, four hours later, when we left the operating room. It was a day so hot and humid I felt steamed-open like an envelope. The woman was sitting on a bench in the courtyard in her dress like a cassock. In one hand she held the piece of cloth the girl had used to conceal her mouth. As we watched, she folded it once neatly, and then again, smoothing it, cleaning the cloth which might have been the head of the girl in her lap that she stroked and consoled.

"I'll do the talking here," he said. He would tell her himself, in whatever Spanish he could find. Only if she did not understand was I to speak for him. I watched him brace himself, set his shoulders. How could he tell her? I wondered. What? But I knew he would tell her everything, exactly as it had happened. As much for himself as for her, he needed to explain. But suppose she screamed, fell to the ground, attacked him, even? All that hope of love . . . gone. Even in his discomfort I knew that he was teaching me. The way to do it was professionally. Now he was standing above her. When the woman saw that he did not speak, she lifted her eyes and saw what he held crammed in his mouth to tell her. She knew, and rose to her feet.

"*Señora*," he began, "I am sorry." All at once he seemed to me shorter than he was, scarcely taller than she. There was a place at the crown of his head where the hair had grown thin. His lips were stones. He could hardly move them. The voice dry, dusty.

"No one could have known. Some bad reaction to the medicine for sleeping. It poisoned her. High fever. She did not wake up." The last, a whisper. The woman studied his lips as though she were deaf. He tried, but could not control a twitching at the corner of his mouth. He raised a thumb and forefinger to press something back into his eyes.

"*Muerte*," the woman announced to herself. Her eyes were human, deadly.

"*Sí, muerte*." At that moment he was like someone cast, still alive, as an effigy for his own tomb. He closed his eyes. Nor did he open them until he felt the touch of the woman's hand on his arm, a touch from which he did not withdraw. Then he looked and saw the grief corroding her face, breaking it down, melting the features so that eyes, nose, mouth ran together in a distortion, like the girl's. For a long time they stood in silence. It seemed to me that minutes passed. At last her face cleared, the features rearranged themselves. She spoke, the words coming slowly to make certain that he understood her. She would go home now. The next day her sons would come for the girl, to take her home for burial. The doctor must not be sad. God has decided. And she was happy now that the harelip had been fixed so that her daughter might go to Heaven without it. Her bare feet retreating were the felted pads of a great bereft animal.

*

The next morning I did not go to the wards, but stood at the gate leading from the courtyard to the road outside. Two young men in striped ponchos lifted the girl's body wrapped in a straw mat onto the back of a wooden cart. A donkey waited. I had been drawn to this place as one is drawn, inexplicably, to certain scenes of desolation—executions, battlefields. All at once, the woman looked up and saw me. She had taken off her hat. The heavy-hanging coil of her hair made her head seem larger, darker, noble. I pressed some money into her hand.

"For flowers," I said. "A priest." Her cheeks shook as though minutes ago a stone had been dropped into her navel and the ripples were just now reaching her head. I regretted having come to that place.

"*Sí, sí*," the woman said. Her own face was stitched with flies. "The doctor is one of the angels. He has finished the work of God. My daughter is beautiful."

What could she mean! The lip had not been fixed. The girl had died before he would have done it.

"Only a fine line that God will erase in time," she said.

I reached into the cart and lifted a corner of the mat in which the girl had been rolled. Where the cleft had been there was now a fresh line of tiny sutures. The Cupid's bow was delicately shaped, the vermilion border aligned. The flattened nostril had now the same rounded shape as the other one. I let the mat fall over the face of the dead girl, but not before I had seen the touching place where the finest black hairs sprang from the temple.

"Adiós, adiós . . ." And the cart creaked away to the sound of hooves, a tinkling bell.

*

There are events in a doctor's life that seem to mark the boundary between youth and age, seeing and perceiving. Like certain dreams, they illuminate a whole lifetime of past behavior. After such an event, a doctor is not the same as he was before. It had seemed to me then to have been the act of someone demented, or at least insanely arrogant. An attempt to reorder events. Her death had come to him out of order. It should have come after the lip had been repaired, not before. He could have told the mother that, no, the lip had not been fixed. But he did not. He said nothing. It had been an act of omission, one of those strange lapses to which all of us are subject and which we live to regret. It must have been then, at that moment, that the knowledge of what he would do appeared to him. The words of the mother had not consoled him; they had hunted him down. He had not done it for her. The dire necessity was his. He would not accept that Imelda had died before he could repair her lip. People who do such things break free from society. They follow their own lonely path. They have a secret which they can never reveal. I must never let on that I knew.

*

How often I have imagined it. Ten o'clock at night. The hospital of Comayagua is all but dark. Here and there lanterns tilt and skitter up and down the corridors. One of these lamps breaks free from the others and descends the stone steps to the underground room that is the morgue of the hospital. This room wears the expression as if it had waited all night for someone to come. No silence so deep as this place with its cargo of newly dead. Only the slow drip of water over stone. The door closes gassily and clicks shut. The lock is turned. There are four tables, each with a body encased in a paper shroud. There is no mistaking her. She is the smallest. The surgeon takes a knife from his pocket and slits open the paper shroud, that part in which the girl's head is enclosed. The wound seems to be living on long after she has died. Waves of heat emanate from it, blurring his vision. All at once, he turns to peer over his shoulder. He sees nothing, only a wooden crucifix on the wall.

He removes a package of instruments from a satchel and arranges them on a tray. Scalpel, scissors, forceps, needle holder. Sutures and gauze sponges are produced. Stealthy, hunched, engaged, he begins. The dots of blue dye are still there upon her mouth. He raises the scalpel, pauses. A second glance into the darkness. From the wall a small lizard watches and accepts. The first cut is made. A sluggish flow of dark blood appears. He wipes it away with a sponge. No new blood comes to take its place. Again and again he cuts, connecting each of the blue dots until the whole of the zigzag slice is made, first on one side of the cleft, then on the other. Now the edges of the cleft are lined with fresh tissue. He sets down the scalpel and takes up scissors and forceps, undermining the little flaps until each triangle is attached only at one side. He rotates each flap into its new position. He must be certain that they can be swung without tension. They can. He is ready to suture. He fits the tiny curved needle into the jaws of the needle holder. Each suture is placed precisely the same number of millimeters from the cut edge, and the same distance apart. He ties each knot down until the edges are apposed. Not too tightly. These are the most meticulous sutures of his life. He cuts each thread close to the knot. It goes well. The vermilion border with its white skin roll is exactly aligned. One more stitch and the Cupid's bow appears as if by magic. The man's face shines with moisture. Now the nostril is incised around the margin, released, and sutured into a round shape to match its mate. He wipes the blood from the face of the girl with gauze that he has dipped in water. Crumbs of light are scattered on the girl's face. The shroud is folded once more about her. The instruments are handed into the satchel. In a moment the morgue is dark and a lone lantern ascends the stairs and is extinguished.

*

Six weeks later I was in the darkened amphitheater of the Medical School. Tiers of seats rose in a semicircle above the small stage where Hugh Franciscus stood presenting the case material he had encountered in Honduras. It was the highlight of the year. The hall was filled. The night before, he had arranged the slides in the order in which they were to be shown. I was at the controls of the slide projector.

"Next slide!" he would order from time to time in that military voice which had called forth blind obedience from generations of medical students, interns, residents, and patients.

"This is a fifty-seven-year-old man with a severe burn contracture of the neck. You will notice the rigid webbing that has fused the chin to the presternal tissues. No motion of the head on the torso is possible. . . . Next slide!"

Click, went the projector.

"Here he is after the excision of the scar tissue and with the head in full extension for the first time. The defect was then covered. . . . Next slide!"

Click.

". . . with full-thickness drums of skin taken from the abdomen with the Padgett dermatome. Next slide!"

Click.

And suddenly there she was, extracted from the shadows, suspended above and beyond all of us like a resurrection. There was the oval face, the long black hair unbraided, the tiny gold hoops in her ears. And that luminous gnawed mouth. The whole of her life seemed to have been summed up in this photograph. A long silence followed that was the surgeon's alone to break. Almost at once, like the anesthetist in the operating room in Comayagua, I knew that something was wrong. It was not that the man would not speak as that he could not. The audience of doctors, nurses, and students seemed to have been infected by the black, limitless silence. My own pulse doubled. It was hard to breathe. Why did he not call out for the next slide? Why did he not save himself? Why had he not removed this slide from the ones to be shown? All at once I knew that he had used his camera on her again. I could see the long black shadows of her hair flowing into the darker shadows of the morgue. The sudden blinding flash. . . . The next slide would be the one taken in the morgue. He would be exposed.

In the dim light reflected from the slide, I saw him gazing up at her, seeing not the colored photograph, I thought, but the negative of it where the ghost of the girl was. For me, the amphitheater had become Honduras. I saw again that courtyard littered with patients. I could see the dust in the beam of light from the projector. It was then that I knew that she was his measure of perfection and pain—the one lost, the other gained. He, too, had heard the click of the camera, had seen her wince and felt his mercy enlarge. At last he spoke.

"Imelda." It was the one word he had heard her say. At the sound of his voice I removed the next slide from the projector. *Click* . . . and she was gone. *Click* again, and in her place the man with the orbital cancer. For a long moment Franciscus looked up in my direction, on his face an expression that I have given up trying to interpret. Gratitude? Sorrow? It made me think of the gaze of the girl when at last she understood that she must hand over to him the evidence of her body.

"This is a sixty-two-year-old man with a basal-cell carcinoma of the temple eroding into the bony orbit . . ." he began, as though nothing had happened.

At the end of the hour, even before the lights went on, there was loud applause. I hurried to find him among the departing crowd. I could not. Some weeks went by before I caught sight of him. He seemed vaguely convalescent, as though a fever had taken its toll before burning out.

Hugh Franciscus continued to teach for fifteen years, although he operated a good deal less, then gave it up entirely. It was as though he had grown tired of blood, of always having to be involved with blood, of having to draw it, spill it, wipe it away, stanch it. He was a quieter, softer man, I heard, the ferocity diminished. There were no more expeditions to Honduras or anywhere else.

I, too, have not been entirely free of her. Now and then, in the years that have passed, I see that donkey-cart cortege, or his face bent over hers in the morgue. I would like to have told him what I now know, that his unrealistic act was one of goodness, one of those small, persevering acts done, perhaps, to ward off madness. Like lighting a lamp, boiling water for tea, washing a shirt. But, of course, it's too late now.

Three Doctors: Watson, Conan Doyle, and Me (Lecture for the New Haven Sherlock Holmes Society, 2003)

When I was first invited some weeks ago to give this talk, I still had enough common decency to decline. It would, I knew, be the most flagrant act of imposturage ever perpetrated on the continent of North America. You see, I had never to my recollection read a story by Conan Doyle, and had only a dim memory of one film with Basil Rathbone as Sherlock Holmes. In my boyhood, when other twelve-year-olds were reading Conan Doyle, I was addicted to the swashbuckling novels of Rafael Sabatini (*Captain Blood, The Sea Hawk, Scaramouche*), but loved even more the horror stories of Edgar Allan Poe. I'm sure this preference played no small role in my choice of a medical specialty. Surgeons love gore, don't you know.

Everyone in the auditorium, I argued, would know more about the subject than I. Whereupon the captain of the New Haven Sherlock Holmes Society proceeded to heap praise upon my head, nor would he hear of my demurrals. So at last o'erswol'n from the flattery, I acquiesced, or perhaps succumbed would be a more fitting verb. Long ago, I became a follower of Tallulah Bankhead who said: "To Hell with criticism; praise is good enough for me!"

Why not? I decided. I shall educate myself in the matter of Sherlock Holmes so as to carry out yet another of my impertinences of the podium. For the last six weeks, I have read nothing but the works of Conan Doyle, and have formed a few opinions which may or may not coincide with those of the aficionados.

First, his name. "Sherlock" in old Norse means fair- or flaxen-haired. But the detective has always been portrayed as dark-haired. A *holme* in Old Norse is an islet in the middle of a fen. A *holm* is also a species of sturdy oak. It is a manly name. Is it mere coincidence, I wonder, that Sherlock Holmes' literary predecessor, Edgar Allan Poe's detective in such stories as "The Murders in the Rue Morgue," is named Auguste Dupin, combining the great Emperor Augustus with another tree, the pine. And Agatha Christie's detective, Hercule Poirot, combines manly strength with yet another tree—the pear. What is at play here is the aligning of the perspicacious man of popular culture (one who observes and is all head and brain) with the archaic heroic spirit. On the other hand, I may have made all that up.

Sherlock Holmes' rooms at 221B Baker Street are known to us all. There is a fireplace with two armchairs, one on either side, where Holmes and Watson conduct their conversations. There is a table with chemical apparatus, a violin, a Persian slipper jack-knifed to the mantel in which Holmes keeps his tobacco, and a bust of Holmes sculpted by one Oscar Meuniere. This bust is, we recall, a decoy for a deadly silent air rifle, and is a means for Sherlock to be in two places at once.

Sherlock's literary predecessor and model, Poe's Auguste Dupin, is a no less strange and enigmatic personage, a man of illustrious family now living in reduced circumstances. Like Holmes and Watson, he and the unnamed narrator of "The Murders in the Rue Morgue" meet, are drawn to each other, and decide to live together in the only vestige of Dupin's patronage—a "time-eaten and grotesque mansion, long deserted through superstitions and tottering to its fall in a retired and desolate part of the Faubourg St. Germain." There the two sit out the day from dawn to dusk behind drawn curtains until nightfall when they sally forth to patrol the city of Paris until dawn.

Compare these quarters and 221B Baker Street with the mansion of Usher in Poe's "Fall of the House of Usher," in which Roderick Usher lived with his sister, Madeline. The mansion of Usher too is in a state of obsolescence and decay, and the death-like pallor of its surface is covered with a web-work of fungi. Roderick's room is profuse, comfortless, antique, and tattered. Many books and instruments lie scattered about, but fail to give any vitality to the scene. From the windows—long, narrow, and pointed—"feeble gleams of encrimsoned light fall on the figure of Usher."

In a deeper sense, the rooms of all three, Sherlock Holmes, Auguste Dupin, and Roderick Usher, are the characters themselves expressed in terms of architecture and interior decoration. They are the dens of men of feeling and sensitivity, the scriptoria of poets, scientists, collectors, amateurs, and dilettantes of all sorts. The contents of each room form a still-life in which the objects are redolent of mystery and the sublime. This paradigmatic still-life is of books, instruments, and the implements of philosophical contemplation—a pipe, a musical instrument (a violin in Holmes' case, a guitar in Roderick Usher's), a coffee or teapot, and often a wineglass and bottle with which to celebrate the triumph of a case. The honorific placing of images and objects in the clutter of a Victorian room takes place in both Doyle and Poe. When Umberto Eco wrote *The Name of the Rose*, he cast the story as a plot by Conan Doyle, and chose for his protagonist (who is a medieval Sherlock Holmes) a typical Norman English name, William Baskerville, which is also the name of the estate that is under a curse.

But let us return to Holmes' bust. The Oscar Meuniere who carved it may well have been a real person. The likelihood, though, is that Conan Doyle invented the name, taking it from a contemporary Belgian sculptor who did busts, and also from his acquaintance with Oscar Wilde, in whose *The Picture of Dorian Gray* a work of art suffers the fate from which its sitter was, for a time, magically excused—just as Holmes' bust died in his stead.

Like Poe's Roderick Usher, Sherlock Holmes is a man of abnormally acute senses, sensitivity, and sensibilities. He is a combination of acumen, analytical genius, and depression, a perennial adolescent—restless, petulant, compulsively inquisitive. Like Roderick Usher, he too has no body; he is all head. I imagine him tall, slim, crisp, acutely intelligent, impatient, and merciless. He has been accused of being dour and humorless—and I must say that a good deal of Sherlock's reported laughter was not out of amusement, but out of triumph, revenge, or plain old *schadenfreude* when his opponents, Inspectors Gregson and G. Lestrade, are proven wrong and so humiliated, and he himself is right. It put one in mind of any number of the faculty of a local university.

In *A Study in Scarlet* we read that Sherlock Holmes was in favor of euthanasia for suffering animals. He willingly murders the sick old dog by offering it the pills found in the murdered Stangerson's room—not out of any feeling of mercy, mind you, but in order to advance his theory that the pills were indeed poison. When the first pill fails to kill the dog, Holmes is aghast. Springing from his chair and pacing wildly up and down, he cries: "Surely . . . my whole train of reasoning cannot have been false. It is impossible! And yet this wretched dog is none the worse." But then he gives "a perfect shriek of delight" and dissolves the other pill in milk and feeds that to the dog, which promptly dies.

Speaking of dogs, it is clear to me that Sherlock Holmes had a good deal of canimosity. (Don't bother looking that word up in the dictionary; I invented it. It means dislike of dogs.) When Holmes and Watson first meet and are becoming acquainted with each other's foibles prior to agreeing to share rooms, Watson declares: "I keep a bull pup." "That dog must go!" responds Sherlock Holmes. The creature is never heard of again. We must remember that Holmes, during his college days, was bitten on the ankle by a bull terrier.

Various theories have been advanced as to the disappearance of Watson's dog. One, that Mrs. Hudson objected to the animal; another that the dog ran away; still another that the dog was accidentally killed when Watson stumbled while carrying it up the seventeen stairs to the sitting room. Personally, I am of the opinion that the dog was the victim of one of Holmes' chemical experiments.

May I dare to mention a few of Conan Doyle's flaws and inconsistencies? In *A Study in Scarlet*, we have Holmes munching silently at his toast, with no explanation how he performed this miracle. Then too here is the matter of Watson's wandering wound, originally sustained in Afghanistan where he was shot with a jezail, an ancient Arabic rifle. Sometimes the wound is described as in Watson's shoulder, sometimes in his leg. And last, we are told that the snake called "The Speckled Band" would crawl through a ventilator and down the bell-rope to the bed where Miss Stoner slept—and then, after being summoned by Dr. Roylott with a low whistle, would crawl back up the bell-rope to its master. This we are told "with certainty." But first of all, snakes are deaf, so this one couldn't have heard the doctor's low whistle. Snakes respond not to noises but to vibrations transmitted to their bodies by contact. Secondly, a snake might conceivably slide down a free-swinging bell-rope, but it certainly could not climb back up. Snakes do not climb, as many think, by twining their coils about an object; they climb by wedging themselves into any crannies and interstices, taking advantage of every irregularity and protrusion upon which to hook themselves. Just so do they rapidly climb up trees. The bite of the viper, we are further led to believe, caused death within ten seconds. Now Sir Arthur! No snake kills in so short a time. The viper in question carried haemotoxic venom, not neurotoxic, and so would take even longer to kill. Either Dr. Roylott was still alive when Holmes and Watson entered his room, or he had died of a heart attack, and the snake had embedded its fangs in a dead man. All this I learned from the family herpetologist.

No more than anyone else can I account for the phenomenon of Sherlock Holmes' survival long after his creator is dead. To this day, hundreds of thousands believe that he was a real person, and some among the benighted actually write letters to him addressed to 2218 Baker Street. The bank situated at that address has to employ someone especially to reply to this correspondence. How did this happen? One falls back upon the sense that urban man has long had a folklore that has flourished with all the energy and success of myth and fable. By urban folklore I mean such characters as Don Quixote, Tarzan of the Apes, and Superman. These figures leapt from their texts instantaneously and entered the public imagination, there to remain. The text has become only a source of classical reference for their reality.

The relationship between two men—one dynamic, charismatic, and colorful; the other subordinate, subdued, and self-effacing—is not new with Sherlock and Doctor Watson. Think of Don Quixote and Sancho Panza, Hamlet and Horatio. Perhaps the most revealing insight into the friendship is when Watson decides to get married, and Holmes complains that Watson is deserting him for a mere wife. It could be said of Watson, the physician, that he narrowed his practice down to one patient, Sherlock Holmes, in order to tag along with him and thereby generate a brand new genre of medical case history—the fevered, obsessive activities of his single patient. Unlike those other writing doctors—Rabelais, Chekhov, William Carlos Williams, Freud, and even Selzer—Watson wrote about only one man who, though he called him "my friend," was really his patient. And has ever patient been accorded more thorough and loving attention from his physician? I doubt that even Queen Victoria's doctor, or Adolph Hitler's, willingly carried their bag and a revolver. Luckily, Watson also carried a notebook. My contention is that it isn't the mystery work, the actual detection, that has kept Sherlock Holmes alive all these years; it is the idealization of a doctor/patient relationship so that it became what is universally seen as a friendship. And every reader knows that if ever Holmes should be taken ill or wounded, there would be Dr. Watson to attend him. There has been some speculation over whether Holmes and Watson loved each other. I think not: Watson had an eye for the ladies and was married at least once. If Holmes ever loved another human being, it would have been his brother Mycroft. He compared Mycroft's visit to a planet leaving its orbit.

If Watson is all bedside manner, Holmes is pure diagnostics. (He is, after all, modeled after Joseph Bell, one of Conan Doyle's professors of medicine.) Much has been made of Holmes' rationality—the science of deduction—based on his famous line: "When the impossible has been eliminated, what remains, however improbable, must be the truth." But Holmes approached a crime the way a good diagnostician approaches a disease, and was really the ultimate inductionist. With a crime as with an ailment, the undertaking is, appropriately, a case. For Holmes, everybody and every place under scrutiny was a patient. He was a great listener, a master at discarding—barely hearing—information that didn't bear upon the case, but able to find significance in the sparsest details. He wasn't (he didn't need to be) a great questioner. For him, witnesses gave themselves away. In the tactical search for clues, a room, a moor, a pocket watch became the signs and symptoms of a disease; he palpated, sniffed, and gazed about with microscopic eyes. For Holmes, as for Poe's Auguste Dupin, most men had a window in their bosom through which he could peer and discover their secrets and thoughts.

Could Arthur Conan Doyle and I ever have been friends? Perhaps. After all, we are both doctors and writers. I admire and trust big strong men with singleness of purpose and great energy. Big he was: over six feet tall and weighing over seventeen stone. At fourteen pounds per stone, that would be two hundred and thirty-eight pounds. But that's where the similarities end. I am a puny nine stone, an old skinful of feathers. Conan Doyle was a good husband, the grimly declared enemy of all lying, unmanly conduct, cowardly shuffling, idle unmerited praise and ambitious self-esteem, in all of which categories I give myself the grade of B-. He is moral and decent; I am chock full of vice. Still another difference between us is that Conan Doyle was a he-man, a man's man, an avid sportsman, good at cricket, soccer, and boxing—about which he said: "The old bare-knuckle fighting of the prize ring is an excellent thing from a national point of view." As someone who has never thrown a punch or even spanked a naughty child, I am at a loss to explain the pleasure such a "sport" as boxing gives to its practitioners, and to those who watch it. Doyle thought that any man worthy of the name would wish to excel in sports and games, while I was a washout except for being a swift runner, which I had to be in order to escape from he bullies and child molesters of Troy, New York, who could not seem to keep their hands off me. No, I don't think Conan Doyle would have had much use for the likes of me.

One similarity between us is that, while still in our teens, both Conan Doyle and I lapsed from the religions foisted upon us from birth. While I have remained in a state of skepticism, Holmes later dove headlong into Spiritualism in which he communed with the dead. This is an example of—what shall I say? It is so very . . . English. Time was, whenever my own eccentricities threatened to get out of hand, I would send myself off to England where they would not be so apt to be noticed among the general oddity.

To his immense credit, Arthur Conan Doyle was not a male chauvinist, and was a strong supporter of women's rights. In "The Doctors of Hoyland," Doyle portrays the young male doctor as priggish, vain, and possessive of his turf. He is austere and of a bland suavity. When a woman doctor moves into town, he is dismissive of her, demeans her abilities, and is openly rude to her. She, on the other hand, turns out to be a gifted practitioner, deft and courageous where he is timid of the scalpel. She is also warm, sympathetic, and honest. Soon she has taken away the bulk of his practice. He is furious and jealous. On the occasion that he is in an accident and has a broken leg, it is she who gives him chloroform and sets the broken bone. In due course, he apologizes to her and proposes marriage, which she wisely refuses.

In the Class of 1953 of Albany Medical College, we were fifty-two graduating doctors of whom only three were women. I am not terribly proud of some of the pranks played upon these courageous three by their loutish and rowdy classmates, of whom I was one. In the fifties and sixties, the specialty of surgery was a male priesthood in which the training involved a good deal of brutality and power delivered from above downward. Ridicule and humiliation were never far away. I'm happy to say that during the last eight years of my sojourn in surgery, women flocked into the field in great numbers. Since

I was known to be the least of all evils among the herd of bullies, many, if not all, of these women interns and residents finagled to be assigned to me. I leave it to your imagination the boost to my masculine self-image. I relished the chance to atone partially for my earlier misbehavior.

I cannot close without thinking of Conan Doyle as Doctor. There has been a concerted effort of late to portray him as a "great physician." But first of all, he was told to become a doctor by his much-adored mother, who felt it would ensure a good livelihood. He was not to the manner born, while I was blooded to it at my father's knee. Doyle's grades in medical school were undistinguished, all but one (in Chemistry) being just "satisfactory." Upon graduating, he opened an office in a small town, where for eight years he engaged in the "terrible occupation of waiting." His practice never was a success—fortunately for the world, as he wrote his stories while waiting.

After eight years Conan Doyle went to Germany for three months to train as an ophthalmologist. Here he is reminiscing on the subject (he was recovering from an attack of influenza at the time of his decision to leave medicine):

> I remember in my delight taking the handkerchief which lay upon the coverlet in my enfeebled hand and tossing it up to the ceiling in my exultation. I should at last be my own master. No longer would I have to conform to professional dress or try to please anyone else. I would be free to live how I liked and where I liked. It was one of the great moments of exultation of my life.

It is true that most of the writing doctors of the past left medicine as soon as their literary talent became known to them—W. Somerset Maugham, Walker Percy, Anton Chekhov, and the others. Only William Carlos Williams continued to practice medicine all his life. I myself remained in surgery for more than thirty years before retiring to try to realize my potential as a writer. And even then, I walked away with great reluctance from my beloved workbench in the Operating Theatre.

Out of his passionate belief in the British Empire, and his loyalty to the throne, Conan Doyle volunteered to serve in the army as a doctor during the Boer War. (He was knighted, not for his literary achievements at all, but for having defended England from the charges of having committed atrocities against the Boers.) He remained in South Africa for three months, not out of any interest in caring for the sick and wounded, but because he craved the adventure of it. He took delight in the physical activity: "The great empty world of the veldt seen fresh in the morning, trains roving through the night, dark groups silhouetted against the flames of campfires. Wonderful is the atmosphere of war," he wrote. During his three months of military service, he reported an epidemic of enteric fever among the British troops. There was no treatment for it, and every day sixty soldiers were buried. On the one real possibility of performing a medical act, Doyle demurred. A soldier had received a bullet wound in the arm. Conan Doyle could not bring himself to extract the bullet, saying: "That had better be left for chloroform and the field hospital." Similarly, when Chekhov was holding a clinic in an outlying village, a woman arrived with a small child who had a large ripe abscess on the neck, needing only a nick to let the pus drain out. But poor Chekhov, undone by the sobs of the mother and the screams of the child, sent for the nearest doctor some thirty miles away. Such, such were the writing doctors of yesteryear. We who have come later were made of sterner stuff. We did not blanch at the sight of blood. On the contrary, we were happiest when "deep imbrued in gore."

No, rather than calling Conan Doyle a "great doctor," I would think of him as a great student of medicine who learned and remembered a vast lore in the field—and made wonderful use of it in his writings.

Reflections on Doctoring (Lecture at the Yale School of Medicine, 1996)

Some people choose to become doctors out of a desire to relieve suffering, or to lead a life in which the possibility of good works is daily present. Some elect out of the fascination with the body, how it is made, how it functions. Who would not be in awe of so marvelous a creation? Any physician, studying anatomy and physiology, would have to echo Marianne Moore's words of wonderment: "What sap went through that tiny thread to make the cherry red?" Besides, by virtue of owning a body, a doctor has a personal interest in the subject. Many is the doctor whose ambition was sparked by an illness or injury sustained early in life. Some are drawn to the profession out of a desire for respectability and financial security; still others out of an attraction toward disease, pathology, the dark side of the body. There is about the unbeautiful facts of blood and wounds something that exhilarates even as it appalls.

I chose to become a doctor when my general practitioner father died suddenly. If I could no longer find him in the flesh, I would find my father through the work that he did. It was a wise decision for a grief-stricken boy, for in the years to come, I grew to know my father more intimately than had we lived together for decades.

During the Great Depression in Troy, New York, the family lived on the second floor of a house, just above Father's office. From my earliest days I sat on the landing and listened to the moan/s and cries that floated up the staircase. No words, only the howled vowels of pain, inarticulate sounds of weeping that rose. Once, attempting to coax me out of a sulk, Father drew me between his knees then gently fit the earpieces of his stethoscope into my ears. He placed the disk over his own heart. All at once, there was the distant muffled thudding of *life* itself.

"Lub-dup," he said, "lub-dup." I listened and was *touched*. Just so is the hound blooded to the hunt at its master's knee. It was a year later at a house call that he again offered me the stethoscope.

"Would you mind?" he asked the elderly man sitting propped in the bed.

"Well, well," said the man, beaming. "Another doctor, is it? Going to follow in your daddy's footsteps?" I went to place the disk on his chest.

"Wait!" said Father. "Warm it with your breath the way I do." I huffed at the disk. "All right, now," he said. And for the first time I placed my hand upon a fellow human being in the diagnostic act and heard the wild irregular beat of auricular fibrillation that has no logical sequence.

Surely the best part of summer vacation was going along with father on house calls, carrying his old black doctor's bag. Scuffed and with its handles drooping like the ears of an old hound, it had accompanied him on his rounds for so long that he had come to treat it as a pet, grooming it with oil or black shoe polish, patching it with adhesive tape or putting in a couple of stitches to reinforce the seam that threatened to give way. Sometimes I would be told to sit on the front stoop where I could hear the outcries of childbirth in a home delivery. In bad weather, I got to wait in a parlor where, through a keyhole, I might catch a glimpse of the solemnities of the sickbed. It was in one of those parlors that I first witnessed death. The door to the sickroom had not stayed shut. Through the crack I could see the bed and its contents. Father leaned over the man who labored there. A rosary had been entwined in fingers that fumbled with the bit of blanket. There was his pointed nose, and the blue toes that had escaped the covers. Rapt, I watched the way he chased his breath until he caught up with it, but only for a moment before it once again broke free and was running away again with quick small steps. Exhausted, the man lay as if deciding whether to mount another chase, then all at once, his ribs started up from the bed and off he went once more, pumping after his wayward breath.

"It is called Cheyne-Stokes breathing," Father told me afterwards. "When they start, you know it won't be long."

"Why does everybody have to die? It isn't fair," I said.

"It is too fair. It's a part of being a person. It would be much worse not to."

While in all other matters Father spoke to me as to a boy, with affection and jocularity, about doctoring he spoke to me as to an adult. As if he knew there would not be any more time. He told me about those kings who could heal a sore just by touching it; how almost at once, the wound would heal. Doctoring was like that, like trying to be a king with a healing touch.

"Some day when you're a man and a doctor, you'll know what I mean." When, years later, I studied the art of taking a patient's history and performing a physical examination, it was as though I had been taught these arts as a child. There was a strange familiarity about them that came, I am sure, from watching my father at work and from listening to him. In the process of the physical examination, whoever else might be present, doctor and patient are alone with each other. No matter how a patient first shows himself to a doctor, it is more diagnostic to watch a man remove his soiled underwear to show his naked affliction. There is something deeply moving about the human body waiting to be examined. Lying or seated, the body has surrendered whatever defensive or acquisitive posture it may have had and presents itself in an attitude of supplication. Palpating the abdomen, the doctor may glance up to see the trust that glows deep within the eyes of the patient. Sparks of it will leap forth to ignite him. For it is trust, not gratitude or worship, that animates the physician. To palm a fevered brow, to feel a thin wavering pulse at the wrist, to draw down a pale lower lid—these simple acts cause a doctor's heart to expand. His own physical condition is altered by the presence of the patient. It is the contagion of the diagnostic embrace. Add to this the possibility of healing and there is no human encounter more beautiful.

It is well known that medicine had its origins in religion. Asklepios, the Greek god of Medicine, passed the secrets of healing on to Chiron, a centaur who, in turn, divulged them to Hippocrates, a mortal. In primitive tribal societies too it has always been the holy man or shaman who emerges from his trances with the power to heal. The shaman has his drum, which is the river of sound through which he can descend to the Kingdom of Shadows to retrieve his tribesfellow from death. The modern doctor listens to the electronic beep of a cardiac monitor and the regulated breathing of a respirator, and is either reassured or warned. Time was, when in order to become a shaman, one had to undergo an initiation of death and resurrection. The aspirant had to be taken to the sky or to the netherworld. Often he would be dismembered by spirits, cooked in a pot and eaten by them. Only then could he be reborn as a shaman. Happily, no such rite of passage goes into the making of a doctor, but there is something about the process of medical training that is reminiscent of the sacred ur-drama after all. A would-be doctor must pass through medical school where the body of a fellow human is dissected and the mysteries of biochemistry and physiology are passed on. Then there is the period of sacrifice and self-denial called internship and residency. Now the will and spirit are subjugated to the discipline of the craft and the art. In some ways, the making of a doctor remains a priestly pantomime marked by a long hard novitiate. What is different is that the doctor practices inherited and learned rites, while the shaman is susceptible to visions. They both perform acts bent upon making order out of chaos. Give me knowledge any day over visions and miracles. It is more reliable.

In Father, the priestly and the sensual existed side by side. His performance of the simplest acts—lighting a fire in the grate, tamping down a cigarette, lathering on shaving cream, trimming his spruce little mustache—partook of these two elements. They were present, as well in his practice of medicine: the way his fingers questioned a pulse, the way he drew down a lower lid or palpated someone's abdomen. Once, he had needed to me to hold a man's leg while he debrided an infected gash. I could not hide my revulsion for the stench, the ugliness of it. Later, on the way home, he spoke of it: "A wound is like a lamp. If all the lights in the house went, you could dress a wound by the light it gives off."

The training of a doctor is long and hard, as it should be. There is no shortcut to the accumulation of wisdom and compassion. A doctor does not slip from his mother's womb with compassion smeared upon him like the drippings of birth. Compassion, rather, is like a sound that drifts up from the numberless wounds, sores, cavities and ulcers the doctor touches and dresses in the course of the years. At first this voice is barely audible to the medical student, hardly more than a whisper as from many mouths. Slowly it gathers, rises from the streaming flesh until at last it is a pure *calling*, an exclusive sound like the cry of certain solitary birds, telling that out of the resonance between patient and doctor there may spring that profound courtesy that is a kind of love. Still, the daily confrontation is a burden that grows heavier with age. The doctor will need all of his wit and humor to defend himself against despair.

"So many times," said Father, "there will be nothing you can do except"—and here his face brightened—"to make sympathetic noises in your throat." From this I have learned not to hesitate to make empty gestures in the face of hopelessness. They can be of immense value to a patient and her next-of-kin. Yes, everything that Father said was a dispatch that would precede me into my life. At intervals, there they would be, waiting for me; I had only to pick each one up and read it in order to find a way to the next message.

One of the blessings for which I am thankful is that all my years of medicine have not robbed me of my awe of the human spirit. I continue to believe that the flesh really is the spirit thickened.

In writing about my patients, I have again and again been drawn to those privileged moments in which there is a sudden showing forth, an epiphany. Here are three—

I stand by the bed where a young woman lies, her face postoperative, her mouth twisted in palsy, clownish. A tiny twig of the facial nerve, the one to the muscles of her mouth, has been severed. She will be thus from now on. The surgeon had followed with religious fervor the curve of her flesh; I promise you that. Nevertheless, to remove the tumor in her cheek, I had cut the little nerve.

Her young husband is in the room. He stands on the opposite side of the bed, and together they seem to dwell in the evening lamplight, isolated from me, private. Who are they, I ask myself, he and this wry-mouth I have made, who gaze at and touch each other so generously, greedily? The young woman speaks.

"Will my mouth always be like this?" she asks.

"Yes," I say, "it will. It is because the nerve was cut."

She nods, and is silent. But the young man smiles.

"I like it," he says. "It is kind of cute."

All at once I *know* who he is. I understand, and I lower my gaze. One is not bold in an encounter with a god. Unmindful, he bends to kiss her crooked mouth, and I so close I can see how he twists his own lips to accommodate to hers, to show her that their kiss still works. I remember that the gods appeared in ancient Greece as mortals, and I hold my breath and let the wonder in.

It is many years since I walked away from my beloved workbench in the operating room in order to become a writer. So complete has been my separation from medicine as to make it seem that I had died and been reborn into another incarnation, only with the singular knowledge of what I had been in my previous existence—a doctor. But now and then it happens that I am brought back with startling clarity to that past life, only seen now through the soft filter of time and with the contemplation of the artist.

I spend the better part of each day at the Yale library where I write and read. Toward evening, I take the shuttle bus home. On one recent day, I boarded the bus and took a seat across the aisle and one row behind the driver, a man I had not seen before. A new bus driver, I decided.

"Where do you want to get off?" he asked

"The Divinity School," I told him. "I live nearby." When he turned to listen, I saw that his chin, lower lip, and the entire front of his neck had been grafted with skin, doubtless to release the contracture of a burn scar. He appeared to be in his late thirties. From where I sat, I could see how easily he turned his head from side to side, raised it, then lowered his chin. An excellent functional result, I thought. Not perfect cosmetically—a ridge here and there, an area of pallor—but of this the man seemed unaware; he made no effort at concealment, wore no scarf or neckerchief. All at once, a mist parted and it dawned upon me that I was the one who had performed that skin graft, that this bus driver as a child had been my patient. A moment later I remembered a small boy, naked, lying on an operating table, his chin attached to his chest by a great purple fan of scar tissue. So dense was this scar that the boy could not extend his head to see but must wrinkle his forehead and peer from the top of his vision. The mouth was pulled open and twisted, the lower lip entirely lost in the wild mass of flesh. I remember leaning over him, holding his hand, his struggle not to cry. Moments later he was asleep with a breathing tube in one nostril.

Now, so many years later, I had an impulse to go up behind the bus driver, to examine, to feel, to ask him to show me the donor site. Perhaps I would recognize it the way one knows his own handwriting. Perhaps he would remember my name? But I remained in my seat.

"Divinity!" he called out. I rose to leave the bus. Best not to trespass upon a previous incarnation.

Sometimes the patient or next-of-kin will turn the tables on you. When that happens they go straight for your soul. I remember one old man baying in his bed . . .

Each breath is a bone he attempts to dislodge from his throat. Such suffering, I think, must atone for any amount of wickedness. This man will die out of debt. Into the sheet each night he looses his saliva, urine, sweat and blood, impregnating the linen with his own oils and gums and resins until the sheets grow heavy while he grows ever lighter. Every morning a nurse comes to change the mummy's bed. But the old man does not die. Day after day, and many times each day, he must be turned in his bed, and lifted, and fed and injected. He has lost the control of his bowels and bladder. Pus drains from openings on his abdomen and thigh.

His wife is small and frail. She, too, is old. "I'm taking him home," the wife tells me.

"But it will be too much for you," I say. "He needs too much tending to. A nursing home would be better . . . for . . . domiciliary care." She smiles at the word.

"His domicile is at 1834 Maple Street. That's our house."

"But what about all the mess ?"

"How much mess can one man make?" she answers. And I am silent. For she has told me what I already knew, but had forgotten. Tending the body of another is an act of infinite loneliness, and carried out alone, a solitary commitment for which one is equipped only from the storehouse of his own heart.

"How much mess can one man make?" I heard her words and I felt that I had been handed a secret letter that one day I must hand on to another. It contained whatever there is to know about the care of the sick.

When all else fails, the old woman teaches, take up reverence and proceed.

Part IV

Illuminations

In 1974, Richard Selzer participated in a Yale lecture series on medicine and religion. Previous speakers in the series had included a Roman Catholic doctor, an evangelical Protestant, and a rabbi. Selzer began: "I speak for the Heathen."

His talk included no gibes at religious belief. In fact, it was most notable for a tone of earnest spirituality: "Even though the thought of Heaven does not console me," Selzer said, "I take comfort in the fellowship of mortality. We are none of us going to make it off this planet alive. We are all at the mercy of necessity and chance. Therefore, we are all brothers and sisters. . . . A doctor is a pilgrim among his pilgrim patients." Selzer did not want to be called a "humanist," because to him that word connoted a rationalistic worldview. Instead, he spoke of intuition and mystery, referring to the flesh as "the spirit solidified" and describing his search for privileged moments of courtesy, courage, and love in daily experience.[1]

Many such moments are captured in Selzer's essays and short stories—and even in brief vignettes like the three encounters that conclude "Reflections on Doctoring." Sometimes the epiphanies become visual, as when a sudden *radiance* illuminates Dr. Bhimjee and Leonard at the end of "Fetishes," or when a brave, dying boy in "Atrium: October 2001" is glimpsed for the last time by the doctor-narrator: "The wheelchair with its contents is already being propelled away. From across the Atrium, I follow with my eyes the radiance that accompanies it."[2]

In "At St. Mary's," that same word is used to make fun of vain surgeons, each of whom "was quite convinced that once he had left the ward his disembodied radiance lingered on." Selzer has never hesitated to portray brusque or self-important physicians, such as the doctor in "Whither Thou Goest" or the anesthesiologist in "Festishes." In "At St. Mary's," however, he once again presents his father, Dr. Julius Selzer, as a model of medical humility. Julius also turns out to have been a good amateur theologian ("he was of the conservative branch of atheism"), and his explanation of the Trinity is profound. Richard, like his father, became a reverent skeptic: "Temperamentally unable to surrender to faith myself, I have remained in a condition of awe at the faith of others. It is what constitutes for me a belief in God, only once removed, like a cousin."

In "Longfellow, Virgil, and Me" Selzer returns to his school days, recalling "an exchange of the heart" that retains its charm across the decades. Comparable moments of grace, generosity, and deep courtesy spark the narratives of "Fetishes" and "Whither Thou Goest," and in the latter case an exchange of the heart is literal. This story began, Selzer told an interviewer, after he read a newspaper account about a murder victim whose organs were transplanted into seven people: "And I thought to myself, gee whiz, *this is a fable of our time*. . . . I'm going to write it. And so, I thought what point of view should I take?"[3] When he decided to make the young widow Hannah the protagonist of his story, and to tell "Whither Thou Goest" as a journey of healing, Selzer worked out his point of view more technically—building scenes of dialogue, advancing the narrative through a series of letters, and relying on a poetic third-person voice to express the nuances of Hannah's epiphanic experience.

Such lyrical omniscience informs many of Selzer's narratives of illumination, as when "Fetishes" conveys the desperation of a patient, Audrey, clinging to her dignity. However, the desperation in "Four Appointments with the Discus Thrower" remains implicit: simply reported by the doctor-narrator without interpretation. Why does the elderly patient in Room 542—a blind amputee, presumably with end-stage diabetes—throw his breakfast against the wall every morning? Selzer has often been asked this question, and in one of his diary entries (the third reprinted here from 2010) he hazards an answer, but the art of the story lies in its open-endedness. The illumination results from the reader's empathy with a sufferer raging futilely against an illness that has taken away his identity.

Selzer's own dire illness in 1991 is chronicled in a chapter from *Raising the Dead: A Doctor's Encounter with His Own Mortality* (Whittle Communications, 1993). After contracting Legionnaires' disease, Selzer was in a coma for twenty-three days. Because he remembered next to nothing about this ordeal, and was writing without reference to his hospital records, he assumed great narrative freedom, splitting his viewpoint—so that the patient becomes both "I" and "he"—and incorporating fictional elements: "Dream, imagination—these are the chariots that the comatose body rides." A later chapter reports a series of hallucinatory episodes (including encounters with monks in thirteenth-century Ireland, and with Father Damien in his leper colony on Molokai), but creative storytelling also colors Selzer's supposedly clinical account of his death and miraculous resurrection.[4] What remains undeniably factual is the affirmation in this work that heralds his recovery: "Saying yes to life, accepting once again the burden and thrill of it."

In "Atrium: October 2001," the line between life and death becomes almost imperceptible, as Selzer turns a real experience into a touching meditation on "the fluidity of things." Reaching out to a precocious cancer patient, the doctor composes a poetic account of death as a return to oneness with nature. "By the end of the story," Selzer says in his explication, "both doctor and Tony experience an epiphany when the continuum of mortality and immortality is sensed." The epiphany is powerfully emotional, and the atrium of the human heart proves far more capacious than the sunlit foyer of a modern hospital.

The doctor in "Atrium" offers the dying boy in the story no comfortable assurance of a personal afterlife. This accords with Selzer's deepest beliefs: "It is not necessary to have a life hereafter," he said in his 1974 speech at Yale. "What is essential is that my life should bear some mark, some insight, if but half-perceived, of the earth of which it is a part." Paradoxically, the earthbound insights in Selzer's writing often illuminate the angelic potential in human nature. •

NOTES

1. The text of this talk, entitled "Not Quite a Humanist," is in Box 31, Folder 55, in the Selzer Papers at the Moody Medical Library, Galveston, TX. Some of the phrasing in the talk is close to Selzer's philosophical reflections in two essays: "Lessons from the Art" in *Mortal Lessons*, Touchstone edition (New York: Simon & Schuster, 1987), 37–48; and "Introduction: The Making of a Doctor-Writer" in *The Exact Location of the Soul* (New York: St. Martin's Press, 2001), 1–15.

2. In some cases, Selzer's descriptions of "radiant" characters are deepened by distinctive word choices. In "Fetishes," for example, the word "gracile" is used to describe Dr. Bhimjee's hands; the same word is used in "Atrium" to describe the neck of the dying boy.

3. Mahala Yates Stripling, "'The Tending Act': An Interview with Richard Selzer," *Composition Studies* 24, no. 1-2 (Spring/Fall 1996), 38.

4. In discussing the controversy over invented material in *Raising the Dead*, Selzer makes no apologies, and in fact regrets having revealed his fabrication later in the book. "Had I been courageous," he says, "I would not have confessed at all"—adding that the mere fact of writing about his supposed death and resurrection made it "almost as real as anything that has happened to me." See his *Diary* (New Haven, CT: Yale University Press, 2011), 2–3.

At St. Mary's (from Chapter 4 of *Down from Troy:A Doctor Comes of Age*)

From early on, I loved going with Father to St. Mary's Hospital. Actually that was its nickname, short for St. Mary, Consoler of the Afflicted. Or as Father liked to say, and made me say it too, Maria Consolatrix Afflictorum; he was of the conservative branch of atheism and insisted on the Latin. The hospital was a three-story redbrick building built in 1914, a long rectangle with two pavilions, or wings, extending from either side. Since it was operated and staffed by the Sisters of Charity, the building was winged in more-ways than one. St. Mary's was situated halfway up the slope of a steep hill, from which you could look down over the town. Ever since, I have always thought that halfway up a hillside is just where a hospital belongs, midway between a cathedral on the top and a jailhouse at the foot, in touch with both the sacred and the profane. Whether it was prophetic or simply a matter of logistics, the cemetery was right up the street. From the hospital's solarium on the second floor you could watch the smoke from the crematorium chimney rise and diffuse over the city as the dead insisted upon mixing with the living. In summer, with the windows open, you could even catch a whiff of it, a compelling early lesson in death, resurrection and ecology. I can still close my eyes and smell that blend of starch, candle wax, ashes and roses that permeated St. Mary's Hospital. It is an odor that I have not smelled since in any of a lifetime of hospitals; it is the odor of sanctity, I think.

The nuns ran the place as though it were the flagship of a fleet on the eve of a naval battle. Here, if nowhere else, cleanliness *was* next to godliness. The polished floors wore a perpetual fanatic gleam; dirt was rooted out as though it were sin. It would take more than mere senility to make me forget

Sister Michael's evening inspection of the long marble corridor. Behind her limped a wretched porter, who had spent the entire day washing and waxing the floor. I remember the stiff white wings of her cornet slicing the gloom, the crusader's curve of her nostrils, her eyes that reconnoitered every corner, then turned upon the miscreant with the glare of black olives as she pointed to a bit of smudge that was invisible to me. I remember how the Nun of Wrath aimed one bony finger at the spot for the poor devil to see, how he stood there with the good-for-nothing look of a dog that has just made a mess on the carpet. With the student nurses, she was equally exacting. Like that precise princess in the fairy tale, the one who was put out of sorts by a rose leaf out of place in the garden, just so did Sister Michael appear in the doorway of a ward, sniff once or twice and go directly to the very bed where one corner of a sheet had not been tucked to ferocity.

The habit of the Sisters of Charity was black, full, and fell to within an inch and a half of the floor. From a cord about the waist, a black rosary hung. The wimple was topped by a starched white cornet with a broad lateral flap on either side of the head. One alone was a sailboat, two side by side a regatta, three a whole armada. These sisters did not walk; they skimmed, they hovered. Free of the drag of gravity by which the rest of us are rooted to the earth, they floated quickly and noiselessly, save for the soft click of wooden beads tossing among the folds of their habits. With each step, the black nose of a shoe would peek from beneath the hem then dart back inside the flaring recesses as though each of them were sheltering a family of mice.

More than once in the springtime I sat in the many-windowed solarium that was filled with vases of lilac and peony and gazed down the long hall in full expectation that the very next thing I would see coming toward me would be Maria Consolatrix Afflictorum Herself, to whom I would, oh yes I would, hold out my wounded heart. One evening Father came to collect me there.

"What were you doing?" I asked him.

"I was bringing a baby boy into the world," he replied. That's the way they used to talk in those days.

"Where did you bring it from?"

"A sealed garden."

"How did you get in if it was sealed?"

"The gate was opened just long enough for me to reach in and take him out. Next subject."

I opened a new line of questioning. "What is the Holy Trinity?"

"It's just an expression."

"No, what is it really?"

"It means the three who are one."

"I don't get it," I told him.

Father thought for a long moment. "Well, look," he said. "Here we are walking this corridor. Do you see those three wall lamps along the way? Let the first one be the Father, the next one the Son, and the third the Holy Ghost. Each lamp gives out its own light, but as we walk down the hall passing from one light to the next we still get some of the light from each one no matter where we are standing. Now do you get it?"

"You made that up."

"Then shut up," he explained. It is fifty years later, and as for the Holy Trinity, I still don't quite get it, but of all the explanations I have been given over the years, Father's makes the most sense.

At St. Mary's, the beds were lined up along the walls of large ward rooms. In time of need, a movable curtain screen could be placed so as to conceal the newly dead or to afford, if not privacy, at least the implication of it. To this day I am of the opinion that private rooms are a wrongheaded idea. Once encaged in a private room, the patient is out of sight as well as alone. This cannot be as safe or as functional as a great ward with fifteen beds lined up on either side, over which one sharp-eyed nurse can keep constant surveillance. To say nothing of the lovely commiseration that prevails in a ward and the hustle-bustle that is the antidote to the boredom of the bedridden. What architects and doctors have lost sight of is the pleasure the sick take in just plain gossiping. It is on a ward, not in a private room, where the craving for gossip is more likely to be satisfied. Besides, unless the gift of prophecy has deserted me, a ward is not one inch farther away from Heaven than a private room. When the time comes for me to be put to bed in a hospital, let it be in a ward, where my sighs and groans can mingle with the sighs and groans of my fellow human beings in the consolation of fraternity, and where it might be given to each of us in turn to utter the most beautiful sentence in the English language: There but for the grace of God go I.

As severe as Sister Michael was with the porter and the students, just so kindly did she move among the sick. Mercy, just before leaving the world of medicine forever, lingered awhile among those nuns. How different those sisters were from the doctors, who stepped importantly among the puddles of patients, especially the surgeons, each of whom was quite convinced that once he had left the ward his disembodied radiance lingered on. Father was the sisters' favorite. Their affection was based on his good-humored teasing, to which they responded with a commotion of cornets and a rolling up of the eyes. With what wit and gallantry he returned to those laborious virgins a glimmer of their long-forsworn sexuality. Temperamentally unable to surrender to faith myself, I have remained in a condition of awe at the faith of others. It is what constitutes for me a belief in God, only once removed, like a cousin. When I was twelve Father lay dying in St. Mary's Hospital. Long before my eyes had had their fill of him. I remember the vigilant nuns grouped like lamps in the darkened room, his face graying away, theirs glowing with an imperturbable golden light.

Years later, during summer vacations from college, I worked as a night orderly at St. Mary's. It was on my first night of duty that I was told to wheel a stretcher from the emergency room to the operating room and to go as quickly as I could, for the cargo in my charge was a young woman who, I was told, was hemorrhaging briskly. With one hand holding aloft a bottle of saline solution and the other pushing, I set off at a speed just short of reckless endangerment, only to find that the single working elevator was in use. When minutes went by, or hours (what does it matter how long?), and still the elevator didn't come, I began to despair for the life of my patient. From the head of the stretcher rose moan after moan to break the heart of Caligula. Was the red stain on the sheet spreading? A sister arrived also to wait for the elevator. At last, from the upper regions of the shaft, I heard the door slide shut, the gears engage and the car set in motion. Like a sentry on the alert, I prepared to storm and capture that elevator and rescue my first patient from certain death—only to watch as the empty car passed sluggishly by without stopping. Its slow disappearance from view remains one of the most sickening events of my life. Again and again I kicked the door and pounded it with my fist and I cursed it much as Jesus cursed the fig tree that bore no fruit. Goddamn elevator! I cried aloud. May your cables rust, your gears be stripped, your door go unhinged so that never again shall you know the bliss of ascension or descent. To all of which the sister responded with one of those sad little smiles those people keep in their repertoire. Then she reached for her beads and began to offer it up. That nun hadn't got past bead one when the elevator appeared out of nowhere, and we all rose to a happy ending.

That was the trouble with working at St. Mary's. You were always at risk of having Her called in on consultation, which kept a permanent sheepish expression on the faces of the heathen.

Longfellow, Virgil, and Me

To search for one's literary forebears is to hunt a genealogy more intimate by far than the identification of the ancient flesh from which one's mere body has come. It is a quest for saints long since lifted to the glory of Heaven, there to sit at golden tables in the vicinity of God. Within my mind, there are two men to whom I remain belted by filaments of the imagination of such a tensile strength as to have withstood the distraction, the wear and tear of thirty years. These are Longfellow and Virgil (*bacia mano*). May Heaven with its endless possibilities have brought them to the same table. And there may they wait patiently, patiently for me.

It was early in my schooling that I was required to lisp from memory the poems of Longfellow. So early that I cannot imagine childhood without him. For the children of Troy, New York, in the nineteen thirties, Evangeline, Minne-ha-ha, the village smith, and the skeleton in armor were the great heroic figures of literature. We knew no others. Nor have these poems left me while all else has either dropped like so many stones beneath the black tarn of forgetfulness or blurred into poor approximation or paraphrase. But then who could forget "Grave Alice and laughing Allegra, and Edith with golden hair"?

And, ah, that intrepid youth "who bore 'mid snow and ice, / a banner with the strange device, Excelsior." Where, we died to know, was he going? What implacable fury hounded him up that mountain, as the shades of night were falling fast? What did it mean, Excelsior? Was it the emblem of a promise given? Some cryptic warning? A terrible cri de coeur? It did not matter. The very syllables drove us mad with yearning. We longed to climb with him, side by side, sharing his passion and his agony, to take from his faltering arm that banner, and to wrap ourselves in Excelsior.

More than one voice quavered and broke, more eyes than mine filled with tears as we spoke that heartrending stanza wherein the brawny village smith, sitting in church with his sons, hears his daughter's voice in the choir, and "needs must think of her mother once more, / How in the grave she lies; / And with his hard rough hand he wipes / A tear out of his eyes." Twenty lumps gathered as one in twenty throats as we surrendered our hearts.

Most dreadful of all was the tale of the *Hesperus*, whose skipper had brought his little daughter to keep him company on the voyage. Her eyes were blue "as fairy-flax," her bosom white "as the hawthorn buds that ope in the month of May." With what commingled terror and grief did we see him lifeless and lashed to the helm, all stiff and stark, with his face turned toward the skies. With what sorrow did we later espy the little girl still tied to the drifting mast. "The salt-sea was frozen on her breast." (O bosom white as hawthorn buds.) "The salt tears in her eyes." (Blue as fairy-flax they were.) And her hair "like the brown sea-weed / On the billows fall and rise." Christ save us all, aloud cried we who had seen no waters more turbulent than those of the viscid Hudson, Christ save us all from the reef of Norman's Woe. It is thirty years later; my hair and brain cells fall from my head in a constant dismal rain. Still I murmur a fervent amen.

Most meticulously studied were the teachers. We scrutinized them like scholarly anthropologists, making observations on their habits, mannerisms, clothing, and dispositions. No fanatic rabbinate ruminating on the Talmud raised more convoluted conjecture. Now and then, rumor, like a madness, would sweep the schoolhouse: "Miss Cleary has a boyfriend." "Miss Feerick wears underpants down to her knees." Frissons of excitement infected from one to the other, leaping across the prurient aisles.

There was Gertrude Vaughn, third grade, her face in a permanent open-lipped smile that, by the addition of no more than a single crease, would have become a captured shriek. And Anna Mahoney, kindergarten, whose giant bosom was so tightly impacted upon her chest as to seem one uncleft tumefaction. Her voice was sweet as the billy club that swung at her brother's leg. Her sister Catherine, the principal, wore flat, laced oxfords with flapping external tongues. With each step her head shook from side to side rejecting every possibility.

From across the sea they had come, fierce Celtic maidens, long, long past their prime, and with a collective hunger that made of the potato famine a mere bagatelle. Such were the schoolteachers of Troy, whose indentured mothers had scoured the bathrooms of the middle class to send their girls to Normal School for the certificates that would ensure that *they* would never take lye and plunger to anyone else's toilet. Like a cloud of rare colored moths they had settled on the blackboards and knee-hole desks of Troy. Oh, let me recall them—their hair marcelled into all the waves of the sea, engulfed in opposing clouds of eau-de-cologne which drifted from each room into the corridors where they fought invisible gaseous battles for supremacy; the reckless prints in which they dressed—here lightning streaked across a sleeve, there Chinese poppies pocked trussed buttocks like some ill-gotten rash, and only lacking was the Spanish Armada in full rout across an abdomen. Thus, tattooed like Zulus, they patrolled, nodding and smiling to each other above the lines of snot, and the pairs and pairs of famished eyes that stared from one to the other in wildest surmise.

In the classrooms, the Palmer Method of Penmanship vied with Civics like princes of the throne. *Silas Marner* was in dread contention with *Santa Lucia*. But it was Latin that was king of Troy. And if Latin was king, his consort was the relentless, the implacable Ethel Houlihan. No bird of paradise she, but drab as a Quaker, her hair a failed bush, her skin and lips of the same leaden hue, with only the eyes ablaze, febrile. When she was angered her rage became almost tangible: it vaporized from her body; it had a smell, like starch. Howling, writhing, breaking chalk, flinging erasers, she gorged us with Latin. We were geese being primed for paté. Over the ridges of vocabulary she led us, scaling the cruelest cliff of grammar only to find another, steeper just beyond. Past ablatives absolute, ut-clauses of purpose, and grievous gerundives she herded us, pausing only long enough to flagellate the laggards. In *Jason and the Argonauts* she was Medea, crazy, abandoned, slaying her children. In *The Aeneid* she was Dido delivering her seaside lament into the head of a typhoon.

Margaret Byrnes sat three aisles away and one behind me. She was the most woebegone person I have ever seen. Everything she did seemed a last desperate effort after the failure of which there would be nothing to do but an act of self-immolation. She it was who each day bore the first brunt of Ethel Houlihan's morning rage. It was ever thus. The one person least equipped, who pretends no concealment of her ineptitude, is the very one who invites the easiest disaster. Lo, the bursting tigress stalks the herd of impala. Confident, restrained, she seeks out the weakest, the slowest, and *finds* her, frail and fainting in the tall grass. Margaret Byrnes labored half the night to translate fifteen lines of *The Aeneid*. In the morning, pale and trembling, came she to class, and to her Calvary. With what a horrid foreknowledge did she cower at her desk, folding and unfolding a hankie long since damp with perspiration, soon to be sopping with tears. Now and then she would be gripped by a shudder most terrible to behold, would socket up her eyes, staring back into that exhausted brain in which datives and genitives tangled and turned helter-skelter.

Had Margaret Byrnes been stupid, ugly, or mean, perhaps I should not have been moved by her passion. But Margaret Byrnes was beauty itself, a pale lamp, a spike of bright yellow. From out the puffs of her short sleeves, thin arms spoke eloquently all the vulnerabilities that she never once put into words. Nor did she look to her classmates for condolence, but suffered alone all the noble dimensions of her battle. Silent, panicky Joan of Arc being led to the stake with the awful premonition upon her. Each day was her martyrdom reenacted, nails, thorns, cross and all.

"Miss Byrnes," came the dread invocation. "Line 110 . . . Tum Dido . . ."

At the first syllable of her name Margaret Byrnes leaped to her feet as though ejected by some dreadful mechanism beneath her chair. Thus sprung and rigid she waited. Soon she would feel that intimate hot breath in the hollow of her neck, the first pressure of fangs, the spurt and run of her blood.

"Well?" urged Ethel Houlihan.

Almost inaudibly Margaret Byrnes cleared her throat. It was an act so piteous as to cramp the bowels of Caligula. The rest of us were become statuary, awaiting its turn beneath the sledgehammer. We could not, had we dared, bleed for her.

"Then Dido . . . ," began the wretched girl.

"Louder," came the fierce commandment. "And faster."

"Then Dido . . ." Margaret Byrnes' voice faltered again, then rallied. " . . . carried back to her palace the souvenirs of her night in the cave with Aeneas, and fondled them with slowly receding passion."

Not even the freest of translations could have produced a less accurate approximation of the text. The very run of all those consecutive words, each one sprung full-grown from the brow of her fancy, was shocking. What followed was the bellow of a stuck buffalo, a "hoyotoho" to deafen Wotan himself.

"Fool. Moron. Stupid. Yes, you *are* beyond hope, beneath contempt. Once again you have not done your homework."

If ever accusation were falsely charged, this was that time. On and on Ethel Houlihan railed; then, as though overcome with sudden boredom, she tossed the carcass abruptly from her jaws, and ordered the whimpering girl to sit. Which Margaret Byrnes did, folding into the seat.

All through this dark night of the soul, the rest of us waited, like Mary, Queen of Scots, for the chunk of the axe. It came.

"Mister Selzer . . . line 110 . . . Tum Dido."

I rose to my feet.

"Then Dido . . . ," I began, paused, looked up from my book, and continued.

" . . . carried back to her palace the souvenirs of her night in the cave with Aeneas, and fondled them with slowly receding passion."

I too had not recited Virgil, nor anything remotely like it, but the words of Margaret Byrnes verbatim. A terrible silence such as I have never known descended upon the classroom. It was as though we were in fact to be present at a beheading.

"What?" whispered Ethel Houlihan, and the wind from that *wh* would have blown Aeneas all the way from Carthage to Italy. Once again the storm rose; the sky turned black; gigantic waves slid beneath my little boat. I yawed; I spun; I lashed myself to the mast, and turned my salt-streaked face heavenward; like the skipper of the *Hesperus*, I made ready to die.

"Answer me, Selzer." She had dropped the mister. It would not go well with me.

"Or it will not go well with you."

But the answer was unspeakable. I had not *planned* to recite the words of Margaret Byrnes, did not know that I would until I had done it. Now I know that it was because they were beautiful and true. They were the words of one who knew the human heart better than Longfellow, better than Virgil, better by far than Christiaan Barnard. Virgil *should* have written them.

At the exact moment that Margaret Byrnes uttered them, I fell recklessly in love with her. Those words were her glove; mine, a vow of fealty, my pledge. In that careening sea, I searched and found her face, and to my everlasting glory, flashed her a smile of such heartbreaking courage as to qualify me for first mate aboard the *Golden Hind.*

What happened next remains one of the half-dozen most important events of my life—for back to me from Margaret Byrnes came slowly, shyly, but undeniably *there*, the pale and lovely reflection of my own smile. Here was no mere gesture of gratitude, but an exchange of the heart. Between those two smiles (O measure them in quanta, in light years) a rainbow arced; there was sealed a covenant, a secret troth plighted. In that moment Margaret Byrnes and I had won no mere present and future, but a past—a past that indeed one day it would be pleasing to remember.

Fetishes

There is Audrey. And there is Leonard. Audrey had waited until she was thirty-two to marry. Not by choice; no one had asked her. But all the time she had never given up hope, so that when Leonard Blakeslee had come along, she had at once reached out her hands for him as though he were an exotic foreign dish whose very strangeness captured her appetite completely. "You'll love me?" she asked him, and never once in all these years had he given her reason to doubt it. The fact that no children had come along was briefly regretted by both of them, then accepted. Somehow, it suited them.

Leonard is an anthropologist. Every so often he goes off to New Guinea on an expedition among the Asmat. It is the only time they are separated. When he is away Audrey feels only half intact, bisected. And Leonard too, as he wrote in a letter (she has saved them all), is "never done with wanting you at my side, where you ought always to be, my darling." She loved that "ought always to be." It was courtly. When he is not going on in that vein, his letters are anthropological, having to do with the language of the tribe for which he is compiling a dictionary, the artifacts he is collecting, the myths and mores of the people, all of which Audrey reads with affection and even genuine interest. Leonard and his artifacts, she would say to her sister, Violet, with an indulgent smile. Not that Audrey is beautiful. No one but Leonard could accuse her of that. But what she had she had, and that was the true love of her husband.

Another thing Audrey has right now is a ten-centimeter cyst on her right ovary which the doctors can't say for certain is benign, and so it will have to come out. Thank heavens Leonard isn't off on one of his expeditions, she thought.

Fifteen years ago, she had been forty-two then, every one of her upper teeth had been extracted while Leonard was in New Guinea. Pyorrhea, the dentist had said. Said it severely. "You've let it go. They are all rotten and ready to fall out on their own."

Audrey was flabbergasted. "I have to think," she had said. "My husband isn't here. He's in New Guinea." She remembered the man's contemptuous little smile. On the way home, she said to Vi, "But . . . Leonard . . ."

"Leonard is not a dentist," said Violet.

And so a few days later Audrey had gone through with it. She hadn't been out of that dentist's office ten minutes when she knew that she had made a dreadful mistake. Vi drove her home afterward. Lying down on the backseat of the car, her mouth numb, her cheeks stuffed with pledgets of cotton, she wondered what Leonard would think, how he would feel. And she recalled something she had heard him say to one of his students, she couldn't remember why: "No one," Leonard had said to the student, "can take your dignity away from you; you might throw it away yourself, but no one can take it away from you." Then and there Audrey decided that Leonard didn't have to know.

"You all right?" Vi asked from behind the wheel, and turned round to see at every red light.

Right from the start, Audrey had refused to take the denture out of her mouth, no matter the pain. There were dark blisters on her gums; she lisped. But she was determined. Leonard would be coming home in two months. Audrey persevered so that with weeks to spare, she had gotten used to the "prosthesis," as they called it, incorporated it. It had become second nature.

Oh, she had had to steel herself against the first times it had to come out, be cleaned, then reinserted. But she had surprised herself. She was calm, curious even, as she turned it over in her hand, examining. Like a pink horseshoe, she decided, and how wise she was to have avoided the vulgarity of pure white. Ivory was more natural. Ivory has endured; ivory has kept faith. In time her palate had molded itself to fit, her gums were snug and secure in the hollow trough. Never, never would she remove her teeth anywhere but in a locked bathroom. She would keep them in at night. It was a myth that you had to take your dentures out at night. Before long, she had no qualms, didn't mind at all. The denture had become for her a kind of emblem of personal dignity, like one of those Asmat artifacts with magic properties, but this having to do with the one thing that mattered most to Audrey: Leonard. "It isn't really cheating," she told Violet.

"You're lucky," said Vi. "You're one of those people who don't show their teeth when they smile."

When at last Leonard burst into the room, gathered her in his arms and kissed her, she smiled as much from triumph as with happiness. "You never cease to charm me," he had said, and she knew then that she had done it. Leonard would never know.

But now it was fifteen years later. "Total abdominal hysterectomy," the surgeon announced. "A clean sweep." As though she were a kitchen floor! "What does that include?" she asked him. "The uterus, both ovaries, both tubes," he told her. "Why my uterus?" She insisted upon the personal pronoun. "Why my left ovary? My tubes?" He then explained, rather too patiently, she thought, that she didn't need her reproductive organs anymore, that the risk of getting cancer in one of those organs was "not inconsiderable." Human beings do not talk like that, she thought. That is not human speech. "And," the surgeon went on, "as long as we are going to be in there anyway . . ." In there! Audrey could not keep her hand from passing lightly across her abdomen.

Then he spoke about the small additional risk of the larger operation, said it was "negligible." But Audrey already knew what it was to go through life missing something. She wished fervently that she had been able to keep her cyst a secret, like her teeth. You would think it would be easier since the ovaries were inside and safely hidden. Imagine having to carry them in a bag between your legs, like testicles. And as for the risk of getting cancer . . . is that a reason to have your organs taken out? All of life is a risk. Living in California is risk; there might be an earthquake. First, her teeth, and now her . . . her womanhood, yes, it was nothing short of that. All at once the operation seemed part of a plot to take her body apart. And she remembered the clink of coins years ago, as that dentist stirred the change in his pocket, stirred it on and on, enjoying the sound of it before he took up the syringe and injected her with novocaine.

On the wall in back of the surgeon's desk was a colored diagram of the female organs. Altogether, it resembled a sweet-faced cow's head rising to the gentle curve of the horns.

"No," she said, closing down. "No, that cannot be. Only my ovary, the one with the cyst. Nothing else, unless there is cancer." She would sign permission only for that. In the end, she had capitulated. "You're doing the right thing, I assure you, Mrs. Blakeslee," said the surgeon as she signed the permission sheet.

At the hospital, Leonard and Audrey followed the nurse into the room. "Get undressed and into this." The nurse held up a knee-length shirt open at the back. She did and over it put on the pale green brocade bed jacket Leonard had given her the night before. It had been arranged that Leonard was to wait in the solarium outside the operating rooms. The surgeon would talk to him there, let him know what he had found. Afterward, he would wait for Audrey to be wheeled from the recovery room a few hours later.

"Visiting hours are over," commanded the page operator. "Will all visitors please leave now."

"Good luck," said Leonard with a smile that was much too bright for him. He's frightened, she thought, and felt tears filming her eyes. After Leonard had left, Audrey lay on the bed, thinking of him—the silky feel of the black hairs on his forearms, his smell of permanence, the sound of his singing. Leonard sang bass. It was her favorite. At sixty-one, his voice was as rich as ever. Sometimes, listening in church to that submarine vibrato, she would have moments of unecclesiastal commotion. Once, when she confessed it, Leonard reproached her with a waggle of his finger. Ah, but his was a magic throat.

*

"I'm Dr. Dowling." The man had knocked and come in at the same time. It is what happens in hospitals, she thought. She was glad to be wearing the green bed jacket. So long as she had it on, there was protection.

"The anesthesiologist," he explained. "I'll be putting you to sleep tomorrow.

"Any questions?"

Audrey shook her head. He had an important sort of face, florid, with jowls made even more congressional by the white political hair that escaped from beneath his green surgical cap. He was wearing a scrub suit of the same color and, over that, a white laboratory coat. The strings of a mask dangled.

"Open your mouth wide as you can." He peered in.

"I see you have an upper plate. Out it comes in the morning before you leave this room. The nurse will mind it for you."

Mute shadows of words trembled at her lips.

"But I never take it out, only to clean . . ."

"Well, you cannot go to the operating room with it in. I cannot put you to sleep with a foreign body in your mouth."

Foreign body! Audrey felt the blood leave her head. Gongs could not have sounded louder in her ears. Then a final cold ticking.

"For how long . . . ?"

"Until you are fully awake. Certainly till evening."

"But you don't understand . . ." she began. Her voice trailed off. The doctor waited, turned his head, looked at her from the corner of an eye.

"Yes?"

"It is . . . My husband does not know that I have a denture. He has been unaware of it for fifteen years. I would not want him to see me without it. Please," she said very quietly. "It is important to me." She waited for the walls to burst.

"Pride," said the man. "No room for it here. Like modesty. Suppose we had to get at your trachea, your windpipe, in a hurry, and then we had to waste time fishing those teeth out. Suppose they came loose in the middle of the operation. There are a hundred 'supposes.'" He started to go.

"It isn't pride," she managed.

"What, then?"

"It's dignity." Perhaps it had been pride at the very beginning, but it had grown. And something else: Audrey understood that the connubial apparatus of a man is more delicate than a woman's. She saw no need to put it to the test.

"Come now. Mrs. Blakeslee, is it?" He consulted the name on the chart to make sure. Audrey struggled to fend off his voice. "You are making too much of it."

All right, then, she would calculate, be a cat.

"Don't you . . ." she began. "Don't you have a little something hidden away that you wouldn't want anyone to know about?" She smiled, laying it on in almost visible slabs. The doctor was taken off guard. "No, actually not." But he had hesitated for the fraction of a second, and so she knew.

"How boring," she said, smiling, giving it to him right in his face. "And, of course, I don't for a minute believe you." This doctor could not know it, but Audrey was fighting for her life. But now she saw that he had retreated a vast safe distance behind his lips.

"In any case, you may not keep them in. And that's that." He stood abruptly and walked to the door.

"Have a good night," he called over his shoulder.

After he had left, Audrey felt her heart go small in her chest. Again there was the clink of coins being stirred in a pocket. With a sudden resolve, she decided that there was no longer any need for tact. The situation didn't call for tact. It called for defiance. I'll sign myself out of the hospital, she thought. Against medical advice, as they say. That cyst on her ovary, it might well be benign. They don't know. Leaving it in would be just one more risk. A risk infinitely smaller than having Leonard see her without her denture. Her mouth caved in, wrinkled like a drawstring pouch. She tried to imagine herself saying to Leonard afterward: "All right, then. You have seen what you have seen. Now accept it. Or not." But she could not. That way lay death. Hers or that of something far more delicate and valuable. No, she thought. No. Never again would she cultivate a belief in inevitability.

Audrey reached for the telephone, dialed.

"Leonard, don't come to the hospital at all tomorrow."

"But why?" He was startled. "Of course I'm coming to see you."

"That's just the point, Leonard, please . . ." She heard her voice flapping about her, out of control. "Please." She was imploring him. "Don't come. Promise me."

"I'm sorry, Audrey. I'm just not going to agree to that. So forget it." His tone was severe, as with a child.

"I don't want you to see me like that."

"Like what?" He smiled with his voice. "I have seen it all before, you know." Oh, but you haven't, she thought. You shouldn't.

"What is it, Audrey? You sound distraught. Shall I come right over? I'll make them let me in."

"I just wanted to spare you," she said harshly. "There are times when people need to be alone."

"No," said Leonard. "I'll be there."

Violet managed the gift shop in the lobby of the hospital. She was two years older than Audrey—a big woman, divorced once, widowed once. Violet did not use makeup. I have nothing to hide, she said. Still, she dyed her hair. For business reasons. When you have to meet the public, gray hair automatically dismisses you. Fifteen years before, they had been closer, when Violet had brought her home from the dentist's office and Audrey had sworn her to a lifetime of silence. But somewhere between then and now Vi had become the kind of woman who sat herself down with ceremony in a deep chair to receive the secrets of others. She would be coming up to the room after she closed the gift shop. Audrey would ask her for a ride home. She would deal with Leonard later.

"I'll do no such thing," said Violet. "Do you mean to lie there and tell me that Leonard still doesn't know about your false teeth?" Vi made a point of never saying "denture." "False teeth" had a balder sound and they had drifted too far apart for softness. The venules on Vi's cheeks dilated with indignant blood. Audrey reached for the light, flicked it off. It was something to do.

"May I turn off the light?" she asked then. In the dark she could see the glossy mound of her sister's hair.

"Listen, Audrey, this has become a sick obsession with you." Her vehemence was reiterated by flashes of gold at neck and earlobes.

"There are madder things," said Audrey. And she lamented the weakness that made her let down her guard before this stranger who was her sister.

"Besides, it's a lie. People shouldn't lie, no matter what."

"Oh, lies," said Audrey. "That's where you're wrong. People don't lie enough. When people tell the whole truth, that's when things fall apart. Most relationships are like some plants, I think. They need to be kept partly in the shade or they wither." A nurse came in and turned on the light. In the sudden glare Violet leaped up at her.

"Now, Audrey, don't be stupid," she said, standing to leave. "Behave yourself." Violet's teeth would never fall out, Audrey thought. They chew words, worry them; the way they buckle up her mouth.

Almost at once there was a hesitant knock at the door. Oh, God. Now who?

"My name is Dr. Bhimjee. I am the intern on this ward." An Indian or Pakistani, she thought. And lame. He limped toward the bed using his head and one arm in the act of locomotion.

"Mrs. Blakeslee, I see that our names both end with two e's." His face was dark, she suspected, more from fatigue than from racial coloring. More than anything else he resembled an ungainly parcel, something bulgy and ill-wrapped. His hair was almost too thick, too black, but relieved by a single swatch of white near the crown. He is not young, Audrey decided. What has he endured and with how much patience? All at once, a fence came down. Who, after all, is to say where, in whom, one places trust?

"I have false teeth," she said, firing the words into his hair. She was shocked at the ease with which the forbidden words had come. The intern gazed down at her.

"Many people do," he said. The slate-colored skin set off the perfection of his own very white teeth. He is beautiful, she thought. And she threw herself further upon his mercy.

"I have had them for fifteen years. My husband has never seen me without them. He doesn't know that I have them. The anesthetist was here. He says I must leave them here in the room tomorrow. My husband will be waiting for me to come back from the recovery room. He will see me. I can't do that. Please, please." The last words rose like echoes. For a long moment they looked at each other, during which something, a covenant perhaps, Audrey did not know, was exchanged. Audrey lashed her gaze to his long gracile fingers. Then, all at once, deep called unto deep. A rush of profound affection came over her. It was nothing like her feeling for Leonard, but for all she knew, it might have been love.

"Do not worry." The r's rolled very slightly. "In the morning, put them in the nightstand. There is a container. I will take them with me to the operation. I am assigned to your case, so I will be there too. Before you leave the recovery room, I will put them back into your mouth. Do not worry."

*

Later, when she awoke in the recovery room, the pain of her incision was the second thing that Audrey felt. The first was the denture which she explored with her tongue. Only then came the pain which, so help her, she did not mind. In spite of it, she curled up like a cat in a basket. Once, when she opened her eyes, she saw, or thought she saw, a dark face above her, a white swatch in a tumble of black hair, like a plume of smoke clinging to the chimney of a snug cottage.

"Don't worry," he was saying softly. "Your teeth are in. Take a deep breath. Again." He listened with his stethoscope. "You will be awake soon." He checked her pulse, and was gone. For a long time his voice lingered, lapsing, returning, drifting into darkness. And then there was Leonard, holding her hand, leaning over the bed to kiss her. "The doctor says it was benign." Audrey smiled up at him within the limits of morphine.

During the days that followed, Audrey found herself thinking about Dr. Bhimjee as much as she did about Leonard. There was a peacefulness about him. Not resignation so much as acceptance. No, definitely not resignation. Resignation suggests defeat. Acceptance, rather. Where had he found it? Wrested it, she supposed, barehanded from a tangle of thorns. He had no need to deceive. It had not been given to him to deceive. She saw him differently now from the way she had that first desperate night. What she had thought was fatigue became the sum total of all the suffering he had experienced. It had worn his face down to the bone. The sockets of his eyes were dark cabins of it. Audrey would have liked to take the bony parcel in her arms, to breathe in his dreams.

And soon it was the hour of Audrey's discharge from the hospital. The intern had come to say good-bye.

"My wife tells me that you have been very kind to her," said Leonard. Audrey could not take her gaze from the two men.

"Not at all."

"I want you to know that I will always remember your"—she saw that Leonard was struggling—"your courtesy."

"Please, it was nothing."

"Nevertheless," said Leonard. "Nevertheless," he repeated, "I want you to have this." He held out a small reddish stone.

"What is that?"

"It is a stone that has been dyed red by the Asmat people of New Guinea. See? It has a monkey carved on one side, a parrot on the other. A shaman gave it to me. He's a sort of doctor too. It wards off melancholy, brings good luck. Please, take it." The doctor hesitated.

"I want you to have it," said Leonard. There was in his voice something vivid, mighty. Maybe it was the sun probing between the slats of the venetian blinds, but from her wheelchair it seemed to Audrey that, at the exact moment when the red stone left the white hand of one and entered the dark hand of the other, something flared up that looked for all the world like fire.

Four Appointments with the Discus Thrower

ONE

I spy on my patients. Ought not a doctor to observe his patients by any means and from any stance, that he might the more fully assemble the evidence? So I stand in the doorways of hospital rooms and gaze. Oh, it is not all that furtive an act. Those in bed need only look up in order to discover me. But they never do.

From the doorway of Room 542, the man in the bed seems deeply tanned. Blue eyes and close-cropped white hair give him the appearance of vigor and good health. But I know that his skin is not brown from the sun. It is rusted, rather, in the last stage of containing the vile repose within. And the blue eyes are frosted, looking inward like the windows of a snowbound cottage. This man is blind. This man is also legless—the right leg missing from midthigh down, the left from just below the knee. It gives him the look of an ornamental tree, roots and branches pruned to the purpose that the thing should suggest a great tree but be the dwarfed facsimile thereof.

Propped on pillows, he cups his right thigh in both hands. Now and then, he shakes his head as though acknowledging the intensity of his suffering. In all of this, he makes no sound. Is he mute as well as blind?

If he is in pain, why do I not see it in his face? Why is the mouth not opened for shrieking? The eyes not spun skyward? Where are tears? He appears to be waiting for something, something that a blind man cannot watch for, but for which he is no less alert. He is listening.

The room in which he dwells is empty of all possessions—the get-well cards, the small private caches of food, the day-old flowers, the slippers—all the usual kickshaws of the sickroom. There is only a bed, a chair, a nightstand, and a tray on wheels that can be swung across his lap for meals. It is a wild island upon which he has been cast. It is room 542.

TWO

"What time is it?" he asks.

"Three o'clock."

"Morning or afternoon?"

"Afternoon."

He is silent. There is nothing else he wants to know. Only that another block of time has passed.

"How are you?" I say.

"Who is it?" he asks.

"It's the doctor. How do you feel?"

He does not answer right away.

"Feel?" he says.

"I hope you feel better," I say.

I press the button at the side of the bed.

"Down you go," I say.

"Yes, down," he says.

He falls back upon the bed awkwardly. His stumps, unweighted by legs and feet, rise in the air, presenting themselves. I unwrap the bandages from the stumps, and begin to cut away the black scabs and the dead glazed fat with scissors and forceps. A shard of white bone comes loose. I pick it away. I wash the wounds with disinfectant and redress the stumps. All this while, he does not speak. What is he thinking behind those lids that do not blink? Is he remembering the burry prickle of love? A time when he was whole? Does he dream of feet? Of when his body was not a rotting log?

He lies solid and inert. In spite of everything, he remains beautiful, as though he were a sailor standing athwart a slanting deck.

"Anything more I can do for you?" I ask.

For a long moment he is silent.

"Yes," he says at last and without the least irony, "you can bring me a pair of shoes."

In the corridor, the head nurse is waiting for me.

"We have to do something about him," she says. "Every morning he orders scrambled eggs for breakfast, and instead of eating them, he picks up the plate and throws it against the wall."

"Throws his plate?"

"Nasty. That's what he is. No wonder his family doesn't come to visit. They probably can't stand him any more than we can."

She is waiting for me to do something.

"Well?"

"We'll see," I say.

THREE

The next morning, I am waiting in the corridor when the kitchen delivers his breakfast. I watch the aide place the tray on the stand and swing it across his lap. She presses the button to raise the head of the bed. Then she leaves.

In this time, which he has somehow identified as morning, the man reaches to find the rim of the tray, then on to find the dome of the covered dish. He lifts off the cover and places it on the stand. He fingers across the plate until he probes the eggs. He lifts the plate in both of his hands, sets it on the palm of his right hand, centers it, balances it. He hefts it up and down slightly, getting the feel of it. Abruptly, he draws back his right arm as far as he can.

There is the crack of the plate breaking against the wall at the foot his bed and the small wet sound of the scrambled eggs dropping to the floor. Just so does this man break his fast.

And then he laughs. It is a sound you have never heard. It is something new under the sun.

Out in the corridor the eyes of the head nurse narrow.

"Laughed, did he?"

She writes something down on her clipboard.

A second aide arrives, brings a second breakfast tray, puts it on the nightstand out of his reach. She looks over at me, shaking her head and making her mouth go. I see that we are to be accomplices.

"I've got to feed you," she says to the man.

"Oh, no you don't," the man says.

"Oh, yes I do," the aide says, "after what you just did. Nurse says so."

"Get me my shoes," the man says.

"Here's oatmeal," the aide says. "Open." And she touches the spoon to his lower lip.

"I ordered scrambled eggs," says the man.

"That's right," the aide says.

I step forward.

"Is there anything I can do?" I say.

"Who are you?" the man asks.

FOUR

In the evening, I go once more to that ward to make my rounds. The head nurse reports to me that Room 542 is deceased. She has discovered this quite by accident, she says. No, there had been no sound. Nothing. It's a blessing, she says.

I go into his room, a spy looking for secrets. He is still there in his bed. His face is relaxed, grave, dignified, as the faces of the newly dead are. After a while, I turn to leave. My gaze sweeps the wall at the foot of the bed, and I see the place where it has been repeatedly washed, where the wall looks very clean and very white in contrast to the rest, which is dirty and gray.

Whither Thou Goest

"Brain-dead," said the doctor. "There is no chance that he will wake up. Ever. Look here." And he unrolled a scroll of paper onto her lap.

"This is the electroencephalograph. It's nothing but a flat line. No blips." Hannah bowed her head over the chart. The doctor cleared his throat, took one of her hands in both of his, and leaned toward her as though about to tell a secret. Hannah submitted to what under any other circumstance she might have considered presumption, submitted because she thought she ought to. It was expected of her. The formality of the occasion and all.

"Hannah, it is three weeks since your husband was shot in the head. The only thing keeping him alive is the respirator."

Hannah waited for the walls of the solarium to burst.

"I'm asking you to let us put an end to it, unplug the machinery, let him go. There is just no sense in prolonging a misfortune." Hannah felt that she should say something, not just sit there, but for the life of her she couldn't think what. The doctor was speaking again.

"But before we do that, we would like your permission to harvest Sam's organs for transplantation."

"Harvest?" said Hannah. "Like the gathering in of wheat?"

"Yes," said the doctor. "That is what we call it when we take the organs. It is for a good cause. That way your husband will live on. He will not really have died . . ."

"Dead is dead," said Hannah.

"I know, I know," said the doctor. And he looked down at his feet for relief. Hannah noticed that he was wearing oxblood wing-tip shoes of a large size. They were the shoes of power.

A week later she received a letter from the doctor.

> Dear Mrs. Owen,
> You will be pleased and comforted to know that because of your generosity and thanks to the miracle of modern science, seven people right here in the state of Texas are living and well with all their faculties restored to them. Your husband's liver has gone to a lady in Abilene; the right kidney is functioning in Dallas; the left kidney was placed in a teenaged girl in Galveston; the heart was given to a man just your husband's age in a little town near Arkansas; the lungs are in Fort Worth; and the corneas were used on two people right here in Houston. . . .

Hannah folded the letter and put it back in its envelope and then into the bottom drawer of the desk without reading to the end. There was no need. She already knew what had become of the rest of Sam. She had buried it in the family plot of the Evangelical Baptist Church cemetery.

*

That was three years ago. And still, she had only to close her eyes to have the whole of the horror spring vividly before her, as though it had been painted on the inside of her eyelids. For Sam's thirty-third birthday they had spent the weekend at the beach. Now they were in the pickup truck on the way back to Houston. Hannah had fallen asleep. It was the sudden stop that woke her up.

"We couldn't be there already," she murmured.

"No," said Sam. "I'm just going to change that lady's tire." Hannah sat up and saw the green Buick pulled off to the side of the road. The right rear tire was flat. An elderly woman sitting behind the wheel looked up and smiled when she saw Sam walking toward her with a car jack in one hand and the tire iron in the other. Hannah got out of the truck and went over to talk. "Bless you," the woman said. Sam hadn't given that jack more than a half dozen pumps when a man—he looked Mexican—appeared out of nowhere with a gun in his hand.

"Sam?" Hannah had said in that low, questioning voice that always made him turn to see if she was upset. For a long moment Sam stayed where he was, crouched over the jack. When at last he stood, he had the tire iron in his hand.

"What do you want, mister?" he said. The Mexican made a gesture as if to turn a key and nodded at the pickup.

"The keys are in the truck," said Sam. The Mexican made no move. Perhaps he did not understand? Sam raised his arm to point. The Mexican fired. It took a long time for the echo of that shot to peter out. When it had, the truck and the Mexican were gone, and Sam lay on his back wearing a halo of black blood. He was still holding the tire iron. Something pink squeezed slowly out of the middle of his forehead.

"Dead is dead," she had told that doctor. But now, three years later, she wasn't so sure. For Hannah had begun to have doubts. Incidents occurred, like the time months ago when she had gone to the butcher's. Just ahead of her at the counter a woman had ordered a chicken. "I want it in parts," she heard the woman say. Hannah had watched as the butcher scooped out the entrails, cleaved the carcass through the middle of the breast, and hacked off its thighs, legs, and wings. The heart, gizzard, neck, and liver he put in a small plastic bag.

"You can keep the feet," said the woman. And then it was Hannah's turn.

"What'll it be?" said the butcher. And wiped the clots from his fingers onto his apron.

"What do you call that?" she asked, trying not to look at his bloody hands. As though they were his privates.

"What do you call what?"

"What you just did, cutting up the chicken. What is the name for it?" The butcher stared at her blankly.

"It's called 'cleaning a chicken.' Why?"

"Cleaning?"

"Look, miss," said the butcher. "I'm real busy. What'll it be?" But Hannah had already turned to leave.

It was after that that she stopped going to the cemetery to visit the grave. It wasn't Sam in that cemetery, not by a long shot. It was only parts of Sam, the parts that nobody needed. The rest of him was scattered all over Texas. And, unless she had been misinformed, very much alive. And where did that leave her? God knows it was hard enough to be a widow at the age of thirty-three, and her sympathies were all with those women whose husbands had truly, once and for all, died. But widowhood, bleak as it might be, seemed preferable by a whole lot to the not-here, not-there condition into which she had been thrust by "the miracle of modern science." At least if your husband were all dead you could one day get over it and go on with your life. But this! This state of bafflement. Maybe, she thought, maybe it was a matter of percentage—if more than 50 percent of your husband was dead, you were a widow. Whom could she ask?

Along with doubt came resentment. Oh, not just at the doctors. They simply do what they want to anyway, without really thinking. Doctors, she decided, don't think. They just *do*, and cover it all up with language. *Harvest. Transplantation.* The soft words of husbandry and the soil. Even they cannot bear to speak the real names of their deeds—dismemberment, evisceration. What was worse, she had begun to resent Samuel. Here she was, living in this sort of limbo, while he, Sam, was participating in not one but seven lives, none of which had anything to do with her. It wasn't fair. Even if he hadn't chosen it, it wasn't fair.

*

Hannah's cousin Ivy Lou was also her best friend. Lately she had taken to bringing her lunch over to eat at Hannah's house. One day when she got there, Hannah was standing at the kitchen window, looking out into the backyard. Over the radio came the pitched monotone of a preacher. The subject was the resurrection of the flesh.

"And it says right here in First Corinthians, chapter fifteen: 'For the trumpet shall sound, and the dead shall be raised incorruptible.'

"And here it is again in Romans, chapter eight, verse eleven: 'If the Spirit of him who raised Jesus from the dead dwells in you, he who raised Christ Jesus from the dead will give life to your mortal bodies. . . .'"

"Turn that damn fool off," said Hannah.

"For goodness' sake!" said Ivy Lou. "What's got into you?" Four years ago Ivy Lou had been born again.

"It's a big lie," said Hannah. "It's the way the preachers swindle you."

"I'm sure I don't know what you are talking about," said Ivy Lou.

"There is no such thing as the resurrection of the flesh," said Hannah. "Just tell me at what stage of life we are supposed to be on the day of resurrection, so-called? Do we look as we did when we were babies? At age forty? Or as we are when we die, old and wasted? And tell me this: What about Samuel Owen on your resurrection day? Here he is scattered all over Texas, breathing in Fort Worth, urinating in Dallas *and* Galveston, digesting or whatever it is the liver does in Abilene. They going to put him back together again when the day comes, or is it to the recipients belong the spoils? Tell me that."

"Well," said Ivy Lou. "I don't have the least idea about any of that, but I do know that you are committing the sin of blasphemy. Hannah, I'm real worried about you. Don't you believe in God anymore?" Hannah looked out the window and was silent for a long moment.

"About God," she said at last, "I have only the merest inkling. That's all anyone can have."

*

Hannah could not have said exactly when the idea first occurred to her. Later, she thought it might have been on the day of the tornado. From the kitchen window her eye had been caught by a frenzy of leaves in the live oak. All that August morning it had been sultry and still, until all at once it turned dark as twilight. Then lightning came to tear open the clouds. And the air, as if desperate to announce great tidings, broke its silence and turned to wind. But such a wind! At the height of the storm Hannah opened the back door and stood to receive the force of the rain on her face, her hair. It stung like pebbles. The violence lasted but a few minutes, after which it settled into a steady drizzle. Then, as abruptly as it had come, the storm passed and the sun came out, leaving Hannah with the feeling that something more than the humidity had been relieved. Something, a pressure that had been building inside her, had boiled its way to the surface, then broke.

That very night she awoke suddenly and sat bolt upright in bed, and she clapped her hand over her mouth as if to hold back what threatened to burst forth from it. A scream? Laughter? She didn't know what. But what she did know, beyond any doubt, as though it had been a revelation, was what it was she must do.

She had been dreaming, and in her dream, she saw two men lying on narrow tables next to each other. One of them was Samuel; the other she could not see clearly. His features were blurred, out of focus. Both of the men were stripped to the waist, and their chests were open in the middle, the halves of their rib cages raised like cellar doors. A surgeon was there, dressed in a blue scrub suit, mask, and cap. As she watched, the surgeon reached his hands into Samuel's chest and lifted forth his heart, held it up like some luminous prize. At that moment, Hannah could see into the chests of both men, see that they were both empty. Then the surgeon turned away from Samuel and lowered the incandescent, glowing heart into the chest of the other man, who promptly sat up, put on his shirt, and walked away.

What was instantly made clear to her—it was so simple—was that she must go to find that man who was carrying Samuel's heart. If she could find him, and listen once more to the heart, she would be healed. She would be able to go on with her life.

In the morning, the idea seemed quite mad. She wondered whether she was losing her mind. And she began to interrogate herself. Why would she do such a thing? What good would it do? To say nothing of the intrusion on the life of a perfect stranger. What made her think he would agree to let her do it? How could she explain it to him when she could not even explain it to herself? What would she say? Would it be like a pilgrim visiting a shrine? No, it had nothing to do with worship. Although, it might be a bit like going to the Delphic oracle for advice. But that wasn't it either. Did she just want to make sure that Sam's heart had found a good home? For God's sake, it wasn't a dog that she had given away. Nor was she the least bit curious about the man himself, other than to know how to find him. "No," Hannah said aloud, addressing the nameless, faceless man of her dream. "Thou shalt be unto my hand as a banister upon a dark staircase, to lead me up to the bright landing above. Once having climbed, I shall most willingly let thee go." The more she thought about it, the more she felt like a woman whose husband had been declared missing in action in a war. What would she have done if that were the case? Why, she would bend every effort to find him—living or dead—even travel to Vietnam or Laos, wherever, and she wouldn't leave until she knew, one way or the other.

Perhaps it was a phantom she was chasing, a phantom that would dissolve when she drew near. But she would have to take that chance. Hannah remembered the time, a year after they were married, when she and Samuel were lying in bed and she had said: "Let's tell each other a secret. You first." And Sam had told her about when he was twelve years old and his father had died suddenly of a heart attack. For a long time afterward he would think that he saw his father on the streets of the city. It was always from the back, so he couldn't be sure. But the man was wearing the same gray fedora and holding the cigarette the same way. The more Sam looked, the more certain he became that it was his father whom he saw walking downtown, that he had not really died, but had gone away or been taken away for some reason, and now here he was. And Samuel would quicken his pace, then break into a run to catch up, calling out "Daddy! Daddy!" in his excitement. And each time, when the man turned around to see, it wasn't, no it wasn't, and there was that fresh wave of desolation. One day, a policeman came to the door and told his mother that Sam had been following men on the street and that one of them had reported him, said he might be a pickpocket, or worse.

"Is it true?" asked his mother. When he didn't answer, she asked him why. But he couldn't or wouldn't say why because no one would believe him or understand, and they would think he was crazy.

"Well, don't you dare do it ever again," said his mother in front of the policeman. But he couldn't stop, because the next day he thought he saw his father again and he followed him. After a year it stopped happening and Sam felt a mixture of relief and disappointment. Relief, because at last he had laid to rest his father's ghost; disappointment, because the wild possibility no longer existed. Sam had never told anyone about this before, he said. It was the first time he had ever mentioned it. When he had finished, Hannah hugged him and kissed him and cried and cried for the young boy who couldn't let go of his father.

"You're so pretty," Sam had said after a while to make her stop.

But Sam had been a young boy, and she was a grown woman. No matter—even if it turned out that she, too, was chasing a phantom.

Hannah went to the cupboard where three years before she had placed the doctor's letter, the one telling her about the seven transplantations. She read it again, this time to the end, and made a list. The kidneys, liver, and lungs, she decided, were inaccessible—hidden away in the deepest recesses of the bodies of those who had received them. How could she get to them? And the corneas just didn't seem right. She didn't think she could relate to a cornea.

That left the heart. A heart can be listened to. A heart can be felt. And besides, there had been her dream. She would seek to follow the heart. But then there was that man, that other, who had lain on the table next to Samuel and whose face she had not been able to see. What if he refused her, mistook her intentions? No, she would explain it to him, write it all in a letter, and then he would agree. He would have to. In the letter she would tell what happened that night on the highway, how Sam had raised his arm to point to the truck, still holding the tire iron, how the Mexican had fired, and what the doctor had said to her in the hospital.

"That way your husband will not really have died," he had said. And that she had said to him, "Dead is dead," but that now she was not so sure. And how, ever since, she had been living in this gray place, unable to grieve or get on with her life because she no longer knew who or even what she was. All this she would tell him in the letter and he would let her come. He must.

*

Once she had decided, it was not difficult to get his name and address, a few of the facts of his illness. Hospital records, she learned, were scandalously accessible to whoever might want to see them, whatever the hospitals swore to the contrary. Anyone who really tried could get to see them—lawyers hunting for malpractice suits, legal assistants, reporters, detectives, graduate students gathering statistics, nurses, insurance companies. It was in this last guise that Hannah called the record librarian of the university hospital and made an appointment. She had followed it up with a letter on official stationery of the Aetna Casualty and Life Insurance Company.

She had had to take Ivy Lou into her confidence; Ivy Lou worked as a secretary for Aetna.

Ivy Lou was appalled. "I don't like it one bit. No good will come of it." And at first she had refused. "I just don't see what you could possibly hope to get out of it." And then, when Hannah didn't answer, "Why? Just tell me why."

"I don't know why," said Hannah. How could she say why, when she really didn't know herself? Perhaps it was something like the way a flower can't help but face the sun, or the way a moth goes to the flame.

"Hannah, you're going to get burned," said Ivy Lou as though she had read her mind. "Besides," she went on, "it's not only sick, it's in the grossest ill taste." Ivy Lou set down her teacup and walked to the door, shaking her head.

But then, there was poor Hannah, and in the end Ivy Lou gave in.

"Just don't tell anyone where you got it," she said when she brought the stationery.

The next week at the hospital, the record librarian welcomed her with a smile and showed her to a cubicle where the chart was waiting for her. POPE, HENRY, she read. AGE: 33: NEXT OF KIN: MRS. INEZ POPE. CHILDREN: NONE. ADDRESS: 8 ORCHARD ROAD, AVERY, TEXAS. DIAGNOSIS: CARDIOMYOPATHY, VIRAL. SURGERY: HEART TRANSPLANT. Reading on, she learned of his “intractable heart failure,” that his prognosis had been “hopeless”—he had been given an estimated life expectancy of a few months “at most.”

And then she came to the part about the operation, which occupied the bulk of the fat chart, and none of which she read. There was no need.

“That didn’t take long,” said the librarian as Hannah walked by her desk.

“No,” said Hannah. “I’m quick.”

*

Avery, Texas. Hannah and Ivy Lou looked for it on a map.

“There it is,” said Ivy Lou. “Way up almost into Arkansas.”

“How far away is that?”

“Maybe a couple of hundred miles, but, Hannah, I’m telling you—don’t. You are making the biggest mistake of your life.”

That night, Hannah sat at her kitchen table with a pen and a blank sheet of paper. “Dear Mr. Pope,” she wrote, then set down the pen. There was something absurd about that *Mr.*, considering that she had been married for seven years to a significant part of the man. But she would let it stand. The situation called for tact, patience, diplomacy. There would be plenty of time for “Dear Henry,” if and when. She picked up the pen and continued.

> My name is Hannah Owen. Could the name mean anything to you? Doubtless not, considering the decorum with which these things are done. I am the wife (some say widow) of Samuel Owen, the man whose heart is even now beating in your chest.
>
> Perhaps you will forgive a woman’s curiosity? I am writing to ask how you are since the operation. Your early discharge from the intensive-care unit, and even from the hospital itself—three weeks! It might be a record of some kind and would seem to show that you had an uneventful recovery. It would follow that you have continued to improve and that by now, three years later, you have completely regained your health? I surely do hope so. It is my dearest wish that the heart is doing as good a job for you as it did for Sam and for me too. Do let me hear from you, please.
>
> Yours truly,
> Hannah Owen

There, she thought. That should do it. Nothing whatever to arouse suspicion or to make anyone wonder. Only the shock of who she was. After that, just an expression of well-meaning concern. When she dropped the letter in the slot at the post office and heard the soft siffle as it went down the chute, she sighed. It had begun.

*

It was two weeks before she saw the envelope in her mailbox written in neat handwriting in black ink. It was postmarked Avery, Texas. How it shook in her hand.

> Dear Mrs. Owen,
> It was very kind of you to write asking after my husband's health. He is not much of a letter writer and has asked me to tell you that he is stronger and healthier than he has been in years. He says he is the luckiest man on earth. By the way, however did you get hold of our name and address? I had thought such information might be protected, under the circumstances, but—I guess not. Thank you for your interest.
> Sincerely,
> (Mrs.) Inez Pope

> Dear Mr. Pope,
> I don't know any other way to say it than to just take a deep breath and come right out with it. What I am going to ask will seem at first quite insane. But I assure you I am no maniac. I want to come and listen to your heart for the space of one hour at a time when it is convenient for you. While I know that at first this request will seem strange to you, I pray that you will say yes. You have no idea how important it is to me.
> Yours truly,
> Hannah Owen

> Dear Mrs. Owen,
> My husband and I have tried to understand your position. But we feel that it would not be at all wise for you to come here. Not that we aren't grateful and all of that, but you have to admit it is a little on the bizarre side. So this is good-bye.
> Sincerely,
> (Mrs.) Henry Pope
> P.S. We have consulted with our doctor, who says it is a terrible idea and perhaps you should get some professional attention to get over it. No offense meant.

> Dear Mr. Pope,
> Your wife does not wish to let me come. I can understand her hesitation. The awkwardness and all. And perhaps it is only human nature, a touch of suspicion. Perhaps I have ulterior motives? I assure you, Mr. Pope, that I do not. As for my interest in you personally, it is limited to you as the carrier of something I used to possess and which I for one reason or another would like to see again. Or rather, hear again. For that is all I want to do—to listen to your heart

for the space of one hour. The way a person would like to go back to visit the house where he had grown up. You are in a sense that house. Your doctor doesn't think it is a good idea? Mr. Pope, the doctors don't think. They are unaccustomed to it. Doctors just do whatever they want to, without thinking. If they had thought, perhaps they might have foreseen the predicament into which the "miracle of modern science" has placed me. No, speak to me not of doctors. They haven't the least idea about the human heart except to move it from place to place.
Yours truly,
Hannah Owen

Dear Mrs. Owen,
I am very sorry. But the answer is still no. And that is final. Ever since I got your first letter, I've been feeling awful. Like ungrateful or something. But I know in my heart it wouldn't be a good thing for you either.
Sincerely yours,
Henry Pope

Dear Mr. Pope,
The circumstances of my husband's death were violent and shocking. In case you do not know, he was shot in the head by a bandit on the highway where he had stopped to help an old lady with a flat tire. I was there. After three weeks on the respirator, they came and told me it was no use, and could they disconnect the respirator? But just before they did that, could they take parts of his body (*harvest* is the word) to transplant to other people? I said yes, and so they took his liver, lungs, heart, corneas, and kidneys. There are seven of you out there. You, Mr. Pope, got the heart, or more exactly, *my* heart, as under the law, I had become the owner of my husband's entire body at the time that he became "brain-dead." Don't worry—I don't want it back. But I do ask you to let me come to Avery for one hour to listen to your heart. It is such a small thing, really, to ask in return for the donation of a human heart. Just to listen. For one hour. That is all, really all. The reasons are private, and anyway, even if I wanted to tell you why, I don't know if I could put it into words. If you see fit to let me come, I will never bother you again, and you will have repaid me in full. Do please let me know when I can come.
Yours truly,
Hannah Owen
P.S. Of course your wife can be in the room all the time. Although, frankly, I would prefer otherwise. Mrs. Pope, what I want to do is no more than what dozens of nurses have done—listen to your husband's heart. Only the reason is different. Couldn't you look at it as just another medical checkup?

Dear Mrs. Owen,
You said there were seven of us recipients. Why me? Or do you plan a statewide reunion with all your husband's organs? And the answer is NO! Please do not keep writing, as it is annoying to say the least, and it is making my wife nervous.
Sincerely,

Henry Pope

Dear Mr. Pope,
You ask "Why me?" And you are right to ask. It is because you have the heart. The others—the liver, lungs, kidneys—are hidden away. I can't get to them. As for the corneas, well, I just can't relate to corneas somehow. But the heart! A heart can be felt. It can be listened to. You can hear a heart. A heart is reachable. That's why *you.*
Yours truly,
Hannah Owen

When there had been no reply for two weeks, Hannah wrote again.

Dear Mr. Pope,
Please.
Yours truly,
Hannah Owen

Dear Mrs. Owen,
No, goddammit, and if you don't stop this business and get the hell out of my life, I'm going to notify the police.
Sincerely yours,
Henry Pope

Dear Mr. Pope,
And so your answer is still No. Oh, can you imagine how sad I am? Now I am the one who is disheartened. Never mind. I will try to accept it, as I have no alternative. You said I can't come and so I won't. I shall not be bothering you and your wife again. You can relax. I can't resist saying one more time, although it doesn't matter anymore, that I was the owner of the heart. It was mine to give. I think I did mention to you that the body of the deceased is the property of the next of kin. It wasn't Samuel who was the donor at all. It was me. But that is all water over the dam. Now may I ask you for a much smaller favor? I would like to have a photograph of you for my scrapbook. Nothing, for goodness' sake, posed or formal. Just a casual snapshot would be fine. Chalk it up to foolish sentiment. Thank you and good-bye.
Yours truly,
Hannah Owen

For three weeks Hannah prowled the house, smoking the cigarettes of disappointment, settling into her despair. Ivy Lou was frankly worried. But she knew better than to suggest a psychiatrist, or a minister, for that matter.

"Hannah," she said. "You have got to pull yourself together and get over it. It was a lousy idea in the first place. What's going to be the end of it?"

"I really don't know," said Hannah and waited for Ivy Lou to go away.

And then there it was, lying at the bottom of her mailbox like a dish of cream waiting to be lapped up. No need to look at the postmark—she could tell that handwriting anywhere. Stifling her excitement, she waited till she was back in her kitchen, sitting at the table, before she opened it. The sole content was a snapshot. No letter.

Hannah studied the photograph. It was three by four inches, black-and-white. The next size up from passport. It showed, at some distance, a thin, dark-haired man slouched against the trunk of a tree, his right knee flexed at right angles, with the sole of his foot braced against the tree. A live oak, she guessed, judging by the girth. His hands bulged the pockets of a zip-up jacket. He wore a baseball cap and was looking off to the left, the head turned almost in profile. The face, what she could see of it, was unremarkable, the eyes, shaded by the peak of the cap, giving away nothing. Only the dark seam of a mouth expressed suffering. Even with the help of a magnifying glass, she could read no more on that face. It was possessed of no mystery. Compared to the large color photograph of Samuel that she kept on the mantel in the parlor, with its generous smile that held nothing back, the snapshot in her hand was of a sick man who had known pain and expected more of it. He looked twenty years older than Samuel, although she knew they were the same age. This was taken before the operation, she decided.

But that he had sent it! Actually looked for and found the photograph, then put it in an envelope and *mailed* it. That heart is *working*, she thought. Hannah smiled and fixed herself a tuna-salad sandwich and a glass of milk.

She waited exactly two weeks—it wasn't easy—before she answered.

> Dear Mr. Pope,
> Thank you so much for the photo. I have put it in my scrap-book. My friend Ivy Lou, who is sort of an actuary, has calculated that your face occupies 2.1 percent of the picture and what with the peaked cap, you are a bit hard to make out. But, still. I like your backyard, is it? Are those azaleas on the right of the live oak you are leaning against? I have a live oak in my backyard too.
> Sincerely yours,
> Hannah Owen

Six weeks later, another letter arrived.

> Dear Mrs. Owen,
> My wife Inez will be in Little Rock visiting her parents on the weekend of October 20th. If you still want to come, I don't see why not, so long as you just stay for one hour. I will expect you at the house at ten o'clock Saturday morning. You know where it is, I'm sure.
> Yours truly,
> Henry Pope

"I wouldn't drive, if I were you," said Ivy Lou. "Not wound as tight as you are. Why, you're as nervous as a bride. See if there's a bus." It was the first piece of Ivy Lou's advice Hannah thought she should take. She didn't trust herself to drive. Besides, she wanted the time to think, to prepare herself. Like a bride, she agreed, but she quickly shooed that notion out of her mind. There was an early-morning bus that got to Avery at nine-thirty, and the next day, before dawn, Hannah was on it. But once on the bus, she couldn't think, only reached up now and then to touch her right ear, which, when the bus stopped in Avery, would become a mollusk that would attach itself to the rock of Henry Pope's chest and cling through whatever crash of the sea.

*

Number eight was one of a dozen identical single-family ranch houses that made up the dead end that was Orchard Road, only this one was ennobled by the big live oak at the back, which fringed and softened the flat roof. At precisely ten o'clock Hannah unlatched the front gate and walked up to the door. Before she could ring the bell, the door opened halfway.

"Come in," he said, keeping himself out of sight until the door was closed behind her. The house was in darkness, every shade and blind drawn and shut. It had the same furtive, tense look she saw on the face of the man standing before her.

"No need to call attention," he said. "It would be hard to explain if anyone saw you come in." He was, she saw, a healthy man who looked even younger than she knew him to be. He had put on at least twenty pounds since that picture had been taken. His hair was light brown, almost blond, and curly. He was wearing jeans and a white T-shirt.

He's nervous as a cat, thought Hannah, and that makes two of us.

Hannah followed him into a small room, a den furnished with a sofa, an upholstered easy chair, and a television set. One wall was lined with bookshelves. She guessed that he had spent his convalescence in this room.

"It's your show," he said. "How do you want me?" When she didn't answer, he reached up with both arms and pulled the T-shirt over his head.

"I suppose you want this off," he said. Then Hannah saw on his chest the pale violet stripe that marked the passage of her husband's heart into this man. She felt her pulse racing. She might faint.

"Well, it's your show," he said again. "How do you want to do this? Come on, let's just get it over with. One hour, you said."

"Best, I think, for you to lie down flat," she said. "I'll sit on the edge and lean over." She had gone over it so many times in her mind.

He lay down and slid a small pillow beneath his head, then shifted as far as he could to give her room to sit. When she did, he rose abruptly to his elbows.

"Where is your stethoscope?"

"I don't have a stethoscope."

"How are you going to listen to my heart without a stethoscope?"

"They didn't always have them," she said. "I'm going to listen with my ear." She gave her right ear two short taps. "I have very acute hearing," she added, because he looked dubious, as though he might call the whole thing off. But he didn't, just lay back down and stared straight up at the ceiling with his arms at his sides, as though he were still a patient at the hospital awaiting some painful procedure.

Then Hannah bent her head, turning toward the left, and lowered first to her elbows, then all the way, lowering her ear toward his left, his secret-sharing, nipple. When she touched his skin, she could feel him wince.

Oh, it was Samuel's heart, all right. She knew the minute she heard it. She could have picked it out of a thousand. It wasn't true that you couldn't tell one heart from another by the sound of it. This one was Sam's. Hadn't she listened to it just this way often enough? When they were lying in bed? Hadn't she listened with her head on his chest, just this way, and heard it slow down after they had made love? It was like a little secret that she knew about his body and it had always made her smile to think of the effect she had on him.

Hannah settled and gave herself up to the labor of listening. Closing her eyes, she drew herself down, down into that one sense of hearing, shedding sight and touch and all her other senses, peeling away everything that was not pure hearing until the entire rest of her body was an adjunct to her right ear and she was oblivious to whatever else might be in the world. She listened and received the deep regular beat, the emphatic *lub-dup, lub-dup* to which with all her own heart she surrendered. Almost at once, she felt a sense of comfort that she had not known in three years. She could have stayed there forever, bathed in the sound and touch of that heart. Thus she lay, until her ear and the chest of the man had fused into a single bridge of flesh across which marched, one after the other, in cadence, the parade of that mighty heart. Her own pulse quieted to match it beat for beat. And now it was no longer sound that entered and occupied her, but blood that flowed from one to the other, her own blood driven by the heart that lay just beneath the breast, whose slow rise and fall she rode as though it were a small boat at anchor in a tranquil sea, and she a huddled creature waiting to be born.

At last Hannah opened her eyes and raised her head. Never, never had she felt such a sense of consolation and happiness. Had it been a dream? Had she fallen asleep? It was a moment before she felt his arm about her shoulders. How long, she wondered, had she lain encircled and unaware? She looked up to see that he was smiling down at her. Angels must smile like that, she thought.

"You were trembling," he explained. "It was like holding a bird."

Gently, Hannah disengaged herself and stood, but listening still, cocking her ear for scraps of sound, echoes. And it seemed to her in the darkened room that light emanated from the naked torso of the man and that the chest upon which she had laid her head was a field of golden wheat in which, for this time, it had been given to her to go gleaning.

Henry Pope followed her to the door.

"Will you want to come again, Hannah?" he asked. How soft and low his voice as he uttered her name.

"No," said Hannah. "There will be no need." And she stepped out into the golden kingdom of October with the certainty that she had at last been retrieved from the shadows and set down once more upon the bright lip of her life. All the way home on the bus a residue of splendor sang in her ears.

Risen
(Part Two of *Raising the Dead: A Doctor's Encounter with His Own Mortality*)

On the evening of March 31, 1991, in a house on St. Ronan Terrace, I sat writing in the room I call my scriptorium. Usually, in Connecticut March is winter hanging by a thread, but this year it had turned hot without any transitional period of moderation; the leaves were already half-size. For most of the month I had been on an extended lecture tour that took me from the island of Kauai to Nova Scotia, then on to Delaware, California, and Texas. Around nine o'clock I left my desk and went to stand at the open window. The branches had begun to stir in a sudden breeze. There was the muffled sound of thunder. Jagged nerves of lightning leaped. In the sultry air the pattern of the wallpaper turned from green to gold; the figures in it grew wavy, they vibrated like heat rising from a pavement. All at once, my legs buckled. From downstairs Janet heard the thud and came running.

"What?" she said.

"I can't think why . . . ," I replied.

"Can you get up?" I tried but could not.

"You'd better call . . ." But she had already dialed. Within minutes two young men in uniform stood over me. I remember being bundled up, the stretcher sliding home aboard the ambulance. One of the men took my pulse and blood pressure, then relayed the information to someone over the phone. I heard the sirens.

"For goodness' sake, don't use the sirens," I told him. "It will disturb the neighbors. Besides, it isn't that serious."

"Take it easy, Pops," said the young man. "It's sporty this way." I remember nothing else until twenty-three days later when I woke up on a ship, I thought; somewhere off the coast of Texas, I thought. Oh yes, there was this: at the emergency room I was placed on a stretcher. All around and above me, a flock of white birds—stooping to peck at my arms, groins, beaking my mouth, rectum, everywhere. Then nothing . . . save for whispers crowding around, leading me deeper and deeper into the darkness. Then they too vanished.

Coma is the state into which he is tumbling. Moment by moment, there is a turning inward of the senses. The sounds, smells, sights, perceptions of the outside world are disappearing. The Milky Way roars across the sky like an army of light. At last, his fall is broken by a soft cushion and he is suspended in a viscous, pearly matrix that is itself both time and space; his vertebrae have melted; he lies here strewn, submerged.

I feel ashamed to pounce upon the page with a narrative that is so open, explicit, so personal. In one sense it is a vivisection, the cutting up of a living creature to see how it works, rummaging among the still-quivering flesh for its soul. As you can see, I am warming up before making a start, rubbing my hands together to summon up courage. If I have written much of it in the third person, well, that is because such an obsessive account of an illness forces one, like Dorian Gray, to confront his own "devilish, furtive, ingrown" self-portrait. The pronoun *he* gives a blessed bit of distance between myself and a too fresh ordeal in which the use of *I* would be rather like picking off a scab only to find that the wound had not completely healed. Still, *I*, the author, will be present throughout, looking on, translating for *him*, the patient.

In writing this journal, I had no overriding wish to educate myself in the subject of Legionnaires' disease, the diagnosis ultimately given to my ailment. Once I had learned that it is caused by the bacterium *Legionella pneumophila*, which thrives in the mist sprayed from air-conditioning ducts, that a building or an airplane having been infested, travelers are especially vulnerable, that it is quite often a massive pneumonia associated with collapse of the respiratory function and therefore fatal; once I had glanced at a few colored photographs of autopsy specimens of lungs and liver and kidney, my curiosity about the disease was exhausted. A writer, like an old-time doctor, prefers impressions to facts. Impressions are what last. Facts, such as the data read from the screen of the computer, have a tendency to change from day to day. But I think it is time to get on with the chronicle of an illness told afterward.

Let us look in upon that cubicle of the emergency room. The stretcher upon which he lies is engulfed in nurses and doctors, each of whom is ministering to him at the same time. In a moment, his clothing is stripped from him. Because he is flailing about, his wrists and ankles have been restrained. From veins in his arms and groins endless ribbons of blood, dark from the cyanosis, are pulled into tubes. His head is steadied, his neck extended by mighty hands; the mouth of the man is pried open and an attempt is made to insert a tube into his trachea. But his agitation is extreme, like that of a man drowning. Or rather, that of a man playing the role of someone drowning in an old-fashioned melodrama. It has that jerky, staccato rhythm. Because of this, the intubation cannot be carried out. Medication is injected into a vein and the doctor at the head of the stretcher tries again.

There. Now the tube is in his trachea, the cuff inflated to keep it from slipping out. Still not fully narcotized, the man shakes his frantic head from side to side, refusing what has been thrust in. He coughs, strains, his neck is a contraption of taut tendons and engorged veins. To the uninitiated it might seem a kind of molestation. At last the morphine reaches his brain; he subsides into flaccidity. His chest lifts, recedes, lifts again at the insistence of the rhythmic, squeezing fist of a perfect stranger. Ointment is squeezed from a tube into his eyes, and his lids are taped shut to protect the corneas. It is the beginning of a long sleep. In the meantime, a catheter has been slid into his bladder, another plastic tube into one of his nostrils to gain access to his stomach. Already, long strings of blackish bile are staining the sheet on which he lies. The cardiogram shows the rhythm of his heart to be precarious—ventricular tachycardia. Drugs are administered, electrodes readied to apply to the chest. An X-ray is taken; one of the doctors remarks that the chest is not expanding symmetrically. The diagnosis is massive bilateral pneumonia with toxic shock. How strange that he had no earlier warning. Despite the administration of pure oxygen, his lips and fingernails remain blue. His temperature, they say, is very high. His pulse too, his blood pressure almost obtainable. Is he going to die? No one knows. But there is more than a hint of death here.

Within minutes, then, he is a preparation, something they have made and whose every flicker and seepage can be measured precisely. In addition to the doctors, nurses and technicians, I, the author, am also there standing, or rather, hovering bodiless above and to the side, out of the way yet able to see, to hear, now and then able to reach down if I wish and touch him, the one lying there on the stretcher who seems to me a small bird perched on an arrow that has been shot from the bow and is flying somewhere. If ever the man wakes up and can speak for himself, I shall have to change pronouns.

The martyrdom of the intensive care unit has begun. It has a certain relentless monotony which would render any such narrative boring. So I shall not proceed day by day through the pestering and goading of the flesh that go by the name intensive care. Suffice it to say that for the next twenty-three days the man in the bed is to be ventilated, dosed, defibrillated, probed, suctioned, and infused. Most of his bodily functions will be taken over. No longer need he swallow, chew, inhale or exhale, cough, urinate, defecate, clear his throat, maintain acid-base balance, cogitate, remember, sigh, weep, laugh, desire. Even the need for making tears has been taken over by the ophthalmic ointment that protects his corneas. For those who will tend him, he is at once the *raison d'etre* and the predicament from which they long to extricate themselves. The doctors are earnest and tireless. They remind me of poor farmers who, year in and year out, turn with their hoes the same exhausted patch of soil, planting and replanting, flogging it, cherishing it. But there will come the day when the pathetic patch of dust will no longer yield. Only then will they let it be. In other words, this man is half-dead, although not quite at the point of no return. For him death would certainly be much easier to achieve than life. The prospect of life regained is like sitting down to a gourmet lunch without the blessing of appetite.

The intensive care unit suggests a blockhouse, a building made of concrete, designed to withstand attack during wartime. Even the patient who is conscious exists here in a kind of reverie. Within the blockhouse twenty respirators, each inhaling at its own pace, make a steady, wet noise like the fall from a fountain. Such a sound goes unnoticed in an intensive care unit beneath the clatter and thump, the footfalls, the calling out, the moaning. So cleverly has the noise of these respirators been woven into the larger fabric of sound that within minutes it cannot be dissected and analyzed for itself. Absolute silence could not be deeper. All the while, in the chimney of his brain, thoughts fly up and, a moment later, waft away, irretrievable.

Dreamer that he is, even in the blockhouse, even from the depths of his coma, he invites the IV pole, the respirator, the whole massive bank of machinery to suggest the background for a story: the hanging bottles of saline become a crystal chandelier; the moans of his sick neighbor are the sound of an oboe being played in another part of the house; the cooing of pigeons on the window ledge becomes the rapturous cries of lovers. Those who enter and leave his room will be characters in a story—there is a nurse, Maureen, with a long, slender neck at the hollow of which rests a tiny gold cross. A chambermaid performs her futile acts of domesticity, fitting her mop in and around the legs of the others. Now and then, she will cast a glance at the wreckage in the bed and sigh. Even to death and beyond, he will be the teller of tales, collecting impressions, defying forgetfulness, and meeting gods all along the road, the way you do when reading Homer or Virgil. He can do all that? In coma? Oh yes, he can. Dream, imagination—these are the chariots that the comatose body rides. It is by these that the flesh extends itself to encompass the whole world.

He had always been thin—a parcel of bones really, stitched together with ligament, strung with nerves and tendons, and with a cap of aluminum hair; his eyes are of that indeterminate color called hazel. But now it is the sixth day. He is swollen like a toad, his flesh cold and soggy, his edematous eyelids at half-mast. You wonder how they could have over-hydrated him so. In their zeal to combat his state of shock, they have given him fifty pounds of excess glucose and saline solution. There is the sadness of a toad in his hazel eyes. The familiar landmarks by which he could once be identified are no longer to be seen: the zygomatic arches surmounting the cheeks, the iliac crests, the tapered phalanges. Where is the squarish mandible that (he has been told) gave his head the look of a Roman senator? Where, the graceful hollow above each clavicle? And all the while, beneath the deceptive fullness of edema, the wasting of his muscles goes on, the congestion of his internal organs. He has become something that even I would not want to touch. Not so the nurses—Maureen, Linda, Heather. Beautifully serene, they continue to stroke and massage him, to wipe away all stains, to bathe and dress him in clean linen. To look at him today you would never guess that he is the same man brought to the emergency room six days ago and set loose at supersonic speed into the void and traveling on remote control.

*

At last, by the tenth day, the diuretic has succeeded in drying him out. Succeeded beyond anyone's expectations. All day and all night, the nurses have emptied the plastic collecting bags suspended from the siderail of the bed, exclaiming. The output of urine is nothing short of heroic. Within four days he has become little more than a skeleton, every bone visible and palpable—the skeleton of a child whose puberty has been delayed. At the same time, he looks ancient enough to have been mentioned in the Old Testament. Oh, let me confess it! Sometimes he seems brave and beautiful to me, although I know that I am the only one who would think so. Look at him! A sprig of chicory blooming between paving stones, indomitable.

Day Fourteen. All the blood that is still in a liquid state has been drawn from his veins; syringe after syringe has glittered with it. The rest is clotted or extravasated into the tissues. Huge purpura, ecchymoses, and hematomas cover the sticks that were his arms. There is a moist rattle in the endotracheal tube. Now and then, a nurse detaches the tube from the respirator long enough to suction it clear, and then the rattle disappears for a while.

I have spent the entire day observing him. The poverty of his body, the way he shivers like a wet dog. The draining away of his flesh and blood. He is like an abandoned cottage in ruins, the eaves of his ribs overhanging the scaphoid belly. His umbilicus, that mute evidence of his ancestry, seems set directly upon the vertebral column. When the narcosis is allowed to lift, he curls up, stretches out slowly like a larva, signaling with the only sound he can make—the faint borborygmi of his bowel. At last I understand the term *embedded*, the way a fly trapped in a chunk of amber must apprehend its plight.

Beneath the sheet he is naked save for his feet, which are encased in brand-new high-top running shoes. His wife has shopped for them at the suggestion of Maureen, who is worried about foot drop. These massive sneakers hold the feet at right angles to the legs. It is ludicrous, and even the anguished members of his family—his children—cannot keep from smiling at the small boy who has taken his new shoes to bed with him.

Day Eighteen. He has been in coma for almost three weeks. What is it like? It is like being encased in a layer of wax that separates him from the rest of mankind. The outer air is a foreign element into which he is unable to break through. Nor should he try, for he could no longer breathe it in. An immense weight holds down his thin bluish eyelids. He could not have raised them. Nor does he want to. He has no need for eyes. Here, there is nothing for him to do but wait and listen to the silences rubbing against each other. Now and then there is a small shifting in the air as if far away, on another continent, a boa constrictor were slowly unwinding from a branch. Could this place have a name? Is it on any map of the world? A decision has been made to wean him from the respirator.

The narcotics and paralyzing agents have been given in lower doses throughout the night. Toward dawn he is lying in the upper berth of a sleeping car; there is no room to sit up or turn over. The train is hurtling across an endless prairie where it is always night. Once in a while the eternal darkness outside the train window is punctuated by something—a forest of bare white birch trees, a herd of cattle, only their white faces showing. A few silvery birds fly. Or are they fish streaming?

There are times when his face seems to contort into weeping; his eyes open and show themselves brimming with a molten sorrow. When it passes, the spasm, there is a relief about the diaphragm as when vomiting or sobbing stops and you can let go of yourself. This morning he even made a gesture as if to reach up and claw from him the skin of wax that is his coma. It is the same gesture made by Lazarus in the painting (School of Rembrandt) when he sits up in the tomb and begins to unwrap his cerements. But unlike Lazarus, the man in bed cannot manage it. By afternoon his arms and legs are once again flailing about, resisting. In the chart his behavior is noted as "combative." Nothing could be further from the truth. What makes him struggle so is not aggressiveness; it is desperation.

The man now is about the size of a small deer lying starved and exhausted in snow. See how he lifts his head, turns it slowly, on his face a look of puzzlement, uncertainty, as he sees me hovering in the corner of the room where wall and ceiling meet. Something passes between us—not quite speech. He opens his mouth as if to eject the tube but cannot. Then with a purposefulness that I did not think he could muster, he reaches one hand up and pulls it, coughing, choking, from his throat with the cuff still inflated. He seems surprised at what he has done, the sounds he is making.

"That was very naughty!" The nurse attaches nasal prongs to deliver oxygen to his nostrils until the doctor can come to replace the tube. Meanwhile, he is rid of the tube and struggles to extrude vowels and consonants from his larynx. Even his eyebrows take part in the effort to speak, the way they arch, lifting as if to encourage his lips and tongue. It gives his face a look of boyish earnestness. But there is no voice, only a thick, gelatinous rasp, as the vocal cords no longer approximate. Minutes later, the anesthesiologist arrives. Just in time, for the cyanosis has darkened. The wrists and ankles of the patient have been secured to the bed. The nurse holds his head as if it were the head of a statue whose sightless eyes have no pupils. The hands that grip him are hard as tongs. In the end he yields to them as though yielding to a strangler's thumbs. The endotracheal tube is replaced, its cuff inflated. The dose of morphine is increased. Immediately, his empty sockets return a gray, stony stare. He must remain paralyzed and unconscious until such time as he no longer needs the respirator. And so he sleeps on.

*

He is like a gardener digging in the earth who makes a decision to lower himself to the underworld. Down and down he goes, swinging from root to root. On either side, worms, rocks, gulches, darkness, eyes like panthers caught in a net of lashes, moisture dripping. Just so does he follow the mushroom scent of hell, and with each fathom grows paler, less opaque, his flesh melting—solid to liquid, until at last there will be only the vagueness of vapor. Once or twice, he looks back up to see how far he has come, but the path behind has closed up, leaving no trace. He would not be able to find his way back. The thick, twisted roots have tapered into fine, hairlike rhizomes that he parts with his hand the way one parts a curtain of beads. His cheeks and arms are coated with cold moisture, more like rot than sweat. The odor of mushrooms grows heavier. Solid ropes of it slide in and out of his mouth, fill his throat. After a long time, the path widens and ends abruptly at the edge of a black river. Here he lies down, not to sleep—in this place there is no need for sleep or wakefulness. Nor is there any need to move.

Day Twenty. The sight of his hands is particularly sad. Those fine muscles between the metacarpal bones and in the web spaces—the interossei and the lumbricals—have atrophied; the mounds of flesh have given way to gullies. The skin is dry and as chaste and beautiful as old paper. But I remember the passion inspired by those fingers, their gifted, sly, infinitely provocative caresses and gestures. No sign of that now.

A doctor turns over first one hand, then the other, searching perhaps for a usable vein. Then he sees the elevated, dimpled scar tissue in each palm that begins to contract and draw down the ring finger. That is the Dupuytren's contracture of which the man has been inordinately proud. He never lost the chance to tell the gullible that these were the stigmata of the Crucifixion. The examining doctor makes a note to show the Dupuytren's contracture to the medical students.

Day Twenty-one. A gray dawn slides through the ill-fitting slats of the venetian blind. From the glum faces of the nurses, it is clear that in the blockhouse things are looking worse. Whatever fragile equilibrium between acid and base, between oxygen and carbon dioxide, between positive and negative that the doctors have managed somehow to piece together has come unraveled. All of the vital signs have taken a turn for the worse. Fever. If it goes any higher, he will burst into flames. A pair of gills would work better than his solidified, liverish lungs. Daedalus! You can make anything! How about it? A pair of gills for the man!

"Let him not die," someone murmurs. The possibility itself lowers the temperature in the room; the patient shivers. With the sheet pulled down, he looks more and more like a winter-starved deer, stricken. *Don't go! Not yet!* Who is that calling out? Then I see that it is I calling out in pursuit of myself. The sheet is drawn smooth up to the armpits (as though he could move) and tucked under the mattress. When the nurse lets his head down, the pillow is scarcely dented by the weight of it. If someone had asked him at that moment what was his dearest wish, it would have been to lie on his stomach with his arms bracketing his head.

Day Twenty-two. All day and night, silt has settled in his veins, turning them solid. Only the bubbles of saliva on his teeth continue to wink bravely in the light. A slow slide of clot advances through his body. It began in the venules of the arms and legs, filled the larger veins, the iliac, the inferior vena cava, flowing slowly toward the heart. By morning, it will have achieved the right auricle. A single muffled thump, and it will be hurled to the lungs. And there it will stay, hardening into a cast of the pulmonary circulation. Should he die, will I too feel the cold mud in the marrow of my bones?

Day Twenty-three. And now it is my sad duty to report to you his death. It occurs at precisely 1:38 P.M. on April 23. He has been in the intensive care unit for three weeks and two days. From far away there comes a drumming so faint and rapid as to be unrecordable by even the most sensitive device in the room. Could it be rain? No, the sound lurches and staggers as though the drummer had slipped and lost his beat.

"Ventricular tachycardia," says the nurse and calls for the doctor. The drumming grows louder and louder until it fills the room. Then all at once it stops as though an arrow had been shot through the throat of the drummer boy. The pace of activity in the room quickens. Maureen pounds vehemently upon his chest, turns up the oxygen flow. Injections are given into the tubing, then directly into his heart (or where she surmises his heart to be), syringes full of calcium and adrenaline. Electrodes are clapped to his chest and a series of jolts delivered which cause the body of the man to jounce hideously in the bed. His lips and fingernails are a deep blue. Minutes go by. The doctor arrives.

"How long has the EKG been flat?"

"Four and a half minutes." For a while they continue their efforts, which are like a pantomime. To no avail. No amount of resuscitation has the least effect. The heartbeat is not restored. At last the efforts are discontinued. There he lies, the sheet having been thrown off in the struggle, his slight body pale, emaciated, childlike were it not for that head like a Roman senator's and his aluminum hair.

"This man is dead."

Maureen, she who had pounced upon him like a cat, jolted him with currents of electricity, seen to the injections into his very heart, sags against a wall. She has given up trying to catch his ghost, which was running away from her. He was already out of her reach and she could not pursue him further. Sorrowfully, Maureen sits by the bed recording the events in the chart, her usually strong, bold handwriting gone shaky. See how she pleats her forehead, draws in her lips, for in spite of all that she has witnessed over the years she cannot bear to be present at this. Time of death, she writes, 1:38 P.M.

It is strange, this painless death. Like stepping through a door held politely open for him. It doesn't seem right, somehow; a trivialization of the event. Death ought to be harder to achieve. Better to be hunted down, rooted out, hurting and bloody. Then death would come as a relief. It would be welcome.

*

It is now ten minutes since the doctor's pronouncement of death. Already the man has taken on that look of dignity that the newly dead have because of their possession of secrets. Or is it that they travel in a beyond that must be entered formally? Maureen is still writing an account of the last minutes of his life, her efforts to resuscitate him—the intracardiac injections of calcium and adrenaline, the jolts of electricity delivered to his chest, the failure of the electrocardiogram to respond. Glancing up, she has noted the characteristic "settling" of his body, the fixity that is incontrovertible; she has seen that so many times. Alone in the room, Maureen pauses in her charting to wipe her eyes with the back of her hand. Bleary with tears, she does not see what I see, that a subtle change is taking place in the contents of the bed, that the utter stillness of the body has been replaced by a calmness of the flesh, that beneath the closed eyelids his eyeballs roll slowly from side to side, then dart the way fish will move in a pond. Look! He shudders as if to shake off something which threatens to cling, and tightens those eyelids; minnows of light rising in the shallows. Then he hears a wingbeat, and feels something fugitive, immaterial, a beige veil being drawn from his face, slowly at first then faster, until the final whisk is like a slap. A moment later he draws the first breath. It is a deep sigh that might be interpreted as one either of sorrow or of satisfaction, as though one precious thing were being relinquished and another embraced. The nurse's incredulous stare! Her galvanic leap to his side! He, blinking in the explosion of light. When he opens his eyes, their color has gone from the ambivalence of hazel to the jubilation of blue.

Again, a breath is drawn, and another and another. A tracing has returned to the electrocardiograph, which the nurse had not yet detached from his arms and legs. The room, which had descended into a subaqueous silence emanating from the corpse, is now fiercely active. All the machinery is back in place, chugging, vibrating, clicking, ringing. Nurses scurry, calling out to one another. They bend over the bed, coaxing, noting and recording each sign of revivification. The intravenous chandelier sends light streaming through his body until he is something radiant and glowing in the bed. From time to time, the nurses turn to look at each other, their faces swept with wild surmise. It is true! After ten minutes of certified death, this man has . . . risen. Risen! Such a word does not belong in an intensive care unit.

Now the man is coughing against the endotracheal tube, he wrinkles his forehead, tears stream from his eyes, he shakes his head slowly from side to side. It is painful to observe the resurrection of a man, to behold a log of inert flesh trying to raise itself. But the pain is all ours. He feels nothing as yet. He is like the bulb of a tulip, probing the earth in which it has lain all winter unaware of its potential, without memory or hope. As we do not ascribe pain to the tulip in its rebirth so ought we not to imagine that he, the man, is torn loose and abraded.

Then he who has performed no purposeful movement in three weeks reaches up one hand and pulls the tube from his throat and mouth. And that is not all: a smile breaks upon his face, but such a smile as has never been seen on the continent of North America. And in a hoarse whisper, but plainly enough, he utters the single word: Yes.

"Did he say yes?"

"What do you suppose he means?"

"I couldn't say. Perhaps he was just answering a question someone had asked him weeks ago before he went into coma."

"Does that happen?"

"More likely it is some odd form of seizure activity."

What he means, what the nurses cannot know, is that everything begins with a yes. That is how the first two bits of energy in the universe greeted each other, collided. Boom! And yes! There was life. So it is with the resurrected. Once again his throat fills with the word until the pressure of it is unbearable and he cries out in the hoarse voice that sticks to his jaws . . . Yes! Saying yes to life, accepting once again the burden and thrill of it.

*

It is the next day. He lies on his back, arms and legs splayed out so as not to disengage any of the needles or tubes. Now and then, he is propped on one side or the other. What he really wants is to curl up so as to give himself a hug, to accept his own warmth. Still, on his face is a strange, far-off look, as if to say, death is easy; it is the return to life that requires courage. When a nurse comes to take his temperature, he follows her solemnly with his eyes that seem to say: I have been to the land of the dead. Do not touch me. From that moment on, his vital signs—pulse, blood pressure, temperature—are normal. His oxygen saturation, 100 percent. There is no longer any doubt that he will recover.

About the consternation of the entire medical staff, there is little to be said. The joy at his reawakening is general, but in each person it is colored with uncertainty.

"You must have been mistaken," they tell the nurses at the weekly morbidity/mortality conference. "It cannot be as you told it . . ."

"The cardiogram was flat," the nurses reply. "The pulse and blood pressure were unobtainable. What else do you need? He was dead."

"Then how . . . ?" The nurses shrug and shake their heads.

Throughout the hospital they can think of nothing else. For weeks, in the laundry, at the coffee shop, in the X-ray file room as in the morgue, every conversation will begin with the words: Did you hear . . . ? On whatever flimsy pretext, orderlies and technicians and next-of-kin will walk past the doors of the intensive care unit just to draw near to the site, each of them taking away a dollop of hope to be saved up for a rainy day. If it happened to *him*, then perhaps . . . It is as if no one who worked at the hospital could go on living without specific knowledge of the event. Just so has it swollen into a legend that even I have come to believe in time. Such is the power of literature, be it written down on paper or passed on from mouth to ear.

*

It is twenty-four days since the night he was taken to the emergency room, well into April. A warm day, with the sun streaming in and lighting up the wall of his room. Torpor envelops him. He hears grasshoppers. They seem to be in the bed with him, all around him, inside his chest. Yes! The noise of the grasshoppers is coming from inside his chest! He gives a soft, flannel cough and the stridulation abates. The ceiling at which he is gazing is made of squares of cork-board. Here and there the expanse of it is interrupted by the handle of an opaque glass panel that can be pulled down. Storage space. Or a hidden compartment like those in the ceiling of a ship's cabin. On board a ship you have to make use of every inch of space. He feels beneath him the gentle rocking of the sea. A coziness comes over him. He is perfectly comfortable. *So!* He thinks, *I am aboard a ship. But where? Perhaps I am in the South?* Yes, he remembers, it is the South; he had been there recently, lecturing in Texas. That's it, Texas! Then he sees the intravenous attached to his arm and he thinks that while in Texas he must have fallen sick, that he is aboard a hospital ship in the Gulf of Mexico. Doubtless soon to be discharged, from the way he feels. So comfortable and drowsy.

From somewhere comes the music of a Strauss waltz. He lies utterly still, letting the light from the intravenous chandelier trickle onto his face and collect there in small glistening pools, while, the mattress takes up the rhythm of the music, scooping, dipping, turning his all but transparent body. He has never felt so graceful, so comfortable in his own flesh. All at once he has an irresistible urge to laugh. Should you ask him the reason for his laughter he would not know, for it is unlike any laughter of his life but something with which he has been infested, a holdover from some almost forgotten glee, now become reflexive and without rhyme or reason. He hears a woman's voice calling.

"Wake up! Wake up, sleepyhead! What's so funny?" It is as though she were summoning him up from a great depth to the surface where he now floats between two sheets, his face visible only in the trough between the waves. He opens his eyes to see his wife, Janet, standing by the bed.

"For goodness' sake!" he says. "What are you doing in Texas, or off the coast of it?"

"This is not Texas," she informs him. "And this is no ship. You are in the intensive care unit of the Yale-New Haven Hospital."

"But the rocking of the waves . . ." He is not ready to give up.

"They have you on one of those newfangled mattresses that inflates here, deflates there. It's run by electricity. That way you won't get bedsores."

"How long have I been here?" It is the only thing he wants to know.

"About three weeks. Twenty-three days of coma to be exact." But he is already hurrying back to sleep.

Atrium: October 2001

It is a seven-block walk from the Yale Sterling Library to the Yale-New Haven Hospital. For thirty-five years, until my retirement from Surgery, I spent each working day and most nights at that hospital, albeit in buildings that have either been renovated so as to be unrecognizable, or razed. For the past sixteen years, I have spent every working day at the library where I read and write. Lately, I have taken to walking down to the hospital for lunch. In a courtyard set among the hospital buildings, there are a dozen tiny ethnic food stands—Thai, Chinese, Mexican, Indian, "Soul," Middle Eastern, and just plain American. In good weather, one can dine *al fresco* on one of the benches. Otherwise, one can take a container of food into the hospital. Which brings me to the Atrium, a vast open, high-ceilinged, bright space, at whose center is a large modernist fountain that, at first glance, seems to be a great ball of water in motion. In fact, it is fed by a stout erect metal pipe at the center and dozens of long narrow-gauge pipes that branch from it at angles. The openings at and near the ends of these secondary pipes are such that from each a circular screen of water issues. These circles of water abut and overlap each other, giving the illusion that the fountain is a gigantic ball of water. The water falls into a moat from which it is drained and recycled. A circle of lamps with copper reflectors illuminates the fountain from beneath the surface of the water in the moat. At any given time, numerous coins lie at the bottom of the moat, where they were tossed by the hopeful and the desperate. The flow of these waters produces a continuous soft, rushing noise.

Six quite tall ficus trees in pots rise well toward the glass cathedral ceiling, which is braced by steel girders. The bark of the ficus is smooth and atrophic, cadaverous. The branches and roots, complex and interwoven, form a mesh at the bottom of the trunk. "What are the roots that clutch, what branches grow . . ." Large planters holding ugly tropical plants—pink bromeliads and white anthurium—serve as a boundary to mark off that portion of the Atrium used for eating from the rest, which is carpeted and made to simulate a hotel lobby, with faux-wooden benches and comfortable chairs and tables. Other large houseplants in tubs—sansevaria, cut-leaf philodendron, and giant dracaena—are placed here and there.

The immediate reason why I began to go there for lunch is that my vision has taken a turn for the worse. If only I could polish my lenses the way Spinoza polished his! I can read for only half an hour at a time without discomfort, and the world has become blurry. An interruption for an hour and a half at noon allows me to resume work later in the day. (Can one go blind from having seen too much?) But that is not the only reason. Perhaps I go to the Atrium to find characters for my stories. I admit that I peer out surreptitiously and eavesdrop, but that, too, is not all. For me, the Atrium is as much a bistro as it is a writer's observation post, a bistro where I go to sit among people I don't know, to enjoy their laughter, their earnestness, the pleasure they take in eating, and in each other. Perhaps I go there to be in the vicinity of the sick and their next of kin. It is with the sick that I feel a sense of belonging. The sick are my kind.

At noon, the Atrium pullulates with people—visitors; doctors in green scrub suits fresh from the Operating Theatre; medical students in short white coats, flaunting stethoscopes about the neck; nurses in white pant-suits, carrying trays of food; patients in pajamas or hospital gowns; pursy, clean-cut, well-groomed medical-equipment salesmen with briefcases, waiting to show their wares to these doctors; maids vacuuming the carpet or cleaning the tables; janitors; orderlies. Each wears the uniform of his calling. And here and there a patient brought there for diversion from the misery and boredom of illness.

At noon, as at any hour of the day or night, the Atrium is never without the distant sound of sirens. Every now and then the voice of the Page announces a "Code 5"—the term for an emergency—and the ward where it is taking place. This, to bring doctors and nurses scurrying to resuscitate. Once I was among those so summoned. And always the soft rushing noise of the fountain.

And then, one day, this:

I have just finished eating lunch and am sitting on a bench in the Atrium, a mere ten paces from the fountain with its murmur and glitter. In a wheelchair, quite near, sits a thin pale boy. He is bald; his lips are crusted, and with a sore at either corner of the mouth. Intravenous fluid drips into his left arm. The bottle hangs from a metal pole attached to the wheelchair over his head. In his lap, a plastic bottle of water with a straw. Now and then the scabbed lips flutter apart, and he takes a sip of air, then another. He looks to be about ten years old and weighs perhaps eighty pounds. His head is all eyes and ears. He seems to be studying me with great interest and without any restraint, the expression on his face one of glacial intelligence. It occurs to me that this boy hasn't the time for shame or restraint, only for honesty. It is inevitable that we should talk.

"What's that you're getting in the IV?" I ask. He glances for a moment at the bottle on the pole.

"It's my pet," he says. "Follows me wherever I go."

"More like your guardian angel." He reacts not at all to this statement. I try again. "Something like a Hospital God. You know, like the ancient Gods of the hearth."

"Lares and Penates," he mutters. "You a doctor?"

"Used to be, long ago. Retired. I got old."

"A condition I won't ever have to face." I am shocked at the tone in which he says this. It is devoid of inflection or irony. I search all over my mouth for something to say. For a long moment we are silent.

"Who told you that?"

"Don't," he says. "I'm way past that."

"How old are you?"

"Fourteen." Another surprise. "And you?"

"Seventy-three. And a half. At my age, you count the halves."

"I'm going to tell you my name," he says, "but first I have to ask if it's OK."

"Of course it's OK."

"Don't be too sure. Now we are strangers, more or less anonymous. By giving you my name, I become somebody who can reach out to grab you, to capture. You could even want to grab me."

"I'll risk it."

"Thomas Fogarty." I see that the crusts on his lips hurt; he barely moves his mouth when he speaks.

"Richard. Richard Selzer," I reply.

"What would you like to talk about?" I ask. "Sports? Music?"

I feel scrutinized by the remorseless blue of his eyes.

"What will you do on your last day on earth?"

"My last day."

"The day when you are going to die."

"Can we talk about something else?" He gives a tiny shake of the head. The huge eyes insist; beneath them are smudges of violet. I'm caught and fluttering in that merciless gaze. He raises the water bottle to his lips and takes a tiny excruciating sip.

"Life hurts," he says. "I measure out the time by sips, see how few I can get along with."

Fourteen. I, who have taken to forgetting everything at an alarming rate, remember my fourteenth birthday when, whispering my own name, I wept.

At that age I was already the man I would become in time, only more honest, braver than I am now. I too had not yet acquired irony. I was as intelligent then as now, as sensitive, as sorrowful. I see at once that this boy is rare, that I must not falsely console or cajole; he wouldn't stand for it. He has already passed through the flames, gone beyond despair and self-pity. He seems enveloped in a shroud of quiet resignation. I see, too, the man he would have become, all intellect and sensibility. I know that his death is the only subject that interests him, this child that is father to the man. And why not? It is his work, his future. All at once I feel ashamed of the good health that has enabled me to live so long, the unfairness of it. Something else too: I feel the stirring of what I can only describe as love for this small skinful of marrowless bones with his mouth encrusted with sores and his gaze that penetrates. Why shouldn't I love him, I who want so much to love?

"You don't have to feel embarrassed for your age. It doesn't matter," he says. My God! He has read my mind! Either he is intuitive or I am transparent.

"What I would do on my last day?" He gives a tiny nod. Above our heads, the leaves of the ficus trees are motionless; there is no breeze to stir them. The swords of the sansevaria slash the motionless air. I have the sense—does he have it too?—that he is the older one, that along with such sickness comes the wisdom, poise, and integrity of years. This boy is ill in every way, but he is not ill at ease. That is my symptom. I hardly dare to speak. I begin.

"On the morning of the day I die, I'll betake myself to the edge of a forest, or be taken there by someone strong enough to carry me deep into the woods. Let it be a forest of great age with huge old oak, beech, and linden trees and a dense canopy above that permits rays of light to slant down to the forest floor. Put me there, I'll tell him, on that bed of shadow. Arrange me upon it. Now wet my lips with a little wine, and then goodbye, with my thanks. I'll go the rest of the way by myself." I see that the boy is listening intently, his eyes feasting on my face. The long gracile neck that lifts his small head toward me—it must take a thousand years to form a neck of such delicacy, and with the power to break one's heart.

"I'll hum or recite, a little of both, maybe, just to hear the sound of my voice. When it stops . . ." All at once, a tuning fork vibrates to a blow. "May I start over?"

The boy, Thomas, nods. I begin again. "It had all been arranged the night before. It is noon when the doorbell rings. Noon, that hour when both hands of the clock are raised up in supplication. From my bed, I can hear his deep voice rumbling. I recognize it as the voice of a former student of mine. Long ago I led him through his first appendectomy, his first herniorrhaphy. Now he is a great surgeon. It is a bond between us. He is big enough to fill the doorway of my room. He bends above the bed and scoops me up against his chest. I feel quite secure in his arms. 'Did you bring it? The wine?' I ask him. 'Oh yes I did. It's in the pickup truck.'

"We ride for a long time. When the truck stops, he gets out and comes around to where I am reclining. Once again he lifts me up against him. And he walks into the woods for a good way, to where great old trees are deeply rooted in the earth and their canopies sway overhead. Here the undergrowth is thicker. There are no paths. Not far away there is a small stream that splashes downward over rocks. A pair of mallards browses among the sad rushes. The iridescent green head of the male! I point down to a shadow on the ground. It is just my size. There, I tell him, put me there. And he does, deposits me gently upon a bed of moss, with fern fronds under my head for a pillow.

"'I'd rather stay with you,' he says.

"'No,' I tell him.

"'Do you mind if I wait in the truck?'

"'No I don't mind, only don't come back until morning. Promise.'

"'All right.'

"'In the morning, when you come, perhaps I'll be gone. Perhaps not. If I'm still here, cover me with earth and leaves so that I won't be cold. If I am gone, then you will know that I have become part of the forest. Don't try to know everything. Some mysteries are not meant to be solved; they are meant to be deepened.'

"Now I am alone in the depths of the pious forest. I feel light, buoyant, partly made of sky, as if an obscure transmutation is taking place, the sort of thing that is probably happening all the time, only we are unaware of it." I glance at the boy in the wheelchair wondering if he has understood me. He seems to be listening with more than his ears, but with his entire body, his flesh and his bones as well. And I know that he has understood fully.

"There is the fragrance of pine tar, mushrooms, and trees. It is so fresh that I cannot stop yawning. But different from the freshness of April. It is October, after all. In this fragrance it is easier to breathe. I inhale deeply and relish the expansion of my chest. How fine it is to fill my lungs with air, using my whole chest. I cannot inhale too much air. Oh yes, I breathe deeply and with a steady rhythm, raising up and lowering with each breath like a bark on a tranquil sea. I am all breathing now. The forest breathes with me. I take part in the breathing of the forest. It is as if I have not yet been born and am in the womb of my mother. I hear noises, the squeaking of a branch, a skittering as of tiny feet running through leaves. A chipmunk, perhaps. Or a fox. I send myself off in different directions. Strange, but I can see myself, the way one sees a mirage. From the truck, I look like a fawn. From the treetops, I am a smudge on the ground.

"I fall asleep and dream that the trees, the rocks, the little stream are peopled by spirits. I am aware of an unknown, unseen splendor. I am happy in the dream of it. To dream so is to be mighty. When I awaken, it is toward dusk. Hour by hour my mind separates itself from my body. I explore my imagination. Now I know that death is just a different kind of existence. Matter can neither be created nor destroyed. Call it whatever you will, it is only the form that changes in death. I become aware of the fluidity of things—not only memory and imagination, but the cells of the body too. There is an inner stream of life composed of blood, cytoplasm, nucleoprotein. It is all flowing."

The boy's lips are parted; his breathing has speeded up, gone shallow; his eyes that never leave my face are shining. Only rarely does he blink or run the tip of his tongue over his crusted, ulcerated mouth. Once or twice I raise the cup to his lips until he takes a tiny wracking sip. All the while I speak in a low murmur that now and then disappears into a whisper so as to underline the privacy of what is passing between us, saying that it is meant only for him. One hand reaches toward me; I surrender a handful of my shirt to it.

"Night is falling and with it comes the feeling of imminence; something is about to happen. Darkness enters my body; I let it. The air around me shifts with the movement of actual angels. Solicitous spiders are weaving me a coverlet. I am the whispering of leaves, more guessed at than seen. Already I am only half flesh and blood, the rest moss, leaf, bark, and oiled fur. Soon I shall be a line of bubbles rising to the surface of life, then winking out. The odor is intoxicating—pine, mushroom, and something herbal. It makes me sleepy. I can hardly keep my eyes open. I yawn. Now I close my eyes, conscious of the world through my hearing alone. It is the deepest kind of repose. Crickets are stridulating, and something curious that chatters and comes and goes as it pleases. I feel the weight of the moonlight upon me like a soft comforter upon the body of a sleeper. I let the forest sprawl across my mind and, all at once, I feel myself inside the vista I have imagined. The night is a confusion of stars and fireflies. I cannot tell which is farther away, the one becoming the other, the here becoming there. It is a painless transition."

"So, Thomas," I say, in the voice of conclusion, "that is how it will be."

"Oh don't stop!" he says. "Tell me more. Please." The thin cotton hospital gown has come untied so that his left clavicle is outlined over its entire length. The slender graceful bone stands out below the fleshless neck, so much older and wiser than all the rest of his body. His expression is vague, yet insistent, as though he has already departed for somewhere else.

"But there isn't any more."

"Then tell it again." Do I imagine it, or has his face taken on a glitter, as with fever?

Suddenly there is a third person present. A nurse in a red pant-suit with a shower cap on her head, a mask hanging loosely at her neck, and white running shoes. Her manner is grimly cheerful, efficient.

"OK, Tony," she says in a loud bluff voice. "Time to go back to bed. We'll be getting a blood transfusion this afternoon." I am appalled by her falsely hearty manner. I am distressed for the boy, who clearly knows that hers is a professional pose.

"It doesn't matter," he says. "I'm used to it. They mean well." Once again he has read my mind.

Tony! So it is not Thomas, after all. He did not give me his real name. Could he have thought that by taking another name, he could unload his illness upon that fictional alter ego? With what reluctance do those fingers release that handful of shirt! The wheelchair with its contents is already being propelled away. From across the Atrium, I follow with my eyes the radiance that accompanies it.

It is the next day, a quarter past twelve. All morning, my mind has been empty of thought other than of him. I am sitting in the Atrium on the same bench. Tony is not there. From across the Atrium, I see the same nurse in the red pant-suit, shower cap, mask, and white running shoes come toward me.

"Tony died this morning. All yesterday afternoon, he dictated this letter to you. I promised I would deliver it." And then she was gone.

> Dear Richard,
> It is just as you said it would be. Already I see myself lying upon a shadow in the forest where you have placed me, my head resting on a pillow of moss. I hear the sound of the waterfall. It is not unlike the sound of the fountain in the Atrium. From the brim of a cup scooped in bark, I drink an ample swallow of pale, icy air. It does not hurt to do so. Like you, I sing or hum *sotto voce* vague melodies, which I compose then and there. All around me there is a labyrinth of shadows. I, too, am "the whispering of leaves, more guessed at than seen." Already I, too, am made half of bark and oiled fur. Only a web of life still clings to my skin. I haven't the strength to shake it off, nor would I want to. Thanks to you, I have been made privy to the mystery of things. Your words move among the shadows, stirring the leaves. They make me think of "The Raven" by Edgar Allan Poe. "The silken sad uncertain rustling of each purple curtain." I wonder if you know that line, and love it as much as I do. My eyes are not entirely shut, like those of a cat sunning itself and drowsing. Between fluttering lids, my fuzzy vision is bordered by a gleam from far away. A moment ago, when the dawn came, it took me by surprise. As if it were the first dawn that ever was—rose yellow and . . .

At that point, the letter ends. I feel my body seated on the bench as the fated Atrium with its cadaverous ficus trees, its penumbra of death, whirls toward infinity. Then I listen to the sound of the fountain and I hear the blood coursing through the atria of my heart.

He was right in saying that by learning his name I could be captured. And so I am writing him down on these pages, not to dispense with him, but in the hope that, by doing so, I will save him, not as a human being, no, but as a character in a story, so that he will not be lost. He will have had conferred upon himself a continuing life. There are characters in the books I have read, and the paintings I have seen, who are more real to me than the people I meet in daily life, who yet wear the futility of flesh and blood. By writing him down in the pages of my notebook, I have given him that stronger reality, turned him into words and rescued him.

I had given him, as well, one of my dreams to play with. It was a ruse, a deception, I know. I, who believe in nothing supernatural, made use of it to prepare this boy for his death. It was as if after years of retirement, I had once again put on scrub suit, mask, and cap, and had taken up my scalpel.

But now I must begin a convalescence from an illness I never had. For no apparent reason, perhaps it is the memory of a leaf trembling, then falling, I will weep. Why do you weep? I am asked. I can only shake my head. There are times when I think that it is he who has entered a new life, and I who am dead.

Oh, let the truth be known—I wanted to keep him for myself. He is unto me like a fountain in my mind, a place where it is always cool and fresh and where I can go to partake of its coolness. Now and then a bit of spray will lay itself gently upon my face. In the days since, again and again Tony is brought back to me with stunning clarity by some errant gust or faint aroma. Then it is that the world trembles around me. The sky above the Atrium quivers, the plants and trees ripple, the whole Atrium founders, until I feel his gaze, clear and true, upon me, and I carry him in my arms, against my chest, and look into the lucid blue of his eyes.

"There," he says, pointing. "Place me there."

As for Tony, I am farther from him than he is from me. I have only to close my eyes to see him again sitting in the Atrium, his Johnny coat having come untied to expose one perfect clavicle. I think I have never seen anything more beautiful than that slender bone beneath his skin. It is for me a relic. I see too how, at the arrival of the nurse to take him away, the IV solution in the bottle trembled as if a train had passed a cottage at night, and a picture on the wall shook gently. I feel him in my arms, against my chest. I see him where I have placed him, in the shadow at the foot of the linden tree. I see his pale hand lying at his side as a leaf might come to rest there. Sometimes I speak to him: "With your eyes," I tell him, "lift this tree up, up, until it touches the sky so that you can climb it all the way to heaven." When I see a fugitive smile play upon his ruined mouth, I know why I was born.

AN EXPLICATION

The Atrium itself is immediately and intensely visual, rendered with a great deal of precise detail—the plants, the skylight, the furnishings, and above all the fountain. Despite the constant activity taking place within it, there is a sense of the inert, the lifeless, as well as a certain vulgarity. It is a product of pretension and interior decoration, as well as an attempt to disguise the true nature and purpose of the hospital. It is a denial of death in architectural terms. Such is the landscape, the theatre where the story takes place. It is the presence of the boy in the Atrium that lends it dignity and taste. Later on, there will be the equally precise portrayal of the forest, and the inevitable contrast between the two places. The forest is clean, pristine, mysterious, subtle. It is devoid of plastic, artificial wood, unnatural vegetation, paint, and varnish. It is also devoid of pus, pain, lesions. It is what a hospice is, in contrast to a hospital—the ultimate refuge, a triumphant place where the imagination reigns and one is free of the agony and terror of mortality.

What are we to make of this short story, if we can even call it a short story? It is hardly more than an encounter between an old doctor and a dying boy, one of those fated moments when two trajectories intersect and there is a sudden moment of revelation. Is the story true? Did it happen? Yes, it is true. It happened. There was just such a coming together of the two in the Atrium of the hospital. But any reliance on narrative is problematical. We cannot be sure how much external reality has become annexed by the author's imagination and transformed by his fantasies. In fact, I suspect he has tinkered with the facts, left out a good deal, accented this, and not that. This is called artistry. In all likelihood, his love affair with the technical ended with his retirement from Surgery. He is no longer a physician, a man of science; he has reverted to a more primitive form of being, one who is receptive to certain subtle influences and to intuition. The doctor in the story knows that he is performing a secret, sacred initiation upon the boy. He hurls himself into this primitive rite recklessly, forgetting himself until that very moment when he hesitates and says to the boy, "That's all there is. There isn't any more." "Then tell it again!" the boy pleads, clutching his sleeve. The doctor's loss of nerve is masked by the arrival of the nurse. The story "Atrium" flies in the face of science. It tries to keep the mysteries of life from being mowed down by the juggernaut of technology.

Is the story sentimental? Of course it is sentimental. Some of the greatest works of art are—all of Dickens, much of Verdi, the paintings of the Virgin and Child. But it is not the false sentimentality that consists of emotions one does not truly feel. It is further saved from sentimentality by the beauty of language. All right, it is a sad piece, one that has brought a lump in your throat. Perhaps you have shed tears. And that is good. I wouldn't want to live in a world where it never happens that one can weep precisely because another wept. Without sorrow, without compassion, the spirit shrivels.

Is it likely that a fourteen-year-old boy would or could write such a letter? No, it is unlikely, but it is possible. At fourteen, I was quite capable of writing such a letter. Let us not forget that, at age fifteen, Rimbaud was writing some of the great poems of rebellion. It is well known that mathematicians reach the peak of their genius in their teens, then quickly decline. Besides, it takes no great leap of the imagination to conclude that the doctor and the boy, Tony, are one and the same, that, in the act of preparing the boy for his death, the doctor has prepared for his own. By the end of the story, both doctor and Tony experience an epiphany when the continuum of mortality and immortality is sensed. Tony is no more and no less than the square root of the doctor. This story was not written with a dry pen, but with one dipped in my body's fluids. Nor was it written easily and quickly, but with a good deal of pain. As the author, I must always be grateful for the improbable gift of the instant when I glanced up to find the boy of the fountain looking at me.

Part V

Being a Writer

When Richard Selzer made a commitment to writing as his second vocation, he realized that it would require a devotion to craft comparable to that which he demonstrated during his surgical training. In conversation with his friend Peter Josyph, Selzer recalled self-imposed homework:

> I began to study it [the English language] as if it were a foreign tongue. I read the dictionary, I read books of syntax and grammar, I learned what the subjunctive really was, I learned what a misplaced nominative was and why not to use it. The way a surgeon would prepare himself for an operation was exactly the way I approached the task of writing. And since words were to be my new instruments, I had to learn them, learn how to use them, put them down in order, suture them together, as it were. [1]

Selzer's love of language is evident in his diary-like meditations on style. These entries also look toward larger issues of structure and meaning, particularly the value of literature to a physician, and such issues are examined more systematically in two essays, "Five-Finger Exercises" and "To a Would-Be Doctor-Writer." The first is a straightforward account of Selzer's own habits and goals as an author; the second purports to be friendly advice to a twenty-five-year-old apprentice, but several references (for example, to the story of Jonah) make it clear that Selzer is really addressing himself. At one point, he seems to be reflecting critically on his early stories of the macabre: "Tell tales of terror, if you must, but tell them sometimes in words of mirth."

In setting standards for himself, Selzer insisted that medical humanities—a field he helped to establish—must look beyond the novelty of writers who happen to be physicians. As *Literature and Medicine* was completing its first successful decade of publication, Selzer offered a "crabby" caution: "If this journal is to remain the voice of criticism in the field for which it is named, it must dispense with the notion that being a doctor is anything but incidental to the making of art. Writers who are also doctors must be held as rigidly to account as all other writers."[2]

Selzer has been anything but crabby in his writing workshops—conducted first at Yale, and then at medical schools and university writing programs all over the United States. The workshop notes reprinted here include writing exercises, suggestions for editing, general observations on craft, and advice about maintaining what might be called "writing morale."[3] The genial spirit of these coaching sessions is crystallized in the final entry, a tribute from a student in Denver.

In his own writing, Selzer told Peter Josyph, "the line is blurry between prose and poetry." In fact, he has published occasional poetry, and one example from 1979 is reprinted here. The interview with Josyph—the culminating chapter in a whole book of revealing conversations—touches on Selzer's favorite writers and on his indifference to literary theory, but it may be most interesting for framing an artistic paradox: an author determined to work within short forms, story and essay, while trying to exploit the full resources of language, even to the point of cultivating a "voluptuous" style.

NOTES

1. Peter Josyph, ed., *What One Man Said to Another: Talks with Richard Selzer* (East Lansing: Michigan State University Press, 1994), 120.
2. Richard Selzer, "An Expostulation," *Literature and Medicine* 10 (1991), 35.
3. Selzer shares other insights about craft in "On Writing," the final section of his *Diary* (New Haven, CT: Yale University Press, 2011), 228–37.

Meditations on Style

As a writer, I am a sensualist. For me, the act of writing is not unlike the palpation of the human body in the act of diagnosis. Even more, it is a sly fingering that invites a response. I love the feel of the prose, its heft of delicacy, its texture. I can taste a word on the tip of my tongue, inhale its very odor.

Were one to find a term that best describes my writing style, I would recommend the use of the untranslatable musical term *rubato*, most often used in reference to the tempo of a piece. The word in Italian means robbery, and has no real relationship to music other than to suggest chaos, or more kindly, flexibility.

*

Why do I use Latin, French, Italian, Japanese, and Korean in my writing? Partly just to show off, but also in an effort to unite the language experience, as a reminder that all language issues from the human need for expression as well as the need for poetical experience. In my next life, I am going to learn Persian. Any language that has given us the words scarlet, peach, azure, lilac, and taffeta is worth learning. And, oh yes, cummerbund.

Even without plot, suspense, rhyme, or logic, I would love language for its own sake, for the way it sounds, the way it looks on a page. Language reaches down into the bones of a human being where the hunger for myth and metaphor is second only to the hunger for food and drink. True communication requires more than straightforward reasoning and easily understood sentences. There is in poetry a lovely mysteriousness that is a form of telling in itself. Nor must every story be told according to the dictates of logic. In my own writing there is a chaos that reflects the chaos that exists in my mind—a certain disconnectedness that I have in fact cultivated. It has become dear to me, as a writer. I never know what will come clattering down the staircase of my brain.

*

Regarding the brevity of my writings—The novels of Scott and Balzac are unreadable by me, because I haven't the patience to swim through three hundred pages of ponderous talk or detailed description in search of a single passage of beauty of truth. In my own work I have a dread of going on too long, of boring the reader, and so I return to the manuscript again and again, to prune and chop until the finished piece is picked clean. It must be done without destroying the lyricism of the prose, which is at least as important as the plot.

At this late date, I hope that I have learned when to take my pen up from the page. The stoppage of ink is no less productive than its spillage. Restraint in creative writing is not easy to acquire, but one must. Too many words are more damaging than too few. There is a value in "unfinish." The sketch is often the more moving and powerful treatment of a subject. Delacroix demonstrated this again and again in his work. His sketch of "Jacob Wrestling with the Angel" is far more moving than his large depiction in oil.

*

The writer puts up a scaffold that is the rough draft of his work. It is a thing of poles, ropes and rigging, and instability. It flaps in the slightest breeze. Here and there a lantern swings. Upon this scaffold he hangs words that decline and conjugate themselves into scenes and characters. Now he stands back and surveys what he has done, then applies a narrative line to give his characters motivation. But the writer must take care lest the scaffold change from a supporting structure into the kind of scaffold upon which he is to be hanged or beheaded.

Oh dear! Something has gone wrong. The plot has turned banal, the characters obnoxious. Now he must climb the flimsy letter to the scaffold, rung after rung, pulling himself up until he has a perspective altogether different from the one he began with. Higher and higher he climbs; wisps of cloud stream in and out. Birds fly about his head, sometimes alighting on the crossbar—pigeons if the story takes place in the city, owls if it is at night, eagles if there is a river full of fish. The scaffolds sways as if it were a treetop. At such a height every movement is risky. A misstep would surely cause him to fall, and it would prove fatal. More than once he loses his footing and hangs by the fingers of one hand until his toe again connects with the reality of the scaffold.

But up so high, he can listen to his characters, converse with them. Together they fashion the work until there comes the moment when it is done. Now he ties a flag to the top-most beam. It bears the words THE END. The story can now stand on its own without the scaffold. The author descends all the way down to the ground. Once there, he gazes up at what he has created. If he has written well, he will have the same pride as God on the seventh day when He looked down upon His creation and declared it good.

*

I think of the text as a *web* (its meaning in Latin). No one's web is more loosely woven than mine, or has more lacerations, folds, stains, most having to do with lapses of memory rather than carelessness.

*

In a venomous review of one of my books, I read that among other sins I am guilty of sentimentality. If sentimentality is what bursts out of the conventions of art and makes a direct attack on the emotions, I confess. That's me, all right.

In a wretched orgy of sentimentality by Louisa M. Alcott called *Good Wives*, a sort of sequel to *Little Women*, Ms. Alcott gathered up all her courage and managed to kill off Jo March. It was a peaceful death. As Beth put it: "The tide went out easily." Reading that at age eleven, I outwept Niobe and doubtless would now if I had the nerve to read it again.

It is upon *Goldie* by Julius Louis Selzer that I cast blame for my acquired vulnerability to sentimentality. That book was what finished me off. Ever since, the only death I can dwell upon without a strangulation of sobs, and a nasolachrymal freshet, is my own. May the tide go out easily.

*

Without putting too much of a gloss on it, I like to think that my little stories are a kind of alms given to the sick and to those who tend them, to give them a transcendent notion of their lives. Such an offering, far from having diminished me, has vouchsafed my life.

*

One of the uses of literature to physicians is the encouragement of tolerance. Bigots and fanatics seldom have any use for literature because they're preoccupied with their prejudices and beliefs. They cannot see their patients as sublime possibilities.

Literature makes it possible for us to look at the sick, and at those who tend them, not as living from moment to disappearing moment, but as "giants immersed in Time." Some of my stories were published more than thirty years ago. Many of the patients, doctors, and nurses upon whom they were based are long since dead. But as characters they live on, and are capable of moving readers—including the young medical students and medical professionals who have read them and who, I like to think, have been partly shaped by them.

*

A writer should not restrain the metaphorical activity of his mind. At the end of a piece of writing, you should be able to say what Chopin said on his deathbed: "My endeavor is as complete as it was in my power to make it." In my story "Atrium" I have striven to make words speak the language of infinity, the way Chopin used the piano. I turn myself into an eye, unblinking, that peers and squints at what it sees.

*

Discovered the word "aposiopesis" in which the speaker drops a sentence in the middle, finishing it after a long pause, with a knowing look. I am glad not to have died before learning this rhetorical device. (Now to make use of it somewhere.)

*

Sat on the back porch watching the icicles committing suicide by *aquarrhage* (their variation of hemorrhage).

*

I am told that art is best achieved by toil, misery, and disappointment. I don't know about that. I know only that writing has made me happy. And happiness has taken a great part in the making of these small creations of mine to which I have the temerity to give the name "art." I love the self-imposed exile of the writer, the giving up of everything else, and the pledging of oneself as a bridegroom or a monk does. To close the door of my scriptorium and turn away from the world, and wait. That is all. Lately, though, it is otherwise. These days, I no longer feel the surge of elation. I am an old empty tin can left out in the yard. Now and then it fills up with rainwater, overflows onto the grass. In the hot sunny afternoons it steams until once again it is empty. Soon, though, there will be a distant growl from the heavens.

*

Like a brave soldier, I extract a metaphor, like a bullet from deep within my own wound.

Five-Finger Exercises

Writing came to me late. I was 40 when I began to teach myself the arachnoid knack of spinning words. My equipment consisted of my discipline—surgery—a relish for language, and a pen. Hardly reason to take off my hospital mask, don tights, and dare the high trapeze of prose. But from that first day, I loved the warmth of the process, the awkwardness, the wobbly first steps of authorship. What emerged on the page was an account of what Jonah must have experienced as he was swallowed by the whale. Since I knew what the gastric mucosa looked like better than the original bible storytellers, the belly of my whale had a good deal more authenticity. That fact alone was thrilling.

I wrote in longhand then and still do. The pen is the writing instrument most congenial to my hand. It has the same length and heft as a scalpel, though one is round and the other flat. Ply either one, and something is shed. From the scalpel, blood; from the pen, ink. I like to watch words issue from my fingers, like a secretion from my body. The word processor does not exist that offers so personal a sense of discharge. Then, too, there are the quick, tiny hisses as the flat of the hand moves across a page from left to right, to say nothing of the long, delicious hiss from right to left when you start a new line. Each time I write a story or an essay in longhand, I feel a triumph over the technological preeminence of the computer keyboard.

In the 1960s, it was rare for a surgeon to become a writer, but I decided to write about what I knew: my work as a doctor. The two careers cross-fertilized each other. My medical situations and portraits were as factual as I could make them, but I learned to betray facts with the "gentle treason of poetry." (Highly suspect behavior for a member of a male priesthood, such as surgery was 30 years ago.)

"Come! Come!" my colleagues scolded. "Stick to your last. Isn't surgery enough for you?" But it was too late. I had succumbed to the irresistible urge to record stories that were being enacted every day at the hospital. Like Ulysses' men, who had melted wax poured in their ears so as not to hear the song of the sirens, I warded off their warnings. I persisted. There was only one person who did not dismiss me outright: myself. From this I learned that a writer must have some measure of will, that he or she must exhibit the requisite courage to put work forward despite any fear of rejection. Something of a trickster's appetite for triumph is necessary in this.

I make rather more use of the English language than less. I'm about as far from a minimalist as you can get. A full-throated ease is what I strive for, not often achieved. Is this outdated? Perhaps. But I doubt that there's any such thing as progress in art. Are the cave paintings at Lascaux more outdated than the paintings of Picasso? I find the former even more compelling for the patina of their 20,000 years.

A good deal of what I do is in the form of a diary. My present project is to prepare my diaries for publication. On the face of it, this doesn't make much sense. First you tell a notebook all your secrets, and then you publish it? In fact, I have come to diaries both by nature and by training. Every doctor is a diarist: You keep a daily record of your patients' illnesses, setting down the vital signs, the physical findings, the patient's "complaints." You order tests, prescribe medications, express disappointment at worsening and joy upon recovery. Such "keeping" seems to me a higher genre than mere storytelling; there is a life at stake at the center of each tale. The best writing I have ever done in my life may have been done in medical charts where the patient is the hero, a character whose very existence is a work of art. It is the only writing I've done that is devoid of vanity and pomp. Still, those were case histories and, as I am now retired from my work as a doctor, I don't write them any more. I write stories that reach for privileged moments of revelation, as when a cleft lip, say, or an ingrown toenail, or a torn rag of flesh takes on a certain radiance. In such moments, flesh becomes the spirit. Unlike a CAT scan or an MRI, these stories don't look for concrete answers. Their aim is more difficult to define; they are apt to be ambiguous. As a writer, I've learned that some life mysteries aren't meant to be solved; they're meant to make us wonder at them.

Writing, for me, is what purring is for a cat. It represents pure pleasure, and there is no purer pleasure than chasing after the nature of a bodily thing and nailing it to a page. To do so, I have often made use of the rich language of medicine. In the 1930s, my father was a general practitioner in Troy, New York. He practiced downstairs. Our family lived upstairs. At night, after office hours, my brother Billy, who was 8, and I, 7, would sneak down to his consultation room and to the glass-front cabinet where he kept his medical texts. Our favorite was the *Textbook of Obstetrics and Gynecology*. It was there that I first became aware of the richness of medical language. There were words such as "cerebellum," "carcinoma," and "sphincter" (which Billy told me was a lady who never got married). Father wanted me to become a surgeon; Mother, who was a singer, hoped I'd become a poet. When I was 12, he died, long before my eyes had had their fill of him. That was when I decided to take up his trade.

Medicine has enlarged the language, offering words such as "cough," "asthma," "hiccup"—all derived from the sounds of the sick. There is a moment of tragic onomatopoeia when old King Lear appears onstage carrying the corpse of Cordelia, and cries like an animal in pain, "Howl, howl, howl, howl!" The symptom of suffering lies outside the precinct of language. It cannot be rendered. In such moments, only howled vowels will do.

After three decades of hurly-burly surgery, I retired. I felt rather like a camel who suspects his master is overloading his poor hump. He turns and looks sadly upon the piled load, sighs at the injustice. All at once, the amperage of my life dropped to 20 watts. I found that dim twilight ideal for entering a writing life. Now there is time to indulge my eccentricities. I carry an amulet in my pocket; I put on my lucky hat, the one that keeps my thoughts from flying off the top of my head. I'm quite sure that I write better by candlelight or if it's raining. That sort of thing.

Unlike surgery, there's a good deal of waiting around in writing. A whole day will go by at my desk, where I sit, instrument in hand, without so much as one keepable word issuing in a tidy, cursive coil. After such a day, I fall into bed like an apple from a tree, with the same thud, only to awaken to an angel holding a perfect sentence out to me on a silver tray.

There seem to be two phases that occur before and after writing. First, there is the mysterious quicksilver of inspiration, an altered state of consciousness that may be biochemical in origin. The second is the tinkering with the text. Both give a good deal of pleasure, although there is such a thing as too much tinkering. A sheepdog that turns obsessive can worry the sheep until they won't graze, only stand huddled and trembling.

Once, I lived for the sense of urgency in surgery. Don't imagine that writing is a more lighthearted pursuit. Nor is it easier to perform, but rather harder to make come out right. The technique in either is intricate, painstaking. In surgery, the body of the patient is opened up and put together again. In writing, the whole world is taken in for repairs and then put back in running order, piece by piece.

To a Would-Be Doctor-Writer

I receive your first literary effort with pleasure, and I take comfort from this further bond between us. You are not the first medical student who has written to tell me that he, too, wanted to be a writer. Most are like Mrs. Pendarvis: "I should like to write," she mused. "Not to publish. Just a few guiltily lovely lines to char in the grate when I am dying." But your first short story marks you as one with a difference.

Do not imagine that this gives you license to abandon the hospital wards to spend all of your time scribbling. A writer must remain rooted in the real world. Only Rilke and Flaubert did not have to. Antaeus wrestled to the death every man who dared to set foot in his kingdom. Whenever he felt himself weakening he would bend to touch his mother, Ge, who was the earth. Taking strength from her, he would rise to vanquish his adversary. In the end, Antaeus was defeated only when Hercules held him aloft in the air and squeezed him to death.

But, my dear Maupassant, the story you sent me lacks kindness. It is what the French call *un conte cruel*. While these may be as fascinating as snakes, they evoke the same single response—horror. Jonah and the Whale, really! If you presume to retell the Bible, you must do more than describe the gastric mucosa of a whale and the physiologic process of vomiting. Else you will be no more than a literary grotesque. A writer, like a doctor, must strive for a kinder heart. A battlefield is not a mere jewelry of beautiful wounds. As you would not lambaste a patient with the grisly details of his impending doom, so ought you not to be cruel or condescending to your characters. It is wrong to lie to a patient in order to encourage him falsely. But, as any gardener knows, it is possible to fool flowers into blooming by keeping a light on all night. In writing, as in medicine, follow Emily Dickinson: "Tell the truth, but tell it slant." There will be plenty of time for horror. There always is.

Nevertheless, Jonah is the quintessential surgical character, and you were instinctive to choose him. In every operation the surgeon is Jonah, albeit not one so reluctant as the original in that he does not say *non serviam*. The patient on the table is the whale into whose body the surgeon enters in the service of God. At the end of the operation, the surgeon is spewed forth onto the dry land, and they are both saved.

I long for the day when you, too, will make rounds and see upon the nightstands of your patients one or the other of your books. This used to cause me anxiety. My God, I thought! It cannot be good for them to read these things. At least, not preoperatively. But now I feel different. Just as the patients expose themselves to me, so do I show myself to them. We are equal.

Some years ago, my first book was published. From my electrocardiogram, you would have thought I had written *Madame Bovary*. The book was a collection of macabre stories (like yours) that no one ought to read after dark. Not long after, I was returning a book to the New Haven Public Library. The librarian there is an old friend. Just ahead of me at the desk stood one of those aboriginal Yankees still found in the cities of New England. Picket thin she was, and with a bun of iron-gray hair impacted at the back of her scalp. I saw at once that she was returning my book! The librarian saw this, too, and thinking to garner for me a compliment within earshot, she said to the woman, "What did you think of that book?"

The woman paused, held my little book between thumb and forefinger as though to avoid contact with something cold and moist. Then, depositing it upon the desk, she said, "I would never let that man operate on me."

I am, and I am not, jealous that you begin to write at twenty-five, whilst my own elephantine gestation took forty years. A person ought not to expect to write oracular books heaving with virile mysticism in a hand still pudgy with baby fat. Who can regret the long rubbing together of two sticks if at the end a pretty flame breaks, and you can warm your hands by it? If I have regrets, they are for the patients I have forgotten. Sometimes, at night, I awaken, sit up in bed, and try to remember a word that one of them said, which if only I could remember, would change my life. But I cannot.

There will be occasions when writing will make you cruel. One night, exhausted and having failed, I came home from the emergency room with red-stained fingers. "What have you have been doing?" my family asked me, their eyes on the hands I had neglected to wash clean. "Picking berries," I replied. "But it's April; there aren't any berries," they said. "Well, then, murder," I said. Ashamed of myself, I climbed upstairs to my desk, still without washing my hands, hoping that the blood would blacken into ink and I would be able to write. No such luck. Nor did I deserve better. At last, I took a shower and went to bed.

While it is possible for a writer to make a story of anything, you are especially blessed. A dozen times a day in the hospital you will encounter a hero or watch a plot evolve. Even to listen to a patient's chest with your stethoscope is to be a child once again listening to a shell for the sound of the far-off sea. Though what comes back to you will be the gossip of the heart, the endless complaint of the lungs' disease, or the dirge and syncopation of death.

There will be a danger of being drawn to the tragic in your writing. I urge you not to ignore the humor that is equally present in the life of a doctor. Tell tales of terror, if you must, but tell them sometimes in words of mirth. Make up for the humorlessness of God. Do this, and you will establish a relationship with your readers. Look, you will say to them, I too am a little child. I love fun, and "shallow foppery." Melville made Queequeg order the construction of his own coffin, then had him try it out for size. And the only one of the crew to survive was Ishmael, who floated away from the wreck on Queequeg's coffin.

Do not be surprised if your writing changes the way your colleagues look at you. "Come! Come!" your colleagues will coax you, in the words of Richard Wilbur: "Forsake those roses of the mind and tend the true, the mortal flower." A doctor who writes is irregular. I am put in mind of the flounder. At birth, the eyes of the flounder, like the eyes of the bass or perch, say, lie on either side of its head. He swims upright, like all the other fish. Then, all at once, something happens to his swim bladder—it deflates or atrophies, whatever, and the flounder can no longer hold himself upright. He tilts to one side and settles to the bottom of the sea. Half of the flounder fall to the right, I suppose, and the other half to the left. Parallel to the sea bottom, the down-eye is no longer of any use to the flounder, and, in fact, is a handicap in that the poor fish must gaze at the sky with one eye and the sand with the other, and as a result it sees nothing. Therefore, the down-eye migrates around the head of the flounder, or right straight through the head, to take its place alongside the up-eye. Now the two eyes of the flounder are on the same side of his head, both looking straight up. You want to be a writing doctor? Be prepared to "flounder." Your colleagues will stare at your migrating eye, and the peculiar way you tilt, but you will not care about that. For you will look about you with dilated pupils, and you will see what no one else can, as though they were blind and only you had vision. You will stand at the operating table just before you are to incise the breast of a young woman, and you will be reminded of the blue-and-white teapots on your grandmother's shelf, which you were told never to touch. And you will think that now, years later, you are about to break one of them.

Best of all, you will have a muse who does not faint at the sight of blood. Take especial care that she not also be bloodthirsty. Sometimes, having been up and working all night, she will be too tired and cranky to sing for you. But you have some power over her as well, and can, if you will, urge her on. Again and again, my own muse has fallen still:

"Come," I call into the shadows, and I strain to listen for her voice. At last she answers:

"When may I stop to rest?" she whines.

"Not yet. Not yet," I tell her, and write another line.

"But when?" comes the petulant cry. She has her tricks. She begs only to rest, but means never to sing again. I do not answer, and write on.

"When?"

"When I finish this sentence," I tell her, and slyly start another page.

Again that awful "When?"

"At the end of the page," and the pen goes crashing along the paper.

"Now," she says. "I shall stop now."

"Don't stop! Don't stop!" I cry like a man being stroked by a lover. With the same hope of delight, with the same fear of abandonment.

If you live with blood enough, you become like it—red, turbulent, restless. When you stop, you clot. To live with ink is no milder a fate. You curl and loop and dot away life, hoping only to pale out. Then, unexpectedly . . . you blot!

Last week I chose medicine over literature. Today, I feel differently. It is what comes of reading Homer. Toward the end of *The Odyssey* we find Odysseus at last deposited upon the shores of his homeland, the kingdom he had left twenty years before. He is the very picture of the vagabond, dressed in rags and with his hair and beard tangled. Trembling with emotion, he makes his way to the gates of his palace and gazes within. What he sees fills him with horror. The suitors of his wife, Penelope, have assumed control of the palace and are conducting orgies and revelry. They are wasting his goods and his cattle; they are squandering his treasure and defiling his house. Penelope and their son, Telemachus, have been helpless to stop them. Now the crafty Odysseus steps inside. He has decided to keep his own counsel, to let the tatters and dishevelment of the years of wandering hide his identity. He is led to Penelope, who engages him in conversation. She likes him well enough, but does not recognize him. She even asks if he has news of her husband, gone so long. He offers none.

Penelope then calls for the old nurse Eurycleia to bathe the feet of the stranger and make him welcome. Now, it happens that forty years before, as a boy of ten, Odysseus had been taken to visit his grandfather on another island. There, during the course of a hunt, he had been gored in the thigh by the tusk of a wild boar. The wound was severe, and quickly became septic. For a long time it was feared that the boy would die. It was this same nurse, Eurycleia, who had then bathed and dressed the wound. I see her applying unguents and herbs, and pressing out the poisons, and cherishing the blood of her little patient as though it were the last of the wine.

At last she saw that the necrotic tissue at the base of the wound had separated and sloughed. New pink buds of granulation tissue appeared. These coalesced to form a healthy bed across which the epithelium raced. And the wound healed. It is forty years later. The old nurse kneels at the feet of the stranger.

> This was the scar the old nurse recognized;
> she traced it under her spread hands, then let go,
> and into the basin fell the lower leg
> making the bronze clang, sloshing the water out.
> Then joy and anguish seized her heart; her eyes
> filled up with tears; her throat closed, and she whispered,
> with hand held out to touch his chin:
> "Oh yes!
> *You are Odysseus!* Ah, dear child! I could not
> see you until now—not till I knew
> my master's very body with my hands!"
> (XIX. 467–76)

It was not his wife or his son who recognized Odysseus. It was his nurse. It was the wound that had awakened the buried past—the wound that was the emblem of all the shared pain and disappointment and exhilaration that are the measure of the tending relationship. As though it had a voice crying out, "hinnen—behold me here!" Homer understood the power of the wound over those who both suffer and tend it.

A critic asks—with boundless impertinence—why a surgeon would write at all. Why he would look for myth and metaphor in the operating room. Isn't the act of surgery enough? No one has the right to dictate to another whether or not he may seek transcendence over the facts of life. It is precisely in the operating room that a surgeon will sing his arias of terror and bravado. The surgeon cuts his patient, and his own flesh must not bleed. He, like the patient, is anesthetized. Only the writer is awake, and listening. Besides, good writing is to be found in unlikely places. Here, from the *Cecil-Loeb Textbook of Medicine*, 12th edition, volume 1 (Philadelphia: Saunders, 1967), 394:

> Tapeworms may be harbored for years and, except for the inconvenience of the gravid segments crawling out of the anus, the host continues in robust health, enjoying both food and drink.

Now show me the writer who would not die to have written that.

Do not artists trespass upon medicine, using differential diagnosis to advance their plots? Shakespeare did it all the time, as when he caused Juliet to say to Romeo: "Ether my eyesight fails me or thou look'st pale." It had to be one or the other. Groucho Marx, too, and with more sangfroid. In *A Night at the*

Opera we see Groucho shamble into a room. He trips over the body of a man lying prone on the floor. He reaches for the man's pulse, at the same time studying his wristwatch. For a long moment he is silent. Then he speaks: "Either this man is dead, or my watch has stopped."

All right, all right, I have not fussed enough with my prose. I have not been logical, orderly—coherent, even. I have only been natural. Accept, please, the awkward words of a doctor writing from the experience of his life. They are truer, at least, than the volumes of twice-cooked cabbage written about the practice of medicine by those who have never taken into their hands the life of a fellow human being.

Notes for a Writing Workshop

Not long after my retirement, I was asked to lead a workshop in creative writing at the medical school where, only weeks before, I had been engaged in the lovely tactile pedagogy of surgery. Creative writing at a medical school? The past decade has been witness to a spate of books by and about doctors. Who, one wonders, is taking care of the sick if everyone who knows how to start an intravenous infusion is in the toils of the Muse?

Not that it is a bad idea for doctors to pause at their labors and the gaze with the third, the pineal, eye of the artist upon the human body and those who tend it. It is high time that Art caught up with Technology. And who am I to murmur, I who spent the final fifteen years of my medical career doing surgery all day, and writing all night? Far be it from me to quench a heart on fire. Still, while the life of a doctor may be a rich source of grist for the writer's mill, the training of doctors ill prepares them for the rigors of vocabulary, grammar, syntax, and punctuation.

And so we seventeen met each Monday evening to write our hearts out. Among other things, we learned that *"No," she hissed* is not really a good idea, and that the distinction between *prone* and *supine* is important to all writers, not just to pornographers. I admit the difficulty here when even a famous doctor-writer who shall remain nameless causes one of his characters (also a doctor) to place a patient in the "prone" position in order to perform a pelvic examination on her. Any woman so positioned would be wise to get a second opinion. We learned, too, that "disembosom" is figurative term having nothing to do with breast surgery. What is art, I asked, but an augmentation of life? It offers surprise, and adds the marvelous dimension of unreality to the real world. It is a short leap from the study of anatomy to the mythopoetic reality of medicine. In one sense my feeble attempts to behold and record what goes on in a hospital are tantamount to the building of a second edifice which is a replica of the first—only this one is made from that most versatile of bodily secretions: words.

*

The writing teacher should arouse and inspire a love of words. To do so, the teacher must know their meaning, origin, and derivation, the way a doctor must know the basic facts of anatomy and physiology before diagnosing and treating patients.

For example, the word "carnivore" is composed of *carnis* (Latin for flesh) and *vore* (Latin for devour, as in "voracious"). In an odd parallel, "sarcophagus" is composed of *sarcos* (Greek for flesh) and *phagus* (Greek for eating), because the ancient Greeks imagined that the stone crypt ate the flesh of the deceased, leaving only the bones.

Consider the word "stethoscope," deriving from the Greek *steth*, which means "chest," and *scope*, from the verb "to look." Stethoscope is thus a misnomer. One does not look with it; one listens.

*

The language of medicine is rich, resonant and alliterative. At least it was until it became reduced to a short-hand that seems more related to the computer than to the human body. Every term is given an acronym or otherwise abbreviated in the interest of speed or efficiency. This new language has an ugly, staccato sound: "V-Tac," for example, instead of "ventricular tachycardia."

I was six years old when I first encountered the beautiful language of medicine from the textbooks on my father's bookshelf: "arteriosclerotic heart," "choledocholithotomy," and so many more.

Were I to choose a medical specialty now, it would be dermatology—for the vocabulary alone: acanthosis nigricans, reticulated lentigo, granular parakeratosis, pyoderma gangenosum. The consistency of these diseases in the mouth is that of pasta cooked *al dente*.

*

My idea of good writing requires that it have two components. First, a sense of masterly ease, spontaneity, a tossed-off flavor that doesn't show the hard work behind it. This is called, in Italian, *sprezzatura*. The second is even more vague. It is like the utterly unconscious repose of an athlete that pervades his whole personality. This is called *disinvoltura*.

*

Be he who he may (I've been looking for a chance to use those five monosyllables. It is English, yes, but with a Hawaiian lilt, something that should be sung while doing the hula), be he who he may, a writer would do well to hone his pen on the stones of the past—the Old Testament, for one. There is no more gorgeous prose anywhere.

*

The secret of art is not verity (the facts), but versimilitude—the illusion of *similarity* to the facts which is the artist's province.

*

Don't regret your sorrows. They may be the wellspring of your best writing. I myself have often, in the depths of melancholy, stumbled over words like cobblestones. All of a sudden, there appears an image I have longed to write for years, but couldn't find the path to it. It is precisely the defeats and disappointments of life that supply the ideal climate of inspiration for a writer. For William Butler Yeats, the writer must be "doom-eager." During the early stages of the creative process, frustration and despair may suddenly give birth to a thought that may change your life for the better. That is when your imagination may go on a rampage, churning up images so fast that you can't write them all down on the page. Here is Joseph Conrad: "My story is there, but in a fluid, an evasive state. I can't get hold of it any more than you can grasp a handful of water."

Conrad felt frustration when paragraphs or phrases refused to crystallize into a finished work of art, but Poe revels in the phantasmagoric in the very shocks and falls that are needed to keep reverie in motion. An example of this is his story "The Pit and the Pendulum." When the narrator learns that the Spanish Inquisition has sentenced him to an agonizing death, he swoons—and this swoon is described as a long fall: "Down, down and still further down, til a hideous dizziness oppressed me." Swoon blurs into a real fall and the narrator finally awakens to find himself in a subterranean chamber on the brink of a circular pit. Dreaming, for some writers, is the ideal state for creation, and that is what you hope to make your reader do: not laugh or cry but dream. Each time the pendulum swings, his imagination is set quivering. And so is that of the reader. In the end, Poe's narrator manages to fall without falling. Just as he totters on the brink of the abyss, he is rescued: "An outstretched arm caught my own as I fell, fainting into the abyss." By this time the reader is half dead from the horror and the suspense.

*

Writing is rather like polishing an old table you've just taken down from the attic. First, you pour some sweet-smelling oil on it. Then, taking a soft cloth, you begin to rub, making circular motions with your arm, leaning into the work, transmitting the energy from brain to shoulder, then down the arm. Soon the surface of the table will begin to light up and glow. What you have done is to liberate the life that had lain dormant in the long-dead tree from which the table had been carved. It is nothing short of a resurrection. The writer polishes his language with the same devotion, until what emerges is a story or a poem.

*

Avoid cliché or redundancy, such the yellow daffodil, gnarled oak tree, or lacy spider web. Seek out new images:

* He traced out the translucent scapulae that rose like hillocks from her back. They are all that is left of our primordial wings, each retaining still the gleam of a bird in flight.

* On his face a look of caged rage.

* The bull turned his head sideward to tear the grass, the huge bulk, the hooved legs, the pizzle all absorbed in the grazing; only the whisking tail with a mind of its own.

* Awoke to a heavy snowfall, with the hemlocks wearing their epaulets proudly.

*

Prune out the little qualifiers: *quite, sort of, kind of, rather, very, too, pretty much, in a sense*, and especially *really*.

*

One difference between traditional craft such as basketry or rug weaving and artistic invention is that traditional craft depends upon repetitious acts while artistic invention depends upon departure from routine. Of course, the techniques of traditional writing—synaesthesia, allusion, onomatopoeia, metaphor and simile are also present in artistic invention. The trick is to use them to stimulate new, original expressions and thoughts.

*

Synaesthesia is the splashing over of one sense into another. In writing, it is a metaphor in which sense-impressions of one kind are transferred to sense-impressions of another kind—an intimate fusion or association of one sensory excitation with another, in such a way that the second is experienced right along with the first, as in "cold light" or "sweet harmonies." Most commonly it mingles the auditory and the visual senses so that sounds seem to have color or texture: "glistening silver laughter" or a "velvet tone of voice." (The singer Mel Tormé was dubbed "The Velvet Fog": a marvelous bit of synaesthesia.)

Synaesthesia is a highly individual experience. The writer must strive to strike just the right note so that the reader will react by thinking: "Yes! That's right!" The timbre of the flute is white, that of the cello is purple or violet, of the violin sky blue, of the clarinet crimson. Brass instruments are said to produce sounds that are gold, yellow, orange or brown.

*

Bases for experiments:

* Use of combined adjectives: the river in winter all cloud-shadowed, ice-fastened. (The Adirondack mountains: be-laked and be-rivered, with slopes, ridges and escarpments.)

* Alliteration and assonance: "the silken sad uncertain rustling of each purple curtain."

* A question that advances a plot or sets a scene: "But had she really understood the hint he had given her?"

*

Allusions enrich a text, and they are economical, allowing a writer to evoke, in just a few words, an atmosphere, a whole period of history, a story. Most allusions should be recognizable, such as those from Shakespeare or the Bible. Here is Lincoln in his Second Inaugural Address: "It may seem strange that any man should dare to ask a just God's assistance in wringing his bread from the sweat of other men's faces, but let us judge not, that we be not judged."

"A just God" is from Isaiah; "the sweat (of their brows)" is from Genesis; and "judge not" from the Gospel of Matthew. Lincoln was slain five weeks after this plea for reconciliation that would have malice toward none and charity for all.

*

Consider the importance of punctuation—for example, the difference between

"Good heavens!" Mr. Sandhill ejaculated.

and

"Good heavens! Mr. Sandhill ejaculated!"

*

The way a word is used causes it to assume substance, take shape. Axe used to carry out a beheading—one hears the *swish* of the blade through the hushed air. Axe used to fell a tree—one hears the *thunk, thunk* of chopping wood.

*

The writer must believe in himself, that he can produce something of value to his fellow man, but at the same time, he must remain humble, avoid vanity and self-love for that is destructive to the latent creativity. These two must remain in balance.

*

A blank page is a freshly made bed awaiting the sleeper and his dreams.

*

And here a page left on the table after the students had left the final session of a workshop in Denver on creative writing:

An Appreciation of Richard Selzer
To a man for whom suffering is as deeply beautiful as vigor and health.
To a man who has lost his faith only to embody it, like a man who has lost his hat but wears it on his head.
To a man who suspects that writing cannot be taught, but who is relentless in inviting his students to improve.
To a man for whom "Colorado" is neither more nor less than a beautiful word, beautiful like "alabaster."
Thank you, thank you, thank you.

It was signed by the student who composed it. His name: James Lough. The date: September 25, 2003.

As evidence that the tribute belonged to *him*, I offered my tears.

Remembrance of Things . . .

A man told me today
That things remember.
The sword, for one,
Remembers the forge, its heat,
The pounding toward sharpness,
And keeps to its shape.
Does it remember too a hot plunge
Through skin, fat, muscle, membrane?
A lick to the hilt?
A slow withdrawal?

The stones of the guard-walk at St. Sophia's
Where Turks have paced out a thousand years,
Those stones, too, remember,
And turn hollow at the thought
Of such heaviness.

The feather recalls its fall
From bird-breast,
And feels nostalgia for that fluttering heart
When it flutters on the wind.

Now I look around at things,
And wonder how they perceive me.
This chair—
Does it welcome the curve of my flesh?
Or will it hold this sitting against me?

And for the ink I let upon this page
Can ever pen forgive
Or paper forget?

Wounded with Wonder

Richard Selzer Interviewed by Peter Josyph

PETER JOSYPH: What can a short story do that a novel can't?

RICHARD SELZER: Well, of course one of the chief goals of a short story is to tell a story quickly and economically—to have the characters change, in some significant way, within a few pages. There is a feeling of compression about it. What it lacks in long, luxurious recounting, it makes up for in its rather bullet-like speed. I think a surgeon is particularly suited by temperament to the short story form as opposed to the novel because the short story is rather like a surgical operation. It has a beginning, a middle, and an end—at least *my* stories do: you make an incision, you rummage around inside for a little while, then you stitch it up.

Writing a short story is like taking out an inflamed appendix. And there is that intimacy with the instrument. When you hold the scalpel, you cannot give it its head: most of surgery is holding back, restraining. After thirty years of restraining my instrument, when I picked up the pen I said: "Go! It's not blood, it's only ink." Suddenly the surrogate was off and I had this marvelous freedom to grab great armfuls of language and run across the page. And in writing, the sheet of paper becomes the patient, in a certain sense. In both cases, you are dealing in wounds. The act of making an incision is the creation of a wound for the purpose of healing the patient. The earliest forms of writing were exactly that: taking up a sharp rock and gouging out hieroglyphs in a flat stone—making wounds, as it were, to tell a story.

The difference is that the surgical wound must heal, eventually, but the writer's wound does not. I'm speaking now not of the wound made on the page, but the writer's *own* wound that he is attempting to heal by the act of writing the story. And yet the writer's wound *must not* heal. He attempts to bridge over that wound with language, but it must not heal—because if it ever did, the result would be the kind of finality of fossilization that would ruin the writer. It would be an act of self-destruction. I think probably what happens to many writers who burn out or who lose the energy or the inspiration to write is that they have healed themselves through the act of writing and there is nothing left to say.

JOSYPH: You once said that one of the problems you have with the contemporary short story is that no blood is shed upon the page.

SELZER: Yes, that's true. And that is why one is often unmoved by even the most accomplished pieces of prose. Blood and ink, at least in my hands, have a certain similarity. When you use a scalpel, blood is shed; when you use a pen, ink is spilled upon the page. Something is *let* in each of these acts, and that is another bond between them. I always wondered why every surgeon didn't write, why I was one of the very few. After all, a surgeon does walk around every day in the middle of a dozen short stories, and it seemed to me that it would be irresistible to write them down as I have done. But I think one of the reasons it isn't so is that the surgeon must remain anaesthetized to the philosophical, the literary, even the human implications of his work, in order to be able to carry it out dispassionately, at the proper remove from the white heat of the event.

JOSYPH: Is there a similarity between the short story and the case history? Does the surgeon himself write the case histories of his patients?

SELZER: Yes, he asks the patient a number of questions and attempts to piece together a diagnosis. Often this is not exact and he is left with two or three possibilities, which constitutes what is called a *differential diagnosis*. Although now, with the new technology, this is most often solved outside of the operating room, when *I* was practicing surgery we were often called upon to do exploratory surgery to find out what was wrong and treat it at the same time. The short story writer, too, is carrying on a diagnostic act. He creates a character, he presents this character with a predicament, with various conflicts, barriers, acts of fate, and then he waits to see how this will develop and what the diagnosis will be.

JOSYPH: Unlike most practitioners of the short form in fiction, you seem content to stay with it.

SELZER: I'm a restless, rather impatient writer: I want to get things done and see what happens. On the other hand, I'm a very slow writer. Each of my short stories takes approximately six months. That is because I write slowly. I write a great deal for each story, and then I boil it down in my laboratory.

JOSYPH: Compare that with Hemingway, who sometimes wrote two or three in a day!

SELZER: I know, and I'm consumed with envy over people who can do that, but for me it is a very painstaking process of writing, rewriting, adding, subtracting—it's like chemistry.

JOSYPH: In the case of your only novel [*Knife Song Korea*], you reversed a common procedure: instead of stretching a story into a novel, you dismantled the novel and published only an excerpt.

SELZER: Well, I realized as soon as I finished my so-called novel that it wasn't a novel at all; it was a series of episodes, all set in the same place and linked together by the narrator, but each event, really, was a short story that stood by itself, and I didn't think it had the sweep and the continuity of a novel. In fact, I don't believe that most so-called novels written today *are* novels. They're *called* novels, but they're really episodic constructs more akin to a series of short stories with the same locale and characters. I much prefer the short fiction of Cheever and Updike to their longer works, I think probably for that very reason. The popular novelists are not really producing novels. I'm not saying that in a negative way, but I don't see them in the same way I see *War and Peace*, or *Anna Karenina*, or *Madame Bovary*, or even *The Magic Mountain*. Many of today's novels seem to have a staccato quality: when you begin a new chapter, it's a new story.

JOSYPH: Isn't it that much more extraordinary, then, that Dickens, or Thomas Hardy, could write novels that are so coherent, and yet they did it weekly, in installments?

SELZER: This is of course a phenomenon. They were both novelists, and both were gifted with immense energy. Robert Louis Stevenson was another case in point. They wrote novels the same way they breathed or ate: it was a physiologic function for these men. For me it isn't; it doesn't flow out of me that way.

JOSYPH: You once quoted a phrase from *Hamlet* to express something key to the author's purpose in writing stories.

SELZER: Yes. It's the point in the play where Hamlet has sneaked back into Denmark from England and is horrified to witness Ophelia's funeral. After they place her in her grave, Laertes leaps in to embrace his sister for the last time, and he begins an oration on his sorrow. Hamlet, offended by this, says:

"Who the hell is *he* to use this kind of high-flown language about *my* tragedy?" Or, as Shakespeare puts it:

> *What is he whose grief*
> *Bears such an emphasis, whose phrase of sorrow*
> *Conjures the wand'ring stars and makes them stand*
> *Like wonder-wounded hearers?*

Well, that is exactly what the writer tries to do, to make of his readers *wonder-wounded hearers*. To do this, the writer will use every stunt he can find in the whole abominable gymnastic of writing. I am constantly aware of that and try never to write a sentence that will not increase by a little bit the temperature of the piece, so that it becomes warmer with each line.

JOSYPH: Are there any contemporary short story writers who wound you with wonder the way some of the nineteenth-century writers can?

SELZER: Of course I am a nineteenth-century writer who somehow got born a hundred years too late. But I can name several: Kay Boyle, Elizabeth Bowen, and V. S. Pritchett. These three are, I would say, my favorite short story writers: they succeed more than anybody. There is also an Irish short story writer named Mary Lavin whom I like very much. Also William Pritchard. You can see that my choices, with the exception of Kay Boyle, are from Great Britain. I don't know why. I do like many of the short stories of Kipling. He's a great short story writer, much underrated. I like the stories of Maupassant, another writer who is underrated these days. D. H. Lawrence wrote about a dozen of the greatest short stories ever written. And I think that Thomas Mann's best works by far were his short fiction. *Death in Venice*, *Mario and the Magician*, and *Felix Krull* were the best things he ever did.

JOSYPH: I have the sense that many contemporary writers feel this pressure that they're not legitimately writers unless they write a novel.

SELZER: Yes, there is this prejudice abroad in the land.

JOSYPH: Editors and agents contribute to that, don't they?

SELZER: They do, they do. I've never had a publisher who didn't urge me to write a novel. They all want THE NOVEL. The short stories, they say, are all right, but you can never finally achieve the kind of wide recognition with short stories that you can with a novel. What these people are overlooking is that true novelists are very rare. Very good short story writers will try to fit themselves into the mold of novelists, and very often they will fail. I know my own genre, and that is the short story.

JOSYPH: But your first book [*Rituals of Surgery*] has three times as many stories as your latest [*Imagine a Woman and Other Tales*], and the average length has increased from ten pages to forty.

SELZER: Do you mean that if I live to be three hundred, I'll write a novel? No, I'm stretching out, I'm looking at more facets of the characters and events, whereas my earlier stories perhaps had fewer dimensions and could be told more quickly.

JOSYPH: You began by writing stories of horror and suspense. What does that enable one to learn as a beginning writer?

SELZER: Surgeons—as you know—we love horror! But when I first began to write, at the age of forty, I realized I had to teach myself this craft, and I chose the horror genre because it seemed to be the simplest. No philosophical implications, no complex characterizations, very little irony. All you had to do was invoke a shoulder in your reader. So I did write horror stories, and they began to be published in *Ellery Queen's Mystery Magazine*. After a few years of that, I had, I thought, achieved a certain level of facility, so that I could reach out and go beyond the horror genre, although *Imagine a Woman and Other Tales* has been referred to by a number of reviewers as a book of horror stories, which horrifies *me*. The themes are dark, but how they can call them horror stories is a mystery to me.

The thing I liked best about both surgery and writing, in the beginning, was the craft. That's what drew me to surgery. I loved learning how to cut and stitch and clamp. The technical side of it thrilled me. Similarly, when I first began to learn to write, it was the suturing together of words into sentences, the selection of these words, the scattering of them on the page, that delighted me. The language was and still is the most important part of my writing. After the work had become incorporated into my body, I could go beyond this intense focus on the language to approach the content, the ideas, the abstractions.

JOSYPH: As you began to draw more closely on your experience as a surgeon, did you begin to explore your own wounds?

SELZER: Yes, every writer does that, don't you think? When you write a story you are, in a way, telling your own. Timidity is the greatest sin. A writer must tell his or her own worst secrets. But there is a difference between an autobiographical work and one which transforms your life into universal terms. A writer's first work is often a matter of getting something off his or her chest. It's the rite of passage that gives one the proper distance, puts one beyond a certain self-indulgence, so that one can write about the world, extracting from that the syrup of transcendence. Nonetheless, as you suggested, it is true that the line between my fiction and my non-fiction is rather blurry, just as the line is blurry between prose and poetry in my works.

JOSYPH: You have told beginning writers to go to the poets for their models and inspiration: Poe, Scott, Dickinson, Moore—

SELZER: And add to that Francis Ponge, who wrote these beautiful, tiny pieces—prose poems, I guess you'd call them.

JOSYPH: It's interesting that you didn't say Hemingway, Steinbeck, Carver—

SELZER: No, I'm not in the minimalist style—

JOSYPH: You're a maximalist?

SELZER: Yes, I'm a nineteenth-century voluptuary. I use as much of the language as I can, instead of as little. I want to enjoy every bit of it.

JOSYPH: But why the poets?

SELZER: Because of their use of simile and metaphor. Metaphor is the secret language of the writer, the gateway to the reader's imagination. Also, poets are very aware of the rhythm and the sound of their lines, and for me, too, that's important in a story. I count a whole lot on the beauty of the language. Marianne Moore, with that marvelous awe she had for Nature, wrote: "What sap went through that tiny thread / To make the cherry red?" That's honesty, that's sincerity, that's humility before the great extravaganza of life. You can't beat that, and in fact it's what I tried to do in writing about medicine, to retain that sense of all she invoked in writing that line.

JOSYPH: I recently read an editor's advice to the aspiring short story writer: "Don't try to be Thomas Hardy." By which he probably meant, *Try to be Raymond Carver*. Then you will read other editors who say: "No minimalism, please." By which they mean, *Do not* try to be Raymond Carver. But whether it's Carver, Hardy, Hawthorne, Hemingway, Poe, Selzer—isn't it that sense of wonder we experience when the work is at its best?

SELZER: Oh, without it you can't achieve anything.

JOSYPH: Look at Carver's "Cathedral." There's nothing minimal about *that*, certainly not in terms of its effect.

SELZER: Marvelous. I am very fond of Raymond Carver's work. That I do not write in that way does not mean that I don't admire him tremendously. He was a master. But it's a matter of style, and a writer does not form or create a style, he discovers it; it is already there in his body, like a fingerprint, and he has to find it. I believe the writer who has a great deal of discomfort writing has not yet discovered his style and is trying to be something he is not.

JOSYPH: What have you learned from reading your critics?

SELZER: I have learned nothing that has helped me. I have only learned by doing the writing itself and by reading. The commentary of the literary critics does not seem to hit the mark, whether it's favorable or unfavorable. I feel that it is written about someone else. I can't relate to it.

JOSYPH: Many of the most revered practitioners of literary criticism are right here in your lap at Yale. Have you gained anything by your exposure to them?

SELZER: Not a bit. Not one bit. I am mystified by all the deconstruction industry. I prefer to read short stories for the pleasure of it. And I do not agree that the criticism of a story is as valuable as the work itself. That is an egotism which is utterly ridiculous. It's monstrous. It's not true. Literary theory doesn't interest me. I'm simple. While I try to write about great themes—love and death, pain, faith or the lack of it—my writing does not swim up from the intellect. My writing is about intuition rather than intelligence. As a reader, I like to hear a good story well told.

JOSYPH: In conversation, you've recounted some of the same events you have written about. What is the difference for you between the oral and the written form?

SELZER: That's interesting. I do see myself in the continuum of writers who were originally troubadours, who sang or spoke their stories. There was an *aural* and an *oral* component to storytelling, as there is to this day in numerous other cultures, in some of the Arab nations, for example, where there is this marvelous tradition of the men—it is usually the men—standing up before the group and telling a story, displaying a great improvisational skill, which we who write everything down seem to have lost. That's one reason I like to read my stories in public. Lending my voice to the written works gives them a dimension they wouldn't otherwise have. I like to *italicize* with my voice; one can *say* an exclamation point if one knows how. I like to get out and confront my readers and make new ones.

There will be fewer readers in the world, perhaps, because of television and the computer, but there will always be that cadre of people who take sensual pleasure in picking up a book and opening it to page one and losing themselves the magical act of reading a story. It is for those people that one writes. Not for fame, not for money. One writes stories to reach out and approach another human being. The other half must come from the reader, of course, or the story doesn't exist. And I am very careful of my readers. When I'm writing a story, some part of my mind is always aware that someone is out there.

JOSYPH: And you never want to cheat them, do you?

SELZER: Never. No cheap shots, no shortcuts, no tricks. I want them to get it, desperately.

JOSYPH: And you make the tacit agreement with your readers which I think relates to your having gazed at the very limits of life as a surgeon: "I will show you something I know about, but you must be willing to follow me all the way." Most of your stories cannot be approached lightly. They aren't written that way.

SELZER: No, they aren't. They're written in blood.

Part VI

Homage

Richard Selzer's affection for certain writers led him to return again and again to their work, as illustrated in his diary discussions of poetry by John Keats, fiction by Robert Louis Stevenson, and essays by Thomas Browne. Selzer never outgrew his youthful enthusiasm for Edgar Allan Poe, whose short stories influenced several of his own early tales of suspense and, in a more subtle way, added atmospheric touches to later stories like "Imelda."[1] Poe is also one of several writers whose work Selzer recast, preserving the shape and tone of the original stories while giving them his own distinctive stamp.

In two cases, Selzer radically amplified his source material. After reading "The Light-house," a fragmentary manuscript discovered after Poe's death, Selzer wrote "Poe's Light-house," narrated by a hospital attendant who has been entrusted with the story by the dying writer. Within the story, the main character's self-isolation is motivated by what is clearly a case of Tourette's syndrome.[2] Earlier, in "The Mirror: A Tale of Aran," Selzer had followed a suggestion by his neighbor in New Haven, the distinguished scholar Richard Ellmann, who relayed a story that James Joyce told but never wrote about an elderly couple in the Irish West, out of touch with civilization, who did not understand that the faces they saw in a hand mirror were their own reflections. With Ellmann's encouragement, Selzer expanded a bare outline into a textured tale.[3]

By contrast, two of Selzer's adaptations have distilled novellas into short stories. "The Whistlers' Room" is based on an obscure book, *Die Pfeiffer-stube* by Paul Alverdes. Set in a German military hospital during World War

I, the narrative deals with soldiers who have suffered severe throat wounds, alleviated by the insertion of metal tubes into their damaged larynxes. Both Alverdes and Selzer use this medical premise as a basis for exploring poignant relationships among the men, including an English prisoner of war and a courageous doctor. "I have justified my act of literary surgery," Selzer writes, "by the certainty that, had I not performed it, *The Whistlers' Room* would have slept unnoticed for centuries, if not forever. What I have done, I have done with gratitude and esteem for Paul Alverdes. This work is an act of homage to him."[4]

Selzer performed a similar act of literary surgery on Thomas Mann's 1954 novella *The Black Swan*, turning it into a twenty-page story, "'The Black Swan' Revisited."[5] Later, when Mann's novella was reissued by the Limited Editions Club, Selzer was invited to give a lecture in New York. In this talk (slightly edited as printed here), he explains the medical background of Mann's story and discusses his own attraction to the work, but adds some artistic misgivings. While exemplifying his incisiveness as a literary critic, Selzer's commentary on *The Black Swan* also offers insight into his own creative process.[6]

"*A Tale of Two Cities* Revisited" offers a lighter kind of literary adaptation. Selzer enjoyed reading his cheeky alternate ending for Charles Dickens' novel from the podium when receiving honorary degrees—for example, from Goucher in 2004, as part of the college's MFA program in Creative Nonfiction. (The Goucher citation described Selzer as "a pioneering artist who has transformed medical writing into literature.")

As a form of literary adaptation, "Crimean Vespers" is unique. It is directly indebted to Anton Chekhov's classic "The Lady with the Small Dog," but Stefan Volkov, Selzer's protagonist, is not based on Dmitri Gurov, the main character in Chekhov's story. Instead, he is modeled on Chekhov himself. Selzer makes that connection clear in his epilogue, which begins with a declaration of deep affection: "Were I to choose the one writer I revere above all others, it would be Anton Chekhov. It is impossible not to love the man for his grace and good will." Quoting from one of his old diary entries, Selzer even entertains the fantasy that his father, Julius, who was born in Odessa, might have been Chekhov's illegitimate son, conceived in a passionate romance similar to the one in "Crimean Vespers."

The story's narration is indeed romantic. Some passages seem to be spoken intimately to the reader; others convey the emotional sweep of a movie. Published late in Selzer's career (2007), "Crimean Vespers" revives several of his familiar tropes: the scene of Ulysses, having returned home in disguise, being recognized by his old nurse when she discovers the deep scar on his leg; the reference to a moth that alights upon the eyelids of sleepers and draws away their tears; and the repetition of "aqualune," a word Selzer invented long ago to describe the path of moonlight on water. All these elements confirm the story's personal significance for the author, enshrining Chekhov as his ideal and offering a literary token of his love.

NOTES

1. Poe's influence on the early stories is evident in "Myself Healed," the final tale in Selzer's *Rituals of Surgery* (New York: Harper's Magazine Press, 1974), in which a man becomes increasingly certain that a plant is growing inside of him. As the first-person narrative becomes more manic, it echoes Poe's "The Tell-Tale Heart." In "Imelda," the next-to-last section uses an underground morgue, illuminated only by torches, as the setting for an operation on a dead girl—as imagined, rather than witnessed, by the narrator.

2. "Poe's Light-house" was originally collected in *Imagine a Woman and Other Tales* (New York: Random House, 1990) and was reprinted in *The Doctor Stories* (New York: St. Martin's Press, 1998).

3. "The Mirror: A Tale of Aran," also reprinted in *The Doctor Stories*, was first collected in *Confessions of a Knife* (New York: Simon & Schuster, 1979). Richard Ellmann gave a fuller summary of the original tale in "The Limits of Joyce's Naturalism," *Sewanee Review* 63 (1955), 567–68. In 1990, long after Selzer had written his short story, he told Peter Josyph about stumbling across Ellmann's article: "I'm glad hadn't seen it before I took up that particular pen. I'd never have had the nerve." See *Letters to a Best Friend* (Albany: State University of New York Press, 2009), 113. In Josyph's *What One Man Said to Another* (East Lansing: Michigan State University Press, 1994), 26, Selzer remembers Ellmann telling him that Joyce had heard the story from John Millington Synge—but the tale is not among those recounted in Synge's *The Aran Islands*.

4. "Epilogue," in *The Whistlers' Room: Stories and Essays* (Washington, DC: Shoemaker & Hoard, 2004), 41.

5. Selzer's version originally appeared in the journal *Grand Street* 5, no. 4 (1986). The story was included in *Taking the World in for Repairs* (New York: William Morrow, 1986) and reprinted in *The Doctor Stories*. Selzer subsequently rewrote *The Black Swan* as a full-length play, which has been performed in various summer venues.

6. The Limited Editions Club volume (New York, 1990) presented Mann's novella, translated by Willard R. Trask, as a large quarto with lithographs by John Hejduk. Because the volume was devoted to Mann's work as a stand-alone "classic," it did not include Selzer's retelling of the story.

Afterlife of *The Black Swan* (1991 Lecture for the Limited Editions Club, New York)

I am delighted by the invitation to mark the publication of Thomas Mann's *The Black Swan* in its Limited Edition reincarnation. My own involvement with the work began in 1983 in Venice. Browsing in a bookstall for something to read, I came upon a battered paperback copy of Mann's penultimate work of fiction. I paid the hundred lire and returned to the Abbey of San Giorgio Maggiore where I was staying, as an impostor in the vicinity of piety. It is an irony worthy of Thomas Mann that so gynecological a novel be read in a monastery.

It was a fated purchase, for from that day to this evening, my life as a writer has been entwined with that book. First I rewrote it as a short story entitled "'The Black Swan' Revisited: Homage to Thomas Mann," and then adapted that story as a full-length play. This is evidence, if any were needed, that a writer must take great care what seeds he lets fall into the soil of his imagination.

Confluent with my discovery of the book in Italy, but preceding it by two years, there occurred another event that triggered my compulsion to retell the story of Rosalie von Tummler. I was at the time teaching surgery at the Yale School of Medicine. One day, in the course of conducting ward rounds, I led a retinue of residents, interns, students, and nurses down a long hospital corridor. Moving briskly along, I glanced in the room of one patient who was not known to me. In the second or two it took to pass by the open doorway, I saw an elderly woman, propped on pillows in a bed, in a state of profound emaciation. She could not have weighed more than seventy pounds. Her hands were spiders at the end of sticks. With arms raised and head bent to the side, she was attempting to pass a long pendant earring through her earlobe. Her head and hands shook with the effort.

This I beheld and then moved on to continue making rounds, but now with the sudden knowledge that I had witnessed something important. From then on, I was to carry with me the image of that woman engaged in her brave act of adornment against what would seem absurd odds. To me it was a revelation about courage, hope, and femininity. Here was a woman who would be beautiful at all costs. Perhaps she wished to please some expected visitor? Or her doctor? Perhaps it was to bolster her self-image? Perhaps, if she were wearing earrings, things could not be so bad. Again and again I was to dwell upon this event and its implications. I suppose I knew from the start that one day I would use it in a story.

Now let us go to the novella by Thomas Mann. Sometime in 1951, Mann was told a true story by his wife, Katia, about an older woman who falls in love with a very young man—and about the deception of her body, which she interprets as undergoing rejuvenation while in reality she is suffering from a fatal illness. In fact it sometimes happens that in the very early stages of serious illness a woman or a man may take on a certain youthfulness: a bit of weight loss, a brightness of the eye perhaps caused by fever, even a delicate pallor.

Mann was seventy-eight and immediately decided to begin a new story, interrupting work on one of his best books, *Felix Krull*, in order to write what he referred to as his little myth about Mother Nature. The story was begun in California, where he was living at the time, and finished in Switzerland in 1953. The title in German is *Die Betrogene* (The Deceived Woman). Its appearance in English was greeted by lukewarm reviews, some of them contrasting the novella with Mann's earlier masterpiece, *Death in Venice*, to which it bears an intriguing similarity. One critic judged the story as evidence of Mann's failing powers. Another, in *Saturday Review*, called it "one of the most repulsive, most devilish works of art that I have looked upon." And in *The New Yorker* Brendan Gill described the novella as "tedious and disgusting." Mann, although hurt, did not defend himself.

What could have offended the reviewers? These were all bourgeois males, it must be said, for whom gynecological topics were taboo. In brief, *The Black Swan* is the story of a post-menopausal woman who is seized by an unseemly passion for a very young man. Widowed for many years, and a leading a quiet, respectable life with her crippled daughter Anna and her son Edouard, Rosalie von Tummler is a lover of Nature in all its facets. Her favorite season is spring, when nature's juices flow at high tide. A young American, Ken Keaton, has come to tutor Edouard in English. Handsome, carefree, casual, very American, Ken soon becomes part of the household. Before long, Rosalie is horrified to find herself in the grip of a sexual desire that she had thought long dead but which has returned with ferocity. She is in despair over her age, which would seem to preclude any response on the part of the young man. At last, she confesses her secret to Anna, to whom love has been denied by her club foot. Anna tries to cajole, then reason with, her mother. When she sees that Rosalie is obsessed, she begins to fear for her sanity. She urges Rosalie to send Ken away. Rosalie refuses.

As time goes by, Rosalie's suffering increases. There are times when she can no longer distinguish passion from pain. But now begins her transformation into a much younger woman, and she notes the signs of change with exhilaration. Her eyes grow brighter, her hair takes on a luster, she loses weight and regains her figure. Love, she rejoices, is making her young again to be worthy of Ken. When at last her menstruation returns, she tells Anna that it is the miracle of love, and Anna too believes that a miracle is taking place. On an outing to a ruined castle, Rosalie and Ken are separated from the two children and find themselves in a hidden lovers' lane overgrown with plants and covered with rotting leaves. The stench is oppressive. It is there that Rosalie throws herself upon the youth, embraces him, and tell him of her passion. He is understandably caught off guard, but in the end acquiesces to an assignation. She will come to his room the next day to consummate their love.

Fleeing the deathly odor of the garden, the two rejoin Anna and Edouard by a pond where two black swans are floating. Ken reaches into his pocket for the bread he has brought to feed them. At the familiar gesture, one of the black swans swims near. But Rosalie, intoxicated with happiness, seizes the bread, still warm from the heat of Ken's body, and begins to gnaw on the crust. Furious at being cheated, the swan lifts its black wings and hisses, frightening Rosalie, who tosses the bread to the bird. On the return trip, Rosalie is rapturous over her coming tryst.

It is a tryst that will never take place. That night she has a massive hemorrhage and is taken to a hospital. An advanced uterine cancer is diagnosed at surgery. What Rosalie had interpreted as a return of her womanhood was in fact a manifestation of the cancer. Just so has her body deceived her. Just so has Nature restored order. While Anna is distraught at her mother's diagnosis, Rosalie finds the transcendent meaning in what has happened. She tells Anna not to pity her. Death has come to her in the guise of love. To how many is that given? She dies peacefully. Her last words: "Nature—I have always loved her and she has been loving to her child." The consummation of Rosalie's love for Ken would have disturbed of the order of Nature and is thus unthinkable. That beautiful black swan with his "blood-red bill, the black beating of his wings" was death, the servant of Nature. Rosalie, snatching the crust of bread for herself, turned her back on Nature to reach for her sexual prize. She must die.

One of the marks of Thomas Mann the novelist was his need to verify the facts. In order to inform himself about gynecology, he wrote to his friend

Doctor Frederick Rosenthal as he had done when he was writing *Doctor Faustus*. In the letter, he outlined the story, insisting that it was based on a real-life incident and questioned the doctor: At what stage of the cancer is it likely that bleeding would occur? What would the operation involve, if one were undertaken? By what signs does the physician recognize uterine cancer? Is post-menopausal bleeding always a sign of cancer? How long does it take for carcinoma to develop from the initial stages to the point where it is no longer operable? Does menstruation cease abruptly at the menopause or does it become irregular and then slowly decrease? "I do hope that answering this barrage of questions will not give you too much trouble. Choose a time for it that is good for nothing else!" Whatever clinical information was given to Mann by Doctor Rosenthal, the explanation of the deceptive bleeding given by the doctor in the novel is rather imaginative: " . . . after the menopause, through heaven knows what process of stimulation, [the cells of the ovaries] begin to develop malignantly. And then the organism, if you likc, is shot through, drenched, inundated with estrogen which leads to hormonal hyperplasia of the internal mucous membranes, with concomitant hemorrhages." The clear implication, if not of the doctor then of the author, is that it was the stimulation of sexual passion that brought on the false menstruation.

Thomas Mann was nothing if not an autobiographical writer. No discussion of *The Black Swan* would be complete without taking into consideration Mann's lifelong, largely suppressed homoeroticism. With the recent an ongoing publication of his diaries, this has become common knowledge. Mann made no effort to conceal from posterity what he took pains to hide from his contemporaries, his seeking out of young men, his offers of money, his repeated rejection and humiliation. It would take no great leap of the interpretive mind to see that the aged writer was telling his own story in the chapter of the aged artist Aschenbach in *Death in Venice*, lusting after the golden youth Tadzio on the beach. In fact, many years later a Polish Count recognized himself as the boy Tadzio. The physical description matched with photographs of himself as a youth, and he remembered sensing that he was being closely observed on the beach by an older man, the real-life author and the fictional Aschenbach.

Thomas Mann, too, was Rosalie von Tummler in *The Black Swan*. Both characters developed a passionate love for a young male, a passion that was never to be realized. Aschenbach dies of cholera; Rosalie of uterine cancer—and each death is the resolution of an erotic passion. And so we can say that the powerful theme of *The Black Swan*, as of *Death in Venice*, is that of liebestod: love/death.

One model for Ken Keaton may have been a young intern named Carlson whom the ill and aging Mann met while a patient at a hospital in Chicago in 1946. Mann was strongly attracted to the doctor, whom he saw as childlike:

"a cheerfully one-sided, capable, simple soul, good to look at" (a description which would fit any number of surgical interns of my own acquaintance). In the novella, Mann embellishes the memory of Carlson. Ken is well-built with broad shoulders, narrow hips, and particularly attractive strong white arms. In addition, he has a charming American style of speech and manner.

Whatever in the world, you may well ask, would prompt anyone to rewrite a story by so acknowledged a master of the craft as Thomas Mann? Was it simply an act of arrogance such as befits the temperaments of a surgeon? Mere cheekiness? A boyish urge to kick over a pedestal? No, I think it was not. It was meant as an act of homage by a far lesser writer to a great one. And the theme was one congenial to my instrument. I was, after all, daily witness to the treason of the body.

Thomas Mann was seventy-eight when he began to write *The Black Swan.* Ill and tired, he felt himself to be already gravid with his own death. The voice in which he wrote was elegiac, elderly. Fascinated and moved as one is by the powerful theme of love/death, Mann in this instance may not have realized its highest potential. There is a perceived chasm between the greatness of the theme and the literary execution of it. In part, this is due to the long dialogues between Rosalie and Anna which comprise a large portion of the text. Stilted, ornate, formal and stylized, the conversations of the two women bear little resemblance to real human speech. Anna and Rosalie thus engage each other in philosophical argument over the questions of Nature and Art in a way that bleeds the narrative of much of its dramatic impact.

> "Victory, Anna, victory, it has come back to me, come back to me after such a long interruption, absolutely naturally and just as it should be for a mature, vigorous woman! Dear child, what a miracle! What a miracle great, beneficent Nature has wrought in me, how she has blessed my faith!" . . . "Dear sweet Mama," said Anna, willing enough to rejoice with her, yet sick at heart, "this is truly a great, a moving event, it testifies to the richness of your nature, which was already evident in the freshness of your feeling" . . . "Say no more, my poor child! What you call my freshness of feeling, and now insist that you enjoyed, you represented to me, more or less bluntly, as sheer folly."

Then, too, there is a certain clumsiness in the way the author insists on providing the reader with the pathological details of the disease. With the only two pages to go before the end, no fewer than three doctors are introduced and given a single sentence or phrase of identification. These three, of whom one is pompous and another craven, discuss the facts of Rosalie's uterus and ovaries in unnecessary detail that is both tedious and unintentionally comical.

> "Just take a look at this mess, Knepperges," said Muthesius. "Presumably it exceeds your expectations." That it also exceeded his own, he gave no sign. "Ours is a noble art," he added, his eyes filling with tears that meant nothing, "but this is expecting a little too much of it. . . . I advise you to adopt my opinion, which is that the whole story started from the ovary—" . . . Knepperges, a thin ambitiously conceited man, made a brief, covertly ironical bow of thanks for the lecture.

And that is the last we ever hear of those three doctors.

Most importantly, it seems to me that Mann was mistaken in his notion that Rosalie must be denied the consummation of her passion, that such would fly in the face of Nature and her intentions. Despite her own acceptance of her fate, I found that to be an act of literary cruelty. Perhaps it is the doctor in me who finds it difficult, if not impossible, to utterly destroy my characters, but must rescue them at the last moment, if not from death then from a fate that is worse than death. In this, I am not alone. You will recall Tennessee Williams' compassion at the end of *A Streetcar Named Desire*. For two and nine-tenths acts of the play, he systematically broke down the defenses of Blanche Dubois, stripping her of every illusion about herself, every bit of dignity. And then . . . she stands alone on the stage awaiting the men who will arrive to take her to the insane asylum. She is the picture of dejection. The men arrive, she straightens, tosses her shawl bravely about her, takes the arm of a doctor and utters what is surely one of the greatest lines of American theatre: "I have always depended upon the kindness of strangers." Tennessee Williams, in that last-minute rescue, returns to his character every bit of her dignity and courage.

Why not, I thought, let Rosalie have her moment of triumph? Would it not lend her death the full bittersweetness that it deserved? After all, Richard Wagner, one of Mann's idols, allows the ill-fated Isolde to realize her passion, and he uses the leitmotif of the famous liebestod to signal subliminally but unmistakably to the audience her physical ecstasy. But Mann had no music with which to convey the act of love. Perhaps, I thought, it could be done with metaphor? And then I remembered that old woman at the hospital and her earring:

> Ken had not visited her at the hospital. At first, she had hoped against all reason that he would, that he would come and take her up in his arms and stroke her back to health. But she knew that he would not come, and she was satisfied with that, forgave him. Why should he come? she thought. He has the innocence of the well. Such innocence must be preserved for as long as possible. There would be plenty of time for death. There always is. And just as she had decided that, there was the nurse telling her that a young man was waiting in the lobby to see her and should she show him up? Yes! Yes! she said in a voice full of longing. The nurse helped her into her bed jacket. Rosalie brushed back her hair with three strokes of a transparent hand. So he has come, she

thought. And waited for the nurse to return with Ken. Oh, God, the dark seam of her lips, her yellow skin?

My earrings, she thought. I must wear them. She reached for the drawer of her nightstand. The effort, or was it the pain she kept hidden beneath the sheets, made her dizzy. At last, fumbling, she had them. Long pendants of gold that hung almost to her shoulders. She must hurry. He would be there within minutes. Rosalie raised one earring to her neck groping shakily for the lobe of her ear. Supporting the working arm out with the opposite hand, she grimaced with the effort. At last, she found the little hole and passed the wire through. Now the other. But try as she might, holding her head to the side, pulling her ear lobe down to searching exhausted fingers, she could do no more than poke the skin with the cold metal. Again and again she jabbed blindly for the hole, all of her strength and will engaged in this act of adornment. At last, she sank back helplessly and gave it up. Her eyes closed on tears of disappointment. She had wanted so much to be wearing them. So that at first she did not see him standing in the doorway. When she opened her eyes and saw, saw not only Ken, but what had settled there on his face, she could not speak.

Ken walked slowly toward the bed. "Here," he said, taking the earring from her hand. "Allow me." His tone was more than solicitous; it was gallant. And, holding her earlobe steady with one hand, he passed the wire through her flesh with a single quick movement. Rosalie felt the casual dexterity of his touch spread from her ear to her neck, then across her cheek until her whole body shivered in the warmth of it. At the same time she saw his large shadow fall across her body. The weight of it made her gasp.

I share her triumph at that moment.

Not content with having stubbed my toe on a monument, I have carried impudence to unheard of extremes by writing a play called *The Black Swan*. Two years ago, it was performed at Williamstown Summer theatre, and last summer again at the Playwrights Institute at Sundance in Utah. On each occasion, I had the playwright's ignoble pleasure of listing to an audience weeping over the fate of Thomas Mann's lovable heroine and rejoicing in her triumph over death. It is my fondest hope that, with the presentation of this talk, *The Black Swan* and I shall disentangle from each other and swim apart once and for all. I have no wish to end my miserable days as a footnote in the bibliography of Thomas Mann.

If I have given the appearance of hesitating to declare Mann's work masterpiece, it is the appearance only. Remember that for seven years the story has captured and held my own imagination. The powerful theme, the endearing heroine, the climactic ending, the evocation of the castle, and the pond with its black swans combined to form a work that deserves to endure. When, the other day, the package arrived and I held this volume in my hand, my old house and everything in it gasped with pleasure. I have never seen a more beautiful book. It is a gift to modern literature that this novella, now graced with the extraordinarily beautiful lithographs of John Hejduk, has been resuscitated and brought back to the full bloom of youth, as Rosalie herself would have wished, and this time without the least bit of deception.

A Tale of Two Cities Revisited

As a doctor, I have witnessed my share of sad endings. Having spent the greater part of my life trying to prolong the lives of my patients, I am now temperamentally unable to kill off the characters in my stories. It is why so few of them get finished. In a review of one of my books, I read that, among my other sins, I am "terminally sentimental." That's me, all right. I come from a family of weepers in whom lachrymation can be brought on merely by saying "Once upon a time . . ." in a lugubrious tone of voice. We know what's coming.

I have even rewritten the endings of other people's stories to give a doomed character another chance. Take *A Tale of Two Cities* by Charles Dickens. As you may remember, Charles Darnay is the handsome young husband of Lucie, the lovely daughter of Doctor Manette. He is also an aristocrat and therefore an enemy of the Revolution. Having been seized and thrown into the Bastille, he is awaiting the guillotine. On the eve of the execution, in an act of excruciating gallantry, Sydney Carton, an English look-alike of Charles, worms his way into the Bastille, and exchanges places with him. For the reason that he does this, I refer you to the original text. Oh well, I'll tell you. For some years, Sydney Carton has been in love with Lucie. Upon being rejected by her, he embarked upon a life of drunkenness, dissipation, and wanton pursuit. Now it is his only wish to secure Lucie's happiness, even at the cost of his own life.

It is the morning of the execution. An axe-colored dawn has broken over Paris. Sydney Carton, posing as Charles Darnay, stands at the foot of the guillotine. He has just delivered his immortal last speech: "It is a far, far better thing that I do than I have ever done. It is a far, far better rest that I go to than I have ever known." Now he kneels to place his neck in the path of the dreadful blade. A hush falls over the crowd . . . All at once there is a commotion on the scaffold. Shouts and curses are heard.

"Zut, alors!"

"Fout le camp!"

"Merde!"

"Sale cochons!" and many other disagreeable accusations are exchanged by the executioners and the revolutionary guards. It seems that the guillotine has broken down. The blade is stuck and cannot be released to fall. It is as though the instrument could not bring itself to kill so heroic a man. Now blows are being exchanged, muskets fired. Sydney Carton, lost in a vision of his own glory, is unaware of the *mêlée.* The crowd, being French, is overcome with emotion at this apparent sympathy of the guillotine for its intended victim. Singing *La Marseillaise*, they swarm over the barricades and onto the scaffold. Sydney Carton feels himself being lifted and carried into the throng. A cloth soaked in chloroform is placed over his face. He inhales deeply—once, twice, three times—and loses consciousness.

When he awakens, he is on board a ship. A beautiful young woman kneels beside him, cradling him in her arms.

"How long have I been here?" he asks.

"Two days," she replies.

"Who are you?"

"*Ma foi!* You do not know me? I am Lucie, the daughter of Doctor Manette and the wife of Charles Darnay, the man whose life you saved." Recognition slowly dawns upon the face of Sydney Carton.

"Lucie! It is you!" he whispers. "But where are you taking me?"

"To England. You will come to live *avec Charles et moi.* We shall have a ménage à trois."

"Vive la France!" cries Sydney Carton as his head falls back upon the soft, soft bosom of Madame Darnay.

And that is how *A Tale of Two Cities* ought to have ended.

I learned later that chloroform hadn't been discovered until 1834, some decades after the French Revolution. Oh well . . .

Crimean Vespers

The year was 1895. Nicholas II occupied the throne of the Tsar. A man of about forty years of age is sitting in a deckchair on the upper deck of the steamboat *Peter the Great*, en route from the port of Odessa on the Black Sea to the town of Yalta at the southern tip of the Crimean peninsula. Stefan Volkov, only days before, had been discharged from the Russian military hospital where he spent eight months recovering from severe gunshot wounds and the ensuing surgery. He is thin almost to the point of being gaunt. Still, he is handsome in a vaguely Asiatic way with black hair now flecked with silver and slightly tilted eyes. Only his eyes are gray, or hazel—that ambiguous color. He is still wearing a military officer's blouse tied around with gold braid. A pince-nez is perched on his nose. It is attached to a long black ribbon. He himself is a doctor, now on the way to a district hospital in the mountains above his native Yalta. Cholera is raging in the neighboring states. It will be his task to stem the tide of it as well as to perform all the duties of a general medical man—surgery, obstetrics, general medicine. But at this moment, he is in the throes of nostalgia as he anticipates a return to the beloved Yalta of his childhood. It is eight hours since the boat departed from Odessa; the coastline of the Crimea has come into view. He is studying it closely—the craggy mountains, the ravines, the caverns into which the sea washes, then retreats. Hours later, looking for diversion from the monotony of the all-but-deserted upper deck, he descends a flight of stairs to the lower level where, it seems, all Russia is in route to Yalta—soldiers on leave, women and children, shopkeepers, construction workers, English tourists, dogs, even. The prevailing ethnic group is Tatar. These men sit cross-legged on the floor of the deck, some eating, some passing a bottle, now and then breaking into song. There are roars of laughter, the gasps of an accordion. A couple is dancing flamenco to bursts of applause. In view of it all, the captain of the steamer stands between two great paddle-wheels, surveying his kingdom.

Stefan's curiosity having been satisfied, he returned to the upper deck where he was again alone save for a young woman at the railing. She was well-dressed and wore a sable cape and green-and-white silk scarf. Under one arm she carried a small white dog. How beautiful she is, he thought, and took a chair on the same side of the boat, not far away. From the very first moment, he could not take his eyes from her, the way she gazed dreamily out over the water, the fur of her cape stirring in the breeze. Now and then, she murmured to the little dog. Only once and only for a moment, she turned her head and gave a quick glance in his direction. For some time, he contented himself with watching her through his pince-nez from behind a newspaper. When an hour had passed without so much as the least acknowledgment of his presence, he thought, all right, he would count on his untried silent strength. The months of his convalescence had left him suddenly famished for femininity. Rising, he went to stand near her at the railing. He was acutely aware of the mass of her honey-colored hair and her delicate features—lightly tanned skin, gray eyes, full lips, long eyelashes and a small, slightly aquiline nose.

"Does she bite?" he asked, nodding at the dog.

"She is a he. And *yes.* He can be jealous."

"May I hold him?"

"At your own risk," and she smiled. As she gave him the dog, it began snapping high-pitched chunks out of the silent air.

"A little Cerberus, is he, only minus the other two heads." When she touched it on the nose in gentle reproach, he saw the green jade ring on the fourth finger of her left hand. So, she is married.

"I am Stefan, and you?"

"You may call me Nina." Adding as an afterthought, "My husband's name is Andre Demiroff."

"Ninotchka! It suits you, somehow." What was she thinking? He died to know. Not that he had the slightest feeling of warmth toward her, he assured himself, only a powerful curiosity. At age forty, he has had no more feelings toward any woman than toward a weathered plank. But within minutes, he felt himself drawn to this one. In answer to her question, he told her of his recent discharge from the army, that he had been wounded. She told him that it was her first visit to Yalta.

"Bravo! You cannot die without having seen Yalta." She gave a small shrug at his obvious pride of place. "Please don't . . . die, that is." All at once, a breeze sent her scarf fluttering across his face. She reached up with one hand to brush it away. He thought he had never seen so graceful a gesture. In making it, she seemed to be declaring herself to him.

"Tell me about it, your Yalta."

"There was an ancient lighthouse at the mouth of the bay. You will see it before long. The waters there are notoriously violent; the sea there really is black. Along the coast, right up to the town itself, are caves carved out the dark water. These are the same ones seen by Orestes when he journeyed here to rescue his sister Iphigenia in the ancient Greek myth. As for the town itself, two small rivers descend through it from the mountains, fertilizing the gardens of the Tatars, offering their limpid tribute before flowing into the bay. All around the town there are fields of buckwheat and tobacco, and herds of sheep. Everywhere there is the odor of carnations, lilies and hyacinths. Fruit and grains are drying alongside each house. The families live mostly on verandahs rather than indoors. In the evening, they call out to their neighbors. The glory of Yalta is its great mosque with an elegant bell tower and an Oriental dome flanked by four minarets."

"I want to hear about Orestes' visit to the Crimea."

"My pleasure. Iphigenia was the younger daughter of the Greek general Agamemnon. In order to achieve victory at Troy, she was to be sacrificed to the gods. At the last minute, she was snatched from the altar by the Goddess Artemis who substituted a fawn, then brought Iphigenia here to the Crimea, then called her Tauris. It was the outer limit of the then-known world. Here she was made a priestess in the cult of Artemis, the Goddess of Fertility and Childbirth. Now when Orestes arrived, he had no idea his sister was still alive, nor did she know of his existence. Theirs was a joyous reunion. Later, they escaped from the brutal Taurians and returned to Attica—a happy ending. Euripides wrote it as a drama—*Iphigenia in Tauris*."

All through the telling of the tale, her gaze never left his face. He felt acutely the intensity of her interest. The afternoon had been warm and placid but at sunset a great red band appeared on the horizon warning of a storm. When night fell, waves washed over the lower decks. The two strangers were not among the seasick.

Night had long since settled over the Black Sea. Where had the afternoon gone? She fell silent, and stood gazing out at the sea.

"Just see how the moonlight lies upon the water," she said.

"An aqualune, it is called: a good omen." All at once, the woman Nina became aware of the lateness of the hour.

"Good Heavens! It is so late, and I am tired. I will go to my cabin. But where will you sleep?"

"Right here, on deck, in this very chair. It will suit me fine."

"But it will not suit me," she answered. "You must come to share my cabin. There is an extra cot."

"Never mind. Remember I am part Tatar, and as a soldier, I am used to such small privations."

"Please, I would like the pleasure of your company. Out here it will be cold, and it has begun to rain." Taking him by the hand, she exerted a gentle but sustained pull. Stefan rose to his feet.

"All right. But you should know that I am already half in love with you."

"Only half?" She dismissed the word "love" with a wave of her hand. "Then am I to be spurned?" Now they were together in the small cabin. For a long moment they were silent. At last she spoke. "Would you show me your wound?" All at once he was deafened by the clapper of his heart.

"But why? Surely you will be offended."

"No, I want to see what you have endured. Does it still show? A wound is the truest measure of a man. A wound does not lie."

"Once again we are in Homer's *Odyssey*."

"How is it like Homer?"

"You have read it?"

"Long ago."

"Toward the end, you may recall, after twenty years of wandering, Ulysses is washed up on the shores of his own kingdom, Ithaca. But he is such a state of dishevelment, and dressed in rags, that he is unrecognized by his wife Penelope or by his son or by anyone else. He is outraged by the presence of his wife's suitors who have taken over the palace and are conducting orgies and revelry. But he is wily and elects to continue his masquerade until the right moment. Penelope tells the old nurse Eurycleia to bathe the stranger and give him fresh clothing. Now it happens that forty years before, when Ulysses was a boy of ten, he was taken on a hunt and had been gored in the thigh by a wild boar. For a long time, it was feared that the boy would die. It was this same nurse, Eurycleia, who tended the wound, pressing out the poisons, applying unguents and herbs until at last new buds of granulation tissue sprang up; new skin raced across and the wound was healed. Now so many years later, Eurycleia, in the course of bathing him, runs her fingers over the stranger's thigh, she feels the wound and knows at once that he is her master, Ulysses. It was not his wife or son who recognized him. It was the wound that announced his presence to the one who had tended it. You, Ninotchka, are like Eurycleia, the nurse in Homer, with one great difference; you are young and beautiful."

"And you are like Homer, a weaver of tales. I am already under your spell. Now, I beg you to show me your wound." All at once, the cabin that had seemed so amicable was full of secrets. Theirs, and the secrets of all those who had occupied it before them.

"Please," she said again. The moonlight was inexorable.

"If you wish it." His mouth was a funnel of dry leather. She was seated on the side of the bed. He went to stand in front of her. Slowly he untied the sash that secured his blouse. It was with no little agitation that he fumbled with the buttons of his blouse. His fingers were stiff and trembling. His hands seemed three sizes too large. He tried to shake them down to normal size as if he were shaking off drops of water. At last, he stood naked to the waist. His white skin gleamed in the moonlight pouring through the oval port-hole. A still-livid scar extended from his right rib cage across the abdomen to disappear beneath his trousers on the left. She ran her fingers lightly over the exposed scar. She could not know that beneath her touch he felt the stirring of something new, an awakening of the long dormant flesh. At that moment, he felt that life was exceeding his capacity to live it. In the silence that followed, he lowered his gaze to his own clenched fingers.

"What is it?" she asked.

"It is usual with me," he replied, "at the very height of pleasure I am melancholy. It is quite absurd."

What she drew down and pressed to her was less a man than a column of fire.

"I have waited too long for you," he said. "I will burn you up." When he lowered his mouth, she was ready for it—the way she took the whole of him upon her tongue! With the joy of discovery, he yielded up his body as he had never done before and let her take hold of him however she pleased. He felt utterly free in her grasp. And she, for her part, engulfed him without hesitation, as if the body she played with was her own.

It is the next morning. The deck steward has just announced that there is to be an overnight stop in the town of Balaclava to make repairs.

"Ah, Balaclava!" he murmured.

"Do you know that place?"

"As a child, I was taken there on vacation. It is very dear to me." While eating breakfast, he told her of a dacha in the woods.

"It is no more than twenty minute ride from the jetty. Will you come there with me?" When she hesitated, he adjusted his pince-nez in her direction. "It is beautifully remote."

"Balaclava, then," she said under her breath. "So that is where I am to go." And she thought, to Tauris, at the behest of the goddess.

At the foot of the gangplank stood a horse-drawn droshky, waiting. Once inside the cab, he could not suppress a quiet laughter. "Why do you laugh?" she wanted to know.

"Because I am happier now than I have been in a long time."

"All right, then, tell me your secret."

"I don't have one."

"I don't believe that for a minute."

"Oh, all right, I wish I had been born a small dog instead of a large person."

"That's your secret? You would prefer to have been a dog?" Her laughter was derisive.

"Why not? A dog is all love; a dog does not fear death; a dog can be carried on the arm of a beautiful woman." When she made no reply, he went on. "All right, tell me what made you say yes when I asked you to come with me to the dacha."

"Oh, intuition, I suppose. Instinct. I can't put it into words without sounding foolish or superstitious. I've learned to answer to these small . . . influences, I guess you'd call them. They tell me what to do, where I should go and with whom. Do you believe in Destiny? I do."

"I could see that in your eyes, the way they swallow one up." He glanced out at the rooftops that climbed so steeply. In the bay, the ships' funnels and masts swayed gently. On one side of the pier, a man carried a pole with a small flame at top with which he was lighting gas lamps. Balaclava consisted of a single road with a number of side streets. These were narrow and uneven. A raised trottoir lay on either side of the main road for the convenience of pedestrians. A clear rivulet ran through the town. At a stone fountain women were washing laundry.

"The trouble with living in St. Petersburg," she said, "is that there is no fountain in the center where women might gather to draw water, wash clothes, gossip and console one another. Women need a fountain."

"Oh, and what do men need?"

"You are better made to speak of that."

"A man needs a bench to straddle, a ball to pitch and catch, something to drink, a pipe of tobacco, another man to brag to."

The houses were low and windowless, but each had its wide verandah where men were smoking hookahs. Nearby each house, a tethered dromedary grazed. Within minutes, they had passed through the town. At the far end of the road, there was an ancient cemetery, the stones tilted every which way in the slow upheaval of resurrection. The path through the forest was wide enough for only a single carriage. So narrow, it seemed to have been torn open by lightning. She wondered what one did if a second carriage were coming in the opposite direction. But the occasion did not arise. Soon enough, the dacha presented itself in the center of a cobbled courtyard. Lightly timbered, airy and floating among its verandahs and many balconies, it was a secretive, secluded place all but enclosed in old cypress and eucalyptus trees. From the moment she stepped down from the carriage, she had the feeling that the place was not of this world but of another where the rules by which she had lived all her life no longer pertained. The room to which they were conducted enhanced this feeling. The innkeeper, a bearded, turbaned Muslim, saluted them in the manner of the Crimea—right hand on his heart, then raised to his lips, head slightly inclined, then led them up a flight of stairs to a large room with a balcony that looked down on the courtyard. In a corner of the room a low round table was surrounded by cushions. It was covered with a profusion of meats, cakes, wine and coffee. The walls and ceiling were of wood paneling. Carpets of brilliant colors covered the floor. Along one side stood a broad low couch. There was a small chimney in the form of a niche in the wall. On another table, a samovar bubbled and steamed. The whole effect was Asiatic. Just before leaving between portieres, the innkeeper lit a scented mosquito coil. The smoke from the coil curled upward. It was more a den than a room, a den in which animals mated and procreated in privacy. Nina knew at once that she had arrived here in accordance with a will other than her own, that here and nowhere else had she been given permission to take hold of her destiny.

"Well, what do you think?"

"It was fated to be," she murmured.

"What do you mean?" But she would say no more about it.

"Come, kiss me," she said instead. For Stefan, she was the embodiment of a desire that had eluded him until now. He felt himself drawn to her lips as to the impossible extreme of experience. It was as if a film that had clouded his eyes had been torn away, and he could see clearly for the first time. For both of them, the night had taken on an unearthly, hallucinatory quality. Was it really happening? When the flame in the lamp on the table burnt out with a sigh, he knew it was real.

In the silence that followed, he glanced up. Her lips were pursed as if she would whistle, her head was bowed, and there were tears in her eyes. It was the portrait of someone trying to stifle pain.

"What?" he asked. He could not connect this woman of sorrow with the one who, only moments before, he had held in his arms. He felt a wave of sympathy for her.

"Listen," he told her, "there is a certain moth that sleeps all day and then flies about after dark until it comes upon someone lying asleep. Whereupon the moth alights on the sleeper's eyelids, inserts its tiny proboscis between the lids and drinks the tears which are its main source of nourishment. Here is a creature that thrives on sorrow. In a better world, suspended alongside every bed, there would be a small wooden cage with a tiny gate. Just before retiring for the night, you would reach up to open the gate, inviting the *consolatrix afflictorum* to emerge. Once you are asleep, out she will come to occupy her benevolent perch upon your eyelids. Hours later, you will awaken, stretch and brush the wingdust from your cheek, then rise to face the new day, unburdened of sorrow."

In the middle of the story, he had removed the pince-nez from his nose, letting it hang from its ribbon. To her, he seemed extraordinarily beautiful at that moment. His voice seemed to come from a great distance. There was an echo in the way he pronounced the words, as though he were translating as he spoke. She was sitting on the bed, looking up at him.

"Would you like to undress me?" The question seemed to him unimaginably obscene, and therefore irresistible. He had an apprehension of her moans of pleasure, of her face at the moment of climax. He understood that this was precisely what was being offered.

"You smell like a Crimean garden." He grasped her hair in his fist. Moments later, deep, deep into her he poured the sweet hot stuff of life, as if obeying her command.

"Tell me what it was that first attracted you." He needed her to say it.

"It is vain of you to beg for praise. Perhaps you will not be pleased when I tell you."

"I'll risk it."

"It was the way the cape hung limply from your shoulders, like desolation itself. And the way you shivered once or twice, not from cold, it seemed, but from something internal that lashed you bone by bone. And oh yes, the pince-nez. I have always had a weakness for a man who wore pince-nez. There, I told you. Are your feelings hurt?"

"I know that I am hardly any young woman's dream of romance."

"The truth? I was just trying to keep from becoming seasick."

"Well, tell me then, at what moment you knew that I was there on the deck watching you."

"Oh, I had noticed you long before you had the nerve to approach me. There was just something about you—a *je ne sais quoi*, as they say. Then, from the moment you spoke, 'What a pretty little dog,' you said, 'does she bite?' From that moment, it was as though we had known each other in a former life, as though what was happening was not for the first time but a coming together after a long separation. I'm afraid you will think me utterly silly. Oh listen! Do you hear it? The sea? It has followed us to this room."

"No, I don't. It is your imagination."

"I hear it rushing in and out of those black caves that frightened Orestes when he first saw them." And as he drifted off to sleep, it seemed to him that the sea, the steamboat, the inn and the whole of the Crimea had blended into a state of intense happiness.

"I love you," he murmured.

"Oh love!" she laughed, dismissing the word with a shrug. Suddenly she bit him on the shoulder, hard enough to make him moan. He sat up and gripped the place where her teeth had left their mark. "That will teach you to speak of love."

Hours later, toward dawn, lying spent in her lover's arms and with the reek of passion in her nostrils, she thought that she would not survive it—the conflagration that had swept through her again and again. She must surely die of it. Even now, the echo of it made her tremble. She shuddered as though far below all of her remaining strength to lie still, to keep from transmitting to Stefan the volcanic eruption, the premonition that she was at last with child. Poor man, she thought, when all he wants is for me to say a word as simple as "love." I have had enough of it, she thought. I need no more; I want no more. Ecstasy was not happiness; it was not from physical bliss that she could reach fulfillment. All at once, she thought of Andres, the husband whom she loved. Oh yes, she loved him, but the need for a child was the greater destiny that propelled her. She could not go on living without that.

Nina lay awake with the weight of the sleeping man upon her. Suddenly the room became unbearable. She could not breathe in it. Gasping, she eased her body from under him, rose, dressed quickly and stepped out onto the balcony. Minute by minute, she felt the ebbing of her passion for Stefan. In its place, there was a new sense of satiation. Until now, she had been ready to die, but no longer. For the first time, she was hungry for life.

Dawn broke, and with it came the far-off whistle of the steamboat announcing the hour of departure. From the balcony, she could see the moonlight glistening on the smooth haunches of the horse that stood motionless save for the automatic swishing of its tail. Again, the hooter sounded. All at once, she was a woman in whom purpose took the place of grace. She stepped to the bed and shook him gently at first, then insistently. And he sleeps on, she thought; I am but a shadow playing across his body.

Again, she pressed his shoulder. "We must hurry. The boat whistle has sounded. We have one hour to go aboard. Come, get dressed." When he sank back upon the bed and made as if to draw her down to him, she slid one arm beneath him and with all her strength pulled him to a sitting position. "Here! I'll help you to dress." She drew down the coverlet and tried to put his arms into the sleeves of his blouse. Soon enough, he was fully awake and finished dressing. "Quickly! The carriage is waiting in the courtyard."

Minutes later, in the carriage, he spread a lap rug over her knees. The little dog nestled in its deep folds between them as though protecting its mistress from him. For long minutes, they rode in silence.

"What are those gunshots?"

"They are hunting thrushes. The little birds fly down here to escape the winter, only to meet those hunters. Nina . . ." He reached for her hand.

"No, please." She withdrew from his touch.

"But . . . last night . . ."

"It was a shadow making love to a shadow. Look Stefan, it is over. I am a different woman from the one who made love to you."

"You look the same to me, just as beautiful, just as desirable. When can I come to see you at Yalta or in St. Petersburg?"

"Never."

"But what have I done? I cannot live without the hope of seeing you again. What in God's name is it that has caused you to . . . dismiss me?"

"My poor Stefan! It is nothing you have done. It's just time to go on living as before. Only for you, I hope there will be a treasured memory to be summoned up for the relishment of your soul. Isn't that enough for you?

Stefan, my Stefan, I may as well tell you that this entire experience has caught me by surprise, at a time when I was not quite myself."

"What do you mean?"

"From the moment I stepped on board that steamboat, I felt that I had entered a strange, unfamiliar land. I had only to wait for it to cast its spell over me. I had no idea that in that land, I would have so immense a pleasure, only that I was free to say 'yes' to everything. It was a land of affirmation. Ever since you told me the story of Iphigenia and Orestes, I have dreamt that the land I entered is Tauris, the ancient Crimea. But all that is over, and it is time to return to our former lives. I am myself again. I am sane."

They were now at the jetty where the steamboat waited.

"Let us part here," she said. "It is for the best."

"But Nina, how am I to remember the time? I want never to forget it."

"I don't agree that permanence has to do with memory. It has more to do with material objects such as are dug up from the ground after centuries, or cups that have been kept in a cupboard by a grandmother for a hundred years."

"No, we are what we remember. There is nothing else. Forgetting is a kind of death. I love you. I will always love you."

"For me, 'love,' as you insist on calling it, is not the foremost need of life. Other things take precedence over it."

"Such as?"

"Hunger, thirst . . . the desire for a child."

"Ah, I begin to see . . ." Stefan reached inside his blouse and removed a gold chain and medallion.

"I want you to have this. Perhaps it will bring about your heart's desire." She studied the medallion which was an ancient coin embossed with the face of a woman. "It is Artemis," he said. "The Goddess of Fertility." Visibly touched, she held the coin to her heart.

Moments later, she had climbed aboard and he lost sight of her. For the duration of the voyage, Stefan remained on the upper deck where he had first encountered her. He had not the courage for another confrontation. It was the hour of arrival at Yalta. A cold rain was falling; the wind was high and the sea turned black and rough. The steamboat lurched toward the jetty, but it soon became clear that it could not dock. In the end, the boat anchored far from shore. They would have to delay landing. Hours later, the rain let up and the wind died down. They would need dinghies, the customs boat to ferry the passengers. Not until the boat had slipped up to the jetty did he dare to stand at the railing. The sailors were putting her to with ropes. He watched Nina waving to an elderly man standing on the pier. He was the epitome of elegance—trim beard, frock coat with velvet lapels, a gold-headed cane in one hand and a bouquet of carnations in the other. He watched as the elderly man took her about the waist, handed her the flowers and led her to a waiting carriage. He was taking possession of his wife. Would she turn around to look at him? No, she would not. Already the carriage was moving away. Stefan suddenly felt the urge to wash his body of her scent, to clean it of the lingering touch of her fingers. There was a bath-house on the edge of the pier. Once inside, he undressed and was directed by the attendant to a bench. On the neighboring bench lay a man with an enormous belly bearing a recent surgical scar. Water streamed from the man's shoulders; steam hung over his head. The attendant, wearing only a loose short robe of toweling, approached with a basin of hot water. A moment later, Stefan, too, was dripping.

Stefan went on to Yalta to assume his post as District Doctor. For five years, he led a circumscribed life. In the morning, he saw patients in his clinic. In the afternoon, he inspected the facilities for control of infectious diseases—cholera, tuberculosis, malaria and the rest. Each evening, on his way home, he stopped in the same bistro for his supper, most often, a bowl of cabbage soup or borscht with boiled beef and potatoes. All this time, he never stopped longing for Nina, nor did he have any romantic affairs or attachments of any sort, as though he were respecting a marriage vow. Then one evening, he stopped at a kiosk to read the front page of a newspaper. There, bordered in black, was the photograph of the man who had met Nina on the jetty, her husband. Reading on, Stefan learned that the man had been a prince in the government of the Tsar, that after serving in a number of foreign embassies, he served as governor of several provinces of the Caucasus. He had recently been named as ambassador to Norway, to which country he had been preparing to depart until his untimely death. The newspaper added that he was survived by his wife and a young son.

A son, thought Stefan!

Three days later, he was on the train from Odessa to St. Petersburg. Once ensconced in a hotel, Stefan set out upon his search. All the first day, he walked the streets of the section of the city used for official residences. Hour after hour he walked on the Nevsky Prospekt, then along Great Morskoy Street and Kovensky Lane. In the afternoon, the fever was upon him. On and on he searched in a blazing delirium. A thick white mist rose from the surface of the Neva. His feet were lost to view beneath the swirl. He felt like a man who has died and is wandering in the hereafter. His black cape hung from his shoulders like a limp flag. At last he stood before a mansion entitled Norwegian Embassy. With his breathing labored and his pulse beating wildly, he climbed the steps and knocked on the door. A liveried servant informed him that the ambassador's wife was in mourning and could not be disturbed. He had only just begun to walk away when, glancing up at the elegant facade of the building, he caught sight of a curtain dropping into place. Someone had pulled it aside. He was being watched! Moments later, she was there beside him. The streetlamp glistened on the rich plumage of her hair that was piled high like that of a woman wading into the sea. She moved easily with the old grace. She had not aged, as he had. Although a mere ten years older than she, from outward appearances it might have been twenty. His hair was generously flecked with white. His complexion was sallow, only heightened to a false ruddiness, she thought, by a fever. Creases furrowed his once-smooth cheeks. At that moment, Stefan felt his own existence lapse. He was a non-being, a spectre who could not come alive to take part in this longed-for, dreamed about reunion. At last, with the residue of life left in him, he spoke in a barely audible voice.

"I had to come, Nina. I could not keep myself away. I pray that you do not take either alarm or offense." Smiling, she took his arm and conducted him down the street.

"Quite the opposite," she said in a voice that stirred him to the very depths. "It is good that you have come. You have grown thinner. Have you been ill?"

"It's nothing." He waved aside the question. "A quartan fever that comes back every once in awhile." In addition to her beauty that had remained intact, she shed a warmth he had not remembered. It was entirely different from the unrestrained passion she had surrendered to in Balaclava. This new warmth was on a gentler stripe; it was familial. From the moment she had taken his arm, she had passed right over the wounded man whose body she had to make use of, and lit upon him as the father of her child. In the five years that had passed, he had become for Nina an abstract force, of nothingness composed, certainly not a creature of the same element as she. But, abstraction or not, he had for one brief night in Balaclava solidified into a flaming arrow that had sought out its mark and touched her to life. This she would never forget. Even so, years later she had only to close her eyes to see the Asiatic town with its two-humped dromedaries, its veiled women in pantaloons washing clothes at the fountain, the small domed mosque with its four minarets. There too, as if painted on the inside of her eyelids, was the path through the forest that was no more than the dry bed of a mountain stream. Until this moment, it was as if she had dreamed the whole experience in answer to her great need.

What she felt she must tell him now—truth—whether he believed her or not, that she had never been unfaithful to her husband either before or since. He, Stefan Volkov, had been the only one. She owed it to him to tell him that. Unbeknownst to her, he too had remained celibate, keeping faith, as if to a marriage vow.

"Nina," his voice trembled. "For months I wrestled with the desire to go find you, first at Yalta, then here at St. Petersburg."

"But you did not, for which I thank you with all my heart."

"No, I did not, but all the while, I had the feeling that I was a coward fleeing from a field of battle. *Ya bezhal ot silnykh osh chuschenii.* I needed to blot you out of my mind or die of it. Throughout those many days and nights, I fought against my longing for you, a longing that has never left me."

"Yes, yes, I understand. Stefan, do you hate me? I think you must. I wouldn't blame you."

"Hate you? On the contrary, I am still in love with you."

"Stefan, have you never thought to marry?"

"Why do you ask?"

"I so much want you to be happy. There is a bond between us that cannot be severed. Aren't you lonely?"

"Not at all. I live on the edge of a dense wood. Inside, the mice keep me company. Out doors, there are nightingales and frogs."

"Then you are impervious to love? You have barricaded your heart?"

"Not at all. I have loved you. I love our son."

"You must know that five years ago in Balaclava I was fighting for my life. I did the only thing I could do." He remained silent. She held up her wrist from which dangled the medallion of the Goddess Artemis. "There is Sergei, the boy. How very much he resembles you, with his slanted sea-colored Tatar eyes and cleft chin."

"Sergei, a beautiful name." He stood very still, his arms at his sides, the jacket now too large for his frame, accentuating the recent loss of weight. He gazed deep into her eyes and saw the sorrow come out of the center of her smile. "You need one of those moths who drink the tears of sorrow." All at once, there was the voice of a child, calling out to his mother.

"Come! Come and see!" The little boy broke away from the hand of his nurse and ran to where they were walking. Stefan saw at once the resemblance to himself—the tilt and color of his eyes. In his excitement, Sergei took, not his mother's hand, but that of the strange man. She watched him go with the boy into the park. Once inside the park gate, Stefan and Nina seated themselves on a bench.

"You may go and play, Sergei," she said. But the boy came to stand between the knees of the man, who closed them about him in a gentle imprisonment. "He has taken a fancy to you. He is never so familiar with strangers."

"It is blood calling unto blood."

"He is not yet aware that his father . . . my husband . . . will not come back to him."

"No, Nina, he knows." The mother's helper came to retrieve her charge. Now Stefan and Nina are alone.

"I must tell you the truth," he began, his voice hardly more than a whispered exhalation. She bent closer and heard the tremor in his voice that could not be quieted. She saw his lips move like those of a man at prayer. "I am sicker than I led you to believe. My chest. There is no possibility of cure, only further wasting. Tomorrow, I shall be leaving, never to return. Nor must you come to Yalta for my sake." When she raised her hand in protest, he went on. "Really, it is the best way. The child has only just lost one father. To inflict upon him another dying man would be quite a legacy of grief. Such a multiplication of sorrow can be damaging. A child can die of it. I know whereof I speak. In the short time we have been together, I have seen how he sighs, how his head droops, how he tries to hide his grief from you. We cannot give him another grave to weep over." Stefan rose to his feet. "I will go to see him for the last time. Stay here, please. But first, can you tell me what has happened to the little dog that brought us together long ago?"

"The dog? Oh, it died."

"I'm sorry. When?"

"Four or five years ago. They don't live very long, you know. That breed."

"No," said Stefan, "we don't." He stood to leave. I'll say goodbye now . . . Ninotchka, don't feel that you have to love me. I have the certainty of that in my dreams. I don't need to see you to feel your presence. Always, at the hour of remembrance, there is the after-hum of your voice and the fire of your eyes. Before you, I was asleep, not yet awakened until you came and tore me from the dark." She too had risen to her feet, but when she tried to take a step toward him, she could not. It was as though there were an invisible barrier that she could not cross. She stood immobile, her eyes streaming.

"Stefan . . . Stefan . . ." was all she could manage.

"Don't weep for me, Nina. I have done no more than fall ill, as one must at last. I do not fear to die. What else could I do, if I am so in love with you? And just think . . ." His voice grew light, bantering. "Perhaps one day you will accept an apparition? I shall always be ready to rise to the occasion. You have only to beckon, and I shall appear."

Then he was gone. Just then, since she herself could not, a gull over the Neva shrieked. But it could not carry away from her the anguish of this parting. It had begun to rain. She continued to stand on the bank of the river, now a sheet of luminosity. What had he called it? An aqualune, she remembered and had to smile in spite of herself. Now the rain had intensified so that she could no longer hear the shrieking of the gull; it had dissolved in the torrent.

Years later, a bit of Schubert in the concert hall would leave her unable to breathe.

EPILOGUE

Were I to choose the one writer I revere above all others, it would be Anton Chekhov. It is impossible not to love the man for his grace and good will. Of his many stories, my favorite is "The Lady with the Small Dog." In it Chekhov characterizes his hero Dmitri Gurov thusly: "Everything in which he was sincere and did not deceive himself, everything that made the kernel of his life, was hidden from other people." In only three ways do I resemble Chekhov: I too am a medical doctor, I too am a writer, and I too feel that my defects and tribulations are no one's business. They are to be borne bravely and in privacy.

It is a cruel irony that in the same year that he completed his medical studies, Chekhov first spit up blood. From that moment, the young doctor must have known that his life would not be a long one. Still, he never once referred to his illness by its name, nor expressed the least pessimism. About his less serious ailments, his hemorrhoids, for one, he did not shrink to tell anyone who would listen.

My affection for Chekhov is not new. The entry in my diary of spring 1990 includes these paragraphs:

> Sometimes, in the prime of my senility, I entertain a fantasy. Dare I confess it? In a Reading Room at Yale's Sterling Library, there is a large globe of the world on a stand. One day I gave it a spin, then braked it with my hand when the Crimea came into view. I located the city of Taganrog on the Sea of Azov where Chekhov was born. I found too the city of Odessa where my father was born. The distance between was an overnight steamboat ride. Next I looked for Yalta where Chekhov, for health reasons, spent so much of his later life. It is but another overnight boat ride from Odessa to Yalta. O let me imagine it!
>
> A man and a woman, previously unknown to one another, stand side by side on the deck of a steamboat departing from Odessa to Yalta. He is a Chekhov, she a Selzer, or whatever we were called over there and back then. Before long, a certain glance would have been exchanged, words spoken. He would have petted the small dog she was holding. She would have gazed down at the strong, well-groomed hand that stroked the dog; perhaps she would have flushed and smiled, ostensibly out of love for her pet. All at once, it is announced that there will be an overnight stop at Balaclava to make repairs. At Balaclava, the two disembark arm in arm. At the waterfront hotel, the woman waits on the verandah while he arranges for a room. Later, between passionate kisses, she whispers,
>
> "What name did you use?"
>
> "Gurov. Dmitri Gurov. Do you like it?"
>
> "For me," she replies, "he is the hero of a romantic novel." The man called Gurov shakes his head and smiles sadly.
>
> "No," he tells her, "not a novel, only a short story."
>
> The reader of Chekhov will recognize the name, Dmitri Gurov, as the character in his story "The Lady with the Small Dog," as well as the steamboat

> and its destination. I offer up my story as an act of homage to the Master. I must rely upon the fame of his story to dissuade the reader from considering mine an act of literary pilferage. In my story, I have given Stefan Volkov the persona of Chekhov as well as his tragic fate. In so doing, I have tried to cement my spiritual kinship with Chekhov as both physician and writer. It is not unlike the kinship felt by Jorge Borges, the blind seer and poet, for Homer, that other blind seer and poet. Edmund Spenser, too, author of *The Faerie Queene*, on more than one occasion hinted that the soul of Chaucer had been transposed into his body, and that he, Spenser, was begotten over one hundred and fifty years after the death of the earlier poet. By insinuating lineal descent from Chekhov, I do no more than perpetuate the vanity. Whether I am at all worthy to harbor these thoughts is not for me to say; only that I have them, and they give my life a larger dimension.

But let me not digress further. It is up to me, the author, to tell what happens next in the story. Let's see . . . where was I? You will recall that at Yalta, Stefan watches from the upper deck as Nina descends the ramp, still carrying the little dog. On the wharf, an elderly man in a top hat and carrying a gold-headed cane is waiting for her. Nine months later, she is delivers a boy with gray eyes and high cheekbones.

"A little Russian!" exclaims the delighted father, "we'll call him Sergei." With those who would deplore Nina's deception of her elderly husband, I do not agree. Speaking both biologically and theologically, a father "begets" a child, calls it forth out of the darkness, as it were. A man is the instrument that a woman uses to create a child. Almost at once, it became clear, to her sorrow, that Nina could not produce enough milk to feed the baby—she, who had wanted so much to become a mother. A young wet-nurse, Masha, was brought into the household for that purpose. Years later, Nina would remember the day she arrived. Masha had just finished feeding Sergei, and had brought him to his mother to hold.

"What a little Tatar he is!" said Masha. "Just look at those big cheeks. All of his face has gone into the making of them. He has a powerful suck. It almost hurts!" And she brought her hands to her breasts.

And then what happens, you want to know. Five years have gone by since Nina's husband Andre died. Stefan, himself mortally ill, had traveled to St. Petersburg to see her. To tell the truth, at this point, I was torn. I had fallen in love with both Nina and Stefan and could not bear to have them part forever, he to his long dying, and she to her widowhood. I should have much preferred them to stay together with their little boy. But no, by this time I was addicted to their anguish. Sorrow may be the only thing in the world one really possesses. Perhaps it would be best to let another six years go by. Stefan's health had continued to fail and he has just died. When news of his death reaches Nina in St. Petersburg, she takes Sergei, now a boy of twelve, to visit his grave in the cemetery at the edge of the forest in Balaclava. It is there that she hears the boy speaking aloud as if to the man buried there.

"I am going to be a doctor, too."

And so it happens that Sergei's ambition is fulfilled; he becomes a doctor. Later, he immigrates to America and settles in the Hudson River town of Troy, midway between Montreal and New York City. In time, Nina goes there to live out her life with her son. From the city of Troy, she would recall how Stefan's eyes had paused, wary as a cat, when he saw her wedding band, how his face grew still, how when he lifted his eyes, she knew not to look into them. One could drown in such a hazel gaze. What she was left with to the end of her days was the scent of carnations, the caves of Orestes that broke up the low shore, and the sound of a balalaika being plucked in another part of the dacha.

And now, another fifty years have passed. Sometimes in a room I call the scriptorium, I close my eyes and imagine my ancestor there with me. I kiss his hands, his eyes, and I stroke the cough from his thin, wracked body as though I were smoothing out a wrinkle in cloth.

Part VII

Diary Entries

When Yale University Press published his *Diary* in 2011, Richard Selzer noted in a preface that, other than the ledger of a business, a diary is the only sort of book that is said to be *kept*: "The word implies faithfulness to the task and preserving at least the appearance of privacy. (The 'keep' is the deepest part of the castle, where its treasures are held at time of siege.) To keep a diary is to tend and marshal thoughts that might wander away the way sheep would were it not for the shepherd who keeps them."[1]

Among the thoughts shepherded in Selzer's *Diary* are personal vignettes, salient memories, philosophical meditations, reflections on literature and art (including the practice of medicine as an art), and fresh expressions of love for the natural world, for cooking, and especially for family. All of those points of focus are evident in the new entries gathered here, but with added concerns about the vicissitudes of age, and about the home in New Haven where his family lived for forty-eight years. Selzer paid tribute to that large house in "St. Ronan Terrace," an essay in his 2004 collection *The Whistlers' Room* (Shoemaker & Hoard). For a good while, Janet Selzer ran the house as a bed and breakfast, but she and Richard eventually came to realize, reluctantly, that they would need to move. The only entry here from 2013 announces their final decision.

Selzer confronts the essential paradox of publishing a diary, acknowledging that "the appearance of privacy" is a literary convention, and that, as a writer, he remains fully conscious of an audience. This means, Selzer says, that "I make use of art and artifice, including metaphor, symbol, allusion, onomatopoeia, irony, and all the 'airy medium of words' that make up the storyteller's instrument." It also means that he maintains a freedom to invent—or at least to embellish—in order to go beyond the facts and arrive at "the real real." As the epigraph for his Yale *Diary*, Selzer chose one of his favorite lines from Emily Dickinson: "Tell all the truth but tell it slant."[2]

None of the following material has been previously published. After an "Undated" section, roughly spanning 1985 to 2008, the entries are arranged by year, but with loose chronology within each section. In this regard, the editing follows Selzer's own practice, as explained in his *Diary* preface: "I have preferred not to insist on exact dates, but to give only years . . . and sometimes even to reverse the calendar and let the past run up to me like an obedient dog."[3]

NOTES

1. Richard Selzer, *Diary* (New Haven, CT: Yale University Press, 2011), xii.
2. Ibid., xii–xiii.
3. Selzer has occasionally published installments not included in the Yale collection, such as "Diaries: 1986–1994" in *Quinnipiac/Schweitzer Journal* 1, no. 2 (Fall/Winter 1994–95), 1–16. Three other diary sections are part of *The Whistlers' Room: Stories and Essays* (Washington, DC: Shoemaker & Hoard, 2004), 86–103, 150–85, and 193–203.

Early Entries, Undated

Friends deplore my "daily grind" at the writing desk. "Why not live a little?" they ask. But I *am* living and nowhere else so fully as here. Let others play golf, have love affairs, take cooking lessons. They will all know where to find me.

*

It is now forty-seven years since I was an intern. While much of that year has slipped into the mist of unremembered antiquity, one incident remains sharply etched. The Chief of Medicine was making rounds on my ward. There was the usual retinue of fellows, house staff and students, straining to catch every word the great man said. The Chief *was* a great man who had made any number of important contributions in the field of cardiovascular disease. As we moved from bed to bed, he listened to my brief outline of the patient's condition, and then began his commentary. A hush fell over the ward, as other patients and nurses were caught up in the occasion.

In the bed next to the one upon which we were focused lay an elderly woman with metastatic breast cancer. She was beyond any known therapy of the time. She began to speak—not words, but sounds that were unintelligible to me. The Chief bent over her, and placed his ear next to her lips. Then reaching into her mouth, he gently removed her dentures and placed them in a cup on her nightstand. She smiled as he rejoined the rounds. She had asked him to remove her teeth. At the time, I marveled at the special qualities of the man that enabled him to have this unique sensitivity. It was the same sensitivity that enabled him to hear and to demonstrate to a student the low-pitched rumble of mitral stenosis on a noisy ward.

If given the choice of blindness or deafness, a doctor would be wise to keep his hearing. Every doctor *must* listen to know the patient in every facet. When the patient speaks, something is revealed that is outside the precincts of vision. The revelation lies not so much in what is said as in the timbre, the echo, the resonance of the voice itself.

*

The word in Greek for butterfly is *psyche*. It is also the word for "soul." The butterfly is the most metamorphic of creatures. By all rights a caterpillar should die, but at the last moment it changes into an entirely different being. Not long ago, I applied my stethoscope to the chest of an elderly woman. From the expression on her face, I could swear I was listening to the beating of Psyche's wings.

*

All night long, sirens so as to make one think that New Haven was under bombardment. For years after my retirement, I would lie awake in bed and listen to the siren of an ambulance carrying someone acutely ill to the Emergency Room. Then I would toss and turn, even sit up, pulse racing, breath coming short and fast, on the alert—like an old race horse, now kept corraled for stud, who trembles and stamps at the thrilling sound of the starting shot, and the cry "They're off!" I'm still kept around, but not for stud.

*

Lunch at Mory's with a young woman I knew when she worked as a secretary in the OR at Yale-New Haven Hospital. From early childhood she has suffered from a most extreme form of epidermolysis bullosa, an hereditary skin disease that makes Dante's eighth circle appealing by comparison. There is a defect in what used to be called the "basement membrane," so that the skin, without the least trauma, will blister and die, leaving a raw surface that must be grafted. The frequent skin cancers to which she is prone must also be excised and grafted. Every few months, she must be brought to the hospital for surgery. She has no full fingers, only on each hand two cone-shaped projections. She has lost all of her teeth and has difficulty in swallowing. Such suffering would be worthy of Job. I guess her age as about 35.

Also present for lunch are the physician's assistant who looks after her, and her physiotherapist. It is they who have arranged this meeting. It seems that for some years the woman has been writing the story of her illness, writing it in longhand in notebooks, two of which she has brought for me to see. She wants to know: Is what she has written worthy? And if so, what should she do now?

The pages of the notebook are covered with a clear, easily legible, delicate girl's handwriting—with all the l's and t's precisely the same height, the bellies and bosoms of the d's and the p's exactly so. The prose is pure and unaffected. Within a minute or two I am caught up in the narrative. The three are waiting in silence while I read. At a nearby table, professors at the Yale Law School are deep imbrued in politics, both national and departmental.

"We have to talk," I begin. I outline a plan whereby the other two will type the notebooks on a computer. There would then be a manuscript we could read to see if there are any gaps that need filling, or what possible turns the story might take. To each of my suggestions she responds with gravity. The heroism of this woman! No self-pity, only a gray-eyed candor. As she speaks about her writing, her otherwise frail voice takes on a firm, authorial tone—the authenticity of having endured, of knowing a secret that the rest of us do not.

We celebrate the enterprise by having dessert. The writer orders a chocolate mousse; the physiotherapist, a chocolate ice cream sundae; the physician's assistant, pecan pie with vanilla ice cream; and I, caramel flan. Didn't we snuff it all down to the final crumb?

In tatters though my memory may be, I think I shall remember this young woman forever, or for as long as there *is* any forever left to me.

*

Read Jesus' statement: "before Abraham I was." And Jehovah's announcement from on high: "I am that I am." In eternity there is no distinction of tenses. Predestination was not what was to come, but the will of God already fulfilled. The last trumpet has already sounded. I may be an atheist, but I do have a religious sensibility.

*

When I was four, Father promised me a silver dollar if I learned to read. Six months later I read aloud the story of Jonah and the Whale from a book of bible stories. For years I kept that silver dollar in a cubbyhole of my rolltop desk, until at 16 and dying of love, I spent it on a harmonica with which I hoped to win a kiss from Emily Jane. Again and again I played for her the only two songs I knew—"Santa Lucia" and "Flow Gently, Sweet Afton." But Emily Jane was not to be blandished. "Don't you know any others?" she asked. And that was that.

"Just as well," consoled Mother. "A kiss given upon demand gives no delight." But I didn't believe that for a minute. Not then and not now.

*

Paid a visit to a sick centenarian, his teeth in a tumbler on the nightstand. While the man lay unresponsive, his teeth looked at me. Teeth can look at you more accusingly than eyes. "It's ridiculous," I said to the submerged dentures, "to take offense at a seventy-year-old man because he is up and around." But the teeth glared on.

"You!" they said.

*

It was Lewis Thomas who told me that he did not dread dying. He felt sure that it would be painless. Somehow the body just knows and releases all sorts of endorphins, enzymes, hormones, somnifacients, and anxiety-suppressants to ease physical and mental distress. This belief is sensible, comforting, and characteristically humane. The photo of Lewis on my desk shows an old sack tied up with string. Only the eyes are still bright blue.

*

In Cleveland a beautiful Irish poet insisted on helping me on with my coat, but she held it so high that I could not find the armholes. After struggling for a while, I stepped out of range. "Here. I'll show you how," I said, then held her coat low, slid it up on her arms, and set it down firmly on her shoulders.

"I get it now," she said, and announced that she'd never done it before. Never to have helped someone on with a coat! It was a fundamental difference between our life styles. "Many thanks for the lesson," she said. "If I'm going to be a good dyke, I have to know how to help a woman on with her coat."

I asked her about the origin of the word "dyke." She thought it might come from Boadicaea, the warrior goddess of the Amazons. Just so is knowledge exchanged to the benefit of one and all.

*

The cumulative effect on the doctor of the suffering and death of patients can be very great. I doubt that many medical students think about this. I know it was not something I thought about as a young doctor. How to deal with the heavy emotional demands? A pediatric neurosurgeon I know deals almost exclusively with tumors of brain and spinal cord. In his office, each week, he talks to half a dozen families who must learn that their child has an incurable, probably fatal illness. I quote him: "Sometimes along with the parents there may be siblings, grandparents, even the sick child. You've got to get the whole family through something. You never lose the sense of the cataclysm they are experiencing. It's emotionally draining. I go to the patients' homes sometimes. I get asked the damnedest questions like 'What is death?' and 'Am I going to die?'"

When I asked what he says to a dying child or to the family, his answer was simple and direct. "Nothing. They know. I am just there, and I let them know I am there."

Here he is about neurosurgery itself: "Fifty years ago there were a few especially talented men in this field. Today the aura and mystique are gone. I can train anyone to be a good surgeon. When they are finished, in a year or two, they'll be as good as I am. I don't come out of the OR saying: 'God, I did that well!' I'm trained to do these operations. After surgery, I say to the family: 'We just don't know. We're just people together. We want the best thing for our kids.' It's all in how you help families, how you get them through it."

How does a doctor deal with the cumulative uncertainty, loss and grief? He does this in accordance with his own life experience. Some do it poorly. They experience burnout, anger, cynicism. Some take to alcohol or drugs. Some do it by drawing closer to their patients and drawing strength and commitment from this personal encounter.

*

Ran into an older Divinity School graduate student who mourned the waste of an afternoon having to do his Greek homework. I gave him a quick lesson in that language: *kalypsos* is Greek for "darkness." If you put *apo* in front of the word, it becomes its opposite—"revelation." Ergo—apocalypse becomes "revelation." He rejoiced at not having to study Greek that day. I did not tell him that his substitute teacher had been born a Jew, and is an atheist by temperament.

*

At Yaddo. Before breakfast, a young poet told me of his "encounter with death" the night before. "I was taking a walk around the lakes late at night, when I heard the great horned owl calling. The sound was both very near and far away. Thus it had a certain simultaneity about it, and a private purpose, as though it were speaking directly to me. I felt fear, and had the profound and palpable sense of something corporeal drawing near. I knew it was Death. Somehow I recognized it. At last, it withdrew."

The poet trembled during the recounting. I tried to reassure him, but who can diagnose such a visitation as benign or malignant?

"It doesn't seem to me laden with foreboding," I said. "Its departure is at least as significant as its coming. That it left you . . . can't you count on that?"

Myself, I'm not so entrenched in the western scientific method as to be closed off to influences beyond the immediately corporeal. I suspect it's a receptivity we've lost or frittered away, much as the ability to withstand pain has been diminished by dependence on analgesics. Perhaps the loss of extra-sensitivity is a price we have paid for civilized life. We are no longer in touch except with each other. Were any such "contact" to occur, it would be by just such a young poet whose brain is teeming with imagery, and whose chemistry is highly charged and resonant.

"It's proof of your poetry," I told him. "Rejoice." But he looked over his shoulder into the distance, as though hearkening.

*

Now 78 years old—but I have only to take up the pen and see the years fall away from that hand. The thick joints lose their knobby bulk; the fingers grow slender and nimble. Gone is all the arthritis and calcification. The Dupuytren's contracture is no longer visible or palpable. It is the hand of a 13-year-old boy. He pauses, and cocks an ear to listen to the larks nesting just outside the window. He dips his pen in their song and writes it in his notebook. The house drowses around him.

Only the handwriting gives evidence of the decades that have passed. It is tremulous, jerky. The l's, t's, and d's tilt every which way, and none are of the same height. The bellies of the b's and p's are either swollen or dented. I read it over, and return to my old age.

*

Strange and marvelous are the ways of our construction. Take urination. After some sixty years of visiting public toilets in airports, train stations, and a hundred away-from-home situations, I have observed that a great many men will spit into the urinal prior to relieving themselves. These are men who, by and large, do not spit elsewhere or otherwise. Spitting, for them, is a ceremonial act that is somehow necessary in order for the upper bladder to contract while the outlet relaxes, allowing for the expression and passage of urine. Without spitting, such men would have to stand there for who knows how long, and with only so-so results. Still other men, fewer in number, whistle or make soft whispery noises in order to initiate the flow. Could there be, somewhere in the autonomic nervous system, an auriculo-vesical pathway (ear to bladder) that transmits the sound of expectoration to the complex mechanism of urination?

*

A great actor knows how to work facial musculature to produce the subtlety of expression desired. Most expressive are the inner extremity of the eyebrow and the angle of the mouth. The *corrugator supercilii* arises from the frontal bone near its union with the nasal bones, and is inserted into the skin of the eyelids, knitting the eyebrows and conveying a mental state or sentiment. The *triangularis oris* or depressor of the corner of the mouth arises from the base of the lower jaw and passes upward to be inserted at the corner of the mouth. It arches the upper lip in contempt or hatred.

*

Numerous reproaches about my decision to donate my body for dissection by medical students. Aside from viewing it as a triumph over death, I adopt a lighter touch: "Better to toss my old bones on the cairn of Medicine, along with other anatomical curiosities."

*

Letter from Mike McCann about a surgeon who was a guest at his B&B and who told Mike that he had been a student of mine at Yale. He said that the most important lesson he learned from me was the importance of touching the patient, that in the act of touching the patient received and the doctor gave what amounted to trust, an absolute necessity in the art of medicine.

I was gratified to be told of this. Thinking about it later, I have to say that I learned the art of touching from my barber, Carl. Whenever he cupped my calvarium in his hand, I *knew* I had been touched. Carl mastered the art of touch, elevating it to the level of a mystical rite. It is just such an infusion of the sacred into the laying on of hands that defines a great doctor as compared with one who is merely learned and careful.

*

In *AIDS and Its Metaphors* Susan Sontag would have us stop viewing illness in metaphoric terms. One sees what she means. The stigmatization of a disease only increases the misery of its sufferers. The efforts of bigots masquerading as moralists to proclaim AIDS as divine retribution for a sinful life is cruel and dastardly.

But it is precisely in terms of metaphors that most of see our serious or fatal illnesses. It is human nature to do so. Metaphor is the best, if not the only, mode of expression by which we can comprehend the unacceptable and the horrific in our lives. Take away from the sufferer his connection with art, myth, and religion—in all of which metaphor is the dominant form of expression—and the physically afflicted is left with nothing but his cold, devastating symptoms. If not metaphorically, how are we to think of our dying selves? Besides, to give metaphoric vent to one's misery does not detract from the understanding that specific diseases are caused by specific bacteria, viruses, or toxins.

Sontag also wants us to avoid military metaphors in speaking of disease. But in fact, it may be impossible for the scientists engaged in AIDS research to think in any terms other than military. The immune system *is*, after all, the defense of the body—and the word defense implies an attacker, the virus, which becomes, by definition, the enemy of the body. It has nothing to do with guilt or blame. It is simply the way it is.

One might be more easily persuaded to listen if Sontag's argument were presented in anything but the clotted prose of the polemicist. A writer who uses the word "culpabilize" (twice) ought to have her word processor washed out with soap. The persistent angry tone of the book, and its roundhouse punches at capitalism, weaken the text. Nor is the author herself able to refrain from the occasional metaphor. In discussing the incidence of AIDS in other countries, she writes: "AIDS is everyone's Trojan horse." How now, Susan Sontag?

*

E-mail from Hank: "Dear Grandpa, I have just invented a new word: PRANTICLE. Can you guess what it means? Love, Hank."

After scratching my scalp raw for an afternoon, I could only come up with this answer: *A pranticle is a long feather used to tickle your horse in order to make it prance, especially in parades and at the circus.*

Never mind: I have enlisted the aid of numerous learned friends. The little scamp must not be allowed to get the better of his Grandpa, all four chambers of whose heart he occupies.

*

Why am I like the Cumaean Sybil? Because every single time I stand up at a podium, having carefully arranged in order all of my notes, I am dismayed to find that they have become disarranged and are to be of no use whatsoever during the talk. It is as Dante wrote:

> *Cosi al vento nellafoglie lievi*
> *Siperdea la sentenza di Sibilla.*
>
> Just so was lost the wisdom of the Sybil
> by the wind on the fragile leaves.

*

Putting me in a tuxedo would be like putting shoes on a rooster. I did have one on once—suspenders, cummerbund and all. Came time to pee but I couldn't find my fly; had to fling off the jacket, unshoulder the suspenders and lower the pants. Swore never again to put one on.

It is the advantage of the average-looking, the plain, that we need never concern ourselves with wardrobe. I have no pressing needs. Everything is allowed to wrinkle and droop. Whatever I put on, becomes me. Everybody says so. A pair of tattered pants, shoes scuffed and down-at-heel, a vest short on buttons, a sweat-stained shirt—hand them all down to me, and I shall look quite the dandy. I never feel so secure as when I have put in new shoelaces. Even an old horse-blanket thrown over my shoulder turns into a stunning *capote de brega.* My friend Reuben Sartorius, himself a Master Tailor, said: "One more hanging thread and you will be taken for John the Baptist."

*

I am almost never seen without the elderly tattered briefcase that has followed me about for thirty years. Far more learned than I, it understands Archimedes' Principle, and is fluent in Hebrew, Latin, French and algebra. It is a descendent of my father's black doctor's bag that could all by itself perform an appendectomy, or so he swore.

*

Janet and I went shopping for clothes! Arrived at the store to find that it was going out of business. Everything was 60% off. I bought two pairs of shoes and a pair of sandals before I made the painful discovery that my right foot is twice as large as my left. Compared to the big dumb clodhopper on the right, my left isn't even a foot. It's a footsie.

"Can you sell me a left seven and a half, and a right ten?" I asked. The saleslady gave me a look. "It's your age," she said. "Sooner or later the other arch will fall, and then they'll be the same."

"Or down will come baby, cradle and all?"

"You're cute," she said, "but all sales are final."

I prepared to chaffer shrewdly despite Janet's gasps. ("You're not! Tell me you're not going to haggle. This is not Baghdad.") Then bought a pair of corduroy pants. "Fits you real nice," said the man in the dressing room, and made a quick pass at my fanny.

"Merry Christmas," I told him.

*

I am just now beginning to emerge from the annual sadness that envelops me during the "holiday season." The words "merry" and "happy" as applied to Christmas and New Year simply do not apply for me. This morning at breakfast I read the program of a concert attended last night by Janet, Gretchen, and Becky. It was performed by the Harlem Girls Chorus. Reading the list of songs performed—some classical, some Negro spirituals, some sacred, some pop, I found myself weeping! Am I so debilitated that I am no longer in command of myself? Why are my tears so ready to spill over? I cannot say. Only that sometimes I must turn away to hide them and to quench a sob.

*

Most of my early works now seem to have been written in a kind of *furor scribendi* in which the pen in my hand broke free of its reins and, heartless and headlong, galloped back and forth across the page. But no more. Age has brought caution and timidity (the worst sin of a writer). Now each line is worried the way a sheepdog can worry a flock so that they cannot graze but only stand in a circle huddled and shivering.

I am reduced to keeping my daily journal, although perhaps "reduced" is not the proper term for the labor of it. There are times when I perceive the Diary to be as worthy a genre as Fiction or the Essay.

*

Up to page 327 of Dawn Powell's *Diaries*. Here is a typical entry (October 31, 1953):

"... furiously and insanely working over novel but so tired I dread sleep for fear I won't be able to wake up and get to work as I hardly sleep and then wake myself with parched eyes to go over book at 6 or 7 am. I never get anywhere no matter how many hours I spend. Another terrible year of fruitless work finally turned aimless. Simply remarkable bad luck—perhaps my just return but let us have some of the luxurious injustice other writers enjoy."

All in all, I admire Powell's writing, but at this point my patience is exhausted—the self-absorption, the pecking at one's own liver and posing as a hard-hitter with a soft heart—it's just too much.

Soon it will be my turn. If there is such a thing as Divine Retribution, the reader will come along who will say the same thing about my diaries.

2009

I should not like to call attention to myself like a frog harrumphing to a bog all day. I am what you see: a small thin delicate-looking man with an unlikely physique. I walk with a cane, without which I would surely tumble to the ground. My wife has tied a circlet of bright red wool around the distal end of the cane so that I would be more able to find it in a coat-rack. Despite her kindly "vaccination," I manage to lose it two or three times a day.

*

Reading the life of Renoir would put any hypochondriac to shame for so much as mentioning his symptoms. Even with his inflammatory arthritis—the constant pain, immobility, sores, abscesses, ulcerations and deformity of the hands—he painted every day to his death. Nor did he ever whine.

Selzer, *faites attention!* To learn of Renoir's martyrdom and courage is restorative. Man is capable of rising above his suffering.

*

This morning I went to the Music Library at Yale, and requested a CD of Verdi's *La Traviata*. The student librarian showed me how to turn it on and I spent a magical hour listening to Act One with Maria Callas, Mario Sereni, and Alfredo Krause. "Un di felice" brought tears to my eyes. I did this to get started on the small piece I would like to be writing. It is a rendering of an actual happening that took place at the Yale gym.

I go to the second floor men's locker room every weekday morning. I pretend to exercise, and then take a shower before I go to the Beinecke

Library. Among the small cadre of gentlemen who go there every morning is, as am I, a small, slight octogenarian with whom I have exchanged no more than a murmured "Good Morning." He goes to the gym to play squash. (This, I have diagnosed from the racket he is never seen without.) Let me be "Shower" and him be "Squash." Neither one of us weighs more than 125 pounds. We are just this side of emaciation. On the day of the happening, Squash and I were each on our way to the shower room. I heard him whistling a melody that I recognized as "un di felice quest anima . . ." from *La Traviata*, an aria I have loved for many years. He was whistling it completely out of tune, but still recognizable. I began to sing under my breath the very aria: "Di quell'amor, quell'amor ch'è palpito . . ."

He was astounded. "You know the libretto!" I went on with it. He stopped, listened, then resumed whistling—and like a polite conductor, he slowed the tempo of his whistling to allow for my need to breathe between phrases:

Dell'universo, Dell'universo intero,
Misterioso, Misterioso altero,
Croce, croce e delizia,
Croce e delizia, delizia al cor.

It was heart singing to heart—two naked old men, under the spell of Verdi, performing a duet of love and passion in the shower room of the Yale gymnasium. I looked up to see an audience of three in front of the shower stalls, beaming, one of them conducting the aria with his arms outstretched.

*

Lay awake last night re-living a childhood experience. The household then consisted of my aged grandfather who spoke no English, my widowed mother, and myself, a boy of fourteen. My mother had married Max, an old friend of the family, and then, not too long afterward, divorced him to marry another man. One day Max appeared at the front door, asking to be let in. I showed him upstairs to the living room. He seemed out of breath. I showed him where to sit, then went to get Mother. The encounter was strained and silent. None of us knew what to say. Suddenly Max crumpled and died. Mother went to phone for the police ambulance. We waited in the living room and heard the siren approaching. My last memory was of the two of us watching from the front stoop, as Max was carried out on a stretcher and slid into the back of the ambulance. A moment later, he was gone.

Mother: "I have been punished."

Me: "For what? For giving the man a room to die in?"

What I did not say was what I thought: that Max had just evened the score.

*

The B&B is full of physicists this week. This afternoon I'll bake my second bread of the week. It is one of the household chores that I like so much to do. It is free of stealth, guile, or ill intent. It touches a primitive nerve that satisfies—like the shoeing of a horse must have been, a century ago.

*

Reading a volume of 17th-century French letters—de Sevigny, de la Fayette, de Maintenon, de la Bruyere, and so forth. I am pleasantly surprised that my French is up to it, and here I bow deeply to Mademoiselle Bouton, my high school French teacher who made all this possible. All praise to her.

Also dipping into letters by Keats, Coleridge, and other English poets. The letter as a genre is worthy of wide readership. A letter is usually comprehensible where a poem may not be. A letter can be informal as well as informative—light-hearted and amusing, where an essay must be arid, or at least rely on high seriousness. I have often written letters that have no basis in fact, but are really a quick passage through the make-believe. The letters of a great scientist, artist, playwright, or governor can reveal the inner personality hidden in other writings. In my own rather uneventful life, I have not located much gold, but have invented episodes in order to entertain, and have sometimes included a letter within the plot of a story when there is a need for dialogue (but not a confrontation) between two characters.

*

Yesterday read a collection of letters written by medieval Jewish traders in the ancient Middle East. One letter was written by a merchant in the tenth century, who had sailed from Alexandria, Egypt, hoping to sell his cargo of pepper and frankincense in Amalfi before continuing on to Tunisia. We are informed in this letter that on the return voyage from Tunisia to Egypt, the ship was pursued by pirates and was forced to flee as far north as Constantinople. The journey, which ordinarily would have taken fifteen days, kept them at sea for more than seventy, during which, in the words of the merchant, "We gulped our blood."

This means, according to the Arabic scholar, that they "lived in utmost dread" with the added implication that "we tried to inspire ourselves with courage." I have never encountered this image anywhere, and I hope to make use of it in my writing in the future.

*

Went to the Kline Science Library to see the drawings of *filodes fulvidorsalis*, the lachcrymophagic moth that I have written about (in "Crimean Vespers") as the siphon of our sorrows, in that it alights upon the cheek of the sleeping human, inserts its long proboscis between eyelid and sclera and sucks off the tears. My trope was that everyone should keep such a moth in a small cage next to his bed in order to wake up every morning cheerful and optimistic. While my trope is fanciful, there really is such a pretty pyralid moth.

*

Letter from Peter Josyph, who recognizes that my most recent works are not conventional stories, but fantasies, figments of imagination that pertain to my own life in some way. In each, I am one of the characters who acts as I would do. These late stories are free from the need to hew to a narrative line: I float, soar, and dive as the spirit takes me.

*

Yesterday, mid-afternoon, after I had just been to see my doctor, Matt Ellman, I became dislocated. Never mind that I had worked at that very hospital for three and a half decades. I couldn't find the Cedar Street entrance. I asked the security guard, a large black man with approachable eyes: "Can you direct me to the Cedar Street entrance, Sir?"

"Your shoe's untied," said a lady walking past. I looked down, and yes it was untied. I made as if to bend down and tie it, but was clumsy and ungainly in my heavy coat and holding my briefcase.

Before I could say "Thanks" to the lady, the security guard was down on one knee, tying my shoe.

"You are the kindest man in New Haven," I said.

"I don't know about that," he replied.

"Well then, make that North America," I said. There was his deep baritone laughter aimed right down on my shoe. I knew right then and there that I was in the company of one of the angels.

On Cedar Street, I caught the Yale Shuttle Bus for home. I only had to wipe my eyes once.

*

On the way to the library at 7:10 A.M., heard the sharp monotone of a cardinal on a branch overhead. It is far more than a whistle or the martial clangor of a trumpet. It is a celebration of the new day, and an announcement of his whereabouts as an invitation to any female that might need seeding. Each time I hear it, the small hairs on my arms tingle and hold themselves upright. I am an Aeolian harp that gladly accepts the impression of a certain sound and tosses it back into the empty air.

*

Spent a long day at the Beinecke, hunched over a blank page with a pen in my hand, turning inward to that molten core where dreams smolder until I reach down and scoop one of them up.

Now who is this tottering by? Why, it is my old Grandpa of childhood whom I have come to resemble in so many ways—especially the tottering, which is all that is left of a once-manly stride. While I am on my way home from the Beinecke, he will be on his way to shul, where he and his cronies constitute the minyan. In memory and imagination I follow him there and listen to the braying of the ten old Yids, none of whom can carry a tune. The sound is unmusical, but all the more beautiful for that.

*

This week I made another jar of pickled green tomatoes (water, salt, vinegar, cloves of garlic, hot red pepper, ground black pepper, bay leaves, and dill weed). It was my Grandpa's favorite. I make it in homage to him. I have extracted from Jon and Danny their promise to help when I next pickle. It is much more satisfying than writing a short story. In my next life, I shall be a preserver—not of lives, though.

*

Turning the pages of an old notebook, I see that nine years ago I was a "wizened, tiny reduction of mankind," weighing 135 pounds and standing 5'8".

Today I am 125 pounds and 5'7". Now that is progress. In another year I shall have gone up in a puff of smoke.

*

I used to be a rock on the shore. Now I have become a wave that washes over it.

This was a melancholy thought to have on Christmas Day, and Janet and I sat in the kitchen looking more like survivors than celebrants. If this keeps up, I thought, I shall be forced to make soup.

Lo! A big pot of it with potatoes, onions, leeks, cabbage, garlic, wine, egg, salt, pepper, lemon juice, tomatoes, sugar, flour, more wine, dill, caraway seed, and bay leaf. I let it simmer all day. Meanwhile baked a bread. Threw a handful of shrimp into the soup. Hollered "Dinner's ready!"

*

What makes all the difference to a writer is where he or she is at the moment of creativity, the actual place. For me, these days, it is the Beinecke Library at Yale. It is there I really live. Outside of the Beinecke I am, like everyone else, terrestial, fleeting, transitory.

No spiritual consolations for me; I prefer the finite to the infinite. Heaven is for the "heavenly": that pale, wispy place populated by insipid, sexless angels. Long ago I shed my religion the way a snake sheds its skin, just as easily and without ever looking back. Nearing the end of my life, I strive to be good-natured, not saintly.

But the Beinecke Library is closed for the holidays, and will not reopen until January 2nd. How will I deal with this calamity? By shedding ink!

2010

Dreamt we had to sell the house on St. Ronan Terrace, where we have lived for 46 years. I awoke with terrible *heimveh* (homesickness). Went out into the garden where the crocuses and daffodils are in bloom, all so hearty and strong.

*

The B&B was stuffed with thirteen guests from all over the world. Parents' Weekend at Yale and the influx of a half dozen physicists from Rutgers, here to use the BEAM in the Nuclear Structure Lab.

Poor Janet! I try to help her as much as she will permit. My duties consist of stripping the beds (but not making them), emptying the dishwasher (but not filling it), making the morning coffee, taking reservations whenever Janet is not home, staying home in order to give her time to vacate the premises for relief, accompanying her to the market to carry packages, load and unload the car, and mainly keeping out of the way and being frugal. Janet is heroic in her determination to keep the family solvent.

*

A royalty cheque for "Discus Thrower" in the amount of $630 came the other day, so I am a bit of help in that direction. The cheque is especially welcome as that story was first published in 1979 in *Letters to a Young Doctor* and written several years prior to that. It has perked up my spirits and hinted that some of my work has a chance of enduring.

"Discus Thrower" is all *contrast*—the blind old amputee set against the antique statue of the Discobolus; the head-nurse's outrage at the patient's violent act (quite natural) set against the quiet understanding of the doctor. It is told in understatement, in contrast to the violence of the act. Although the story is only four pages, it has engendered voluminous commentary over the years. To me, the man's outrageous behavior appears as a tragic expression of defiance against the cruel fate that has left him blind and legless, isolated from all others. His act is not insane or senseless. It is what every deathly ill patient might want to do: to even the score—and even more, to triumph over the grotesque fate that has afflicted him. His is a noble rebellion.

As for his laughter, I chose not to explain it, but to leave it indistinct, a mystery. Even if I understood it myself, as a writer I know that the mind of the reader is more likely to return to the inexplicable in search of further meaning.

*

A red-letter day. I was introduced to Susan Howe at the Beinecke Library by Nancy, curator of modern American literature. It seems that Susan's husband had died suddenly two years ago. A pulmonary embolism. When the autopsy report was given, it became known that the eyes had been removed. Susan has wondered why all this time. I was asked to meet with her to think about it. In the thirty-eight years of my practice of surgery, I had never encountered such a thing. But then, when I was a surgeon, organ transplantation had not yet been a commonly performed procedure. The only possibility that came to me was that the man had been a registered organ donor, and that this was noted on his driver's license or some other document, and that might constitute written permission to harvest the corneas for transplantation.

From that, we embarked on what I can only call a meditation on the event, and that the eyes were seeing still, beyond death. We also exchanged thoughts on the life of a writer. She is an esteemed poet and essayist. I liked her at once, an attractive youthful slender woman, modest and so affable. We have arranged for more meetings to come. I am grateful to Nancy for bringing us together.

Now it has happened that I have made two new friends within a couple of days of each other—I who do not have a talent for friendship, and have spent almost all of my time seeking solitude and anonymity. Nancy has lent me three of Susan Howe's books, one of which is *My Emily Dickinson.* This after I had announced to them both that ED was my favorite poet, and quoted "I heard a fly buzz when I died . . ."

*

A preacher has put it abroad that tomorrow will be the end of the world. That will not keep me from baking a bread in the afternoon, as I had planned. I'll take it with me on the voyage to Hell.

*

Reading in the correspondence of Harold Nicolson and Vita Sackville-West. Most enjoyable, and a revealing peek at English aristocratic attitudes. Here is Harold on life in our Long Island: "I cannot conceive how these people endure the life they lead. Nobody ever seems to know who is lunching with whom and whose house is which. They drift in and out of those white porticoes howling at each other in merriment and neighborliness." And a bit later, playing tennis with the Roosevelts at a neighboring house: "As always in this country a terrible sense of UNREALITY robs it of all meaning. It has just been bought with money. It has never grown an inch by itself. There is none of that sense of children having played among the woods . . . which gives our houses the aroma of continuity. Something horribly provincial mars this continent even at its most lovely."

A reader can get mighty fed up with this sort of blather after a couple of letters. But they are great fun to read in spite of that snobbery.

*

Every chance I get, I walk to East Rock Park. From the footbridge by the waterfall two elderly willows, all knobs and varicosities, are fording the stream. The way they hold up their skirts and throw themselves about!

*

Awoke during the night with the song "I'll take you home again, Kathleen" in my mind, and my cheeks wet with tears. The song seems to me to be an unhappy melody. In my dream it was being sung by a clear Irish tenor in the Troy Music Hall. I was a small boy weeping in the front row.

I'll take you home again, Kathleen,
To where your heart is ever turning,
To where the fields are bright and green,
I will take you to your home, Kathleen.

But the Kathleen of my dream was a young girl who has just died of tuberculosis at the Pawling Sanatorium in Troy. This may be the origin of the story "Tom and Lily," which is my own poor version of *Romeo and Juliet.* I lay awake the rest of the night with the song in my mind.

*

A hectic day at the library where I had meant to get a bit of writing done. When I arrived at 9 A.M., there were already two students waiting to discuss my work, especially some pieces from *Mortal Lessons* they'd been assigned in Yale English classes. They had the energy for it. I did my best. Had to ask for a helping hand to stand up. I'm sure it will be included in their essays, along with my other infirmities.

Then there were the members of the library staff with medical questions. One of the security guards had been bitten by a tick, and part of the bug was in her yet. That sort of thing. I have become the de facto house doctor at the Beinecke Rare Book Library. Not much writing gets done, but so what?

Home to help Janet with the B&B. Took out trash, emptied dishwasher, stripped beds, and took a couple of reservations. Then came my turn. I poured a glass or two of wine, then went out into the garden, picked lilies-of-the-valley and something lavender that I can't name, for an arrangement. Also a large bunch of viburnum in full bloom. That was fun. It was also medicinal. I missed my true calling; I should have been a florist.

*

Sunday was one of the two most egregious American sentimentalities—Father's Day. You know the other one. I take no part in either "celebration." All three of my get phoned to utter the conventional greeting, despite that they know my objection to the commercialization of fatherly love. To my credit, I maintained a discreet silence while they each wished for me Happiness, whatever that is.

I did make Gretchen laugh: "To think that half a century ago, I gave a squirt, and before I knew it, there you were!" She opined that no other father in North America would say such a thing to his daughter. She was right about that.

*

There is a new deliveryman at the library, and we have become friends. I correct the letters he writes to his customers. He is reading *The Rise and Fall of the Third Reich* (pronouncing the *ch* as in "church"), and now wants to tell his own story—"nothing special, mediocre, you know, for the eleventh and twelfth graders." Everyone has a story to tell, he says, whether it is "oral, plural, or written." (Could he have meant pleural?) More and more, he sounds presidential.

*

Went for hot and sour soup for lunch at the Great Wall, a Chinese restaurant on Whitney Avenue, where the food is excellent but the servers, with one exception, are sullen and cold. You have to decide ahead of time if the soup is worth the rudeness. While I was eating, a middle-aged black man came up, greeted me by name, and reminded me that he was the singer who used to work at the library. He let me know that he is still singing—modern jazz, the Tijuana Brass type—whereupon he launched into a falsetto delivery of Herb Alpert's famous orchestration and libretto of "A Taste of Honey" without the least shyness. On and on he sang in a high pure falsetto that might have been the voice of a 12-year-old boy imitating the brasses and piano. At last, he left me to finish my soup. Later at the Beinecke, everyone knew who it was: one of the three Hopkins brothers. They said how lucky I was to have heard him again in person. So there you are: for lunch, hot and sour soup with "A Taste of Honey." It was not listed on the menu.

*

Read the Book of Ruth in the Old Testament. The most beautiful part of the story, and justly famous, is the commitment of Ruth to Naomi, her mother-in-law, to go with her to Bethlehem rather than return to the house of her own mother in Moab—this after the death of Naomi's husband and her two sons: "Entreat me not to leave thee. Whither thou goest, I shall go. Thy people shall be my people, thy God shall be my God. Where you die, I will die, and there will I be buried . . ."

As for the rest, it is a portrait of Naomi as a sly, cunning, schemer who advises Ruth how to attract the attention of Boaz, to go gleaning in his fields after the reapers, to place herself in full view of the man, to lie nearby him when he sleeps then wait for poor Boaz to act, which of course he does in order to carry out the will of God, as implored by Naomi. There is altogether too much about ephahs of barley and purchase of land all in the name of the God of Israel. But the story is redeemed by Ruth's entreaty.

I could not resist using Ruth's commitment to Naomi ("Whither Thou Goest") as the title of my story about the widow of a man whose heart was used for transplantation. Unable to overcome her grief, the widow locates the recipient, then goes to visit him in order to listen once more to her husband's heart. When she presses her ear to the man's chest and hears the beating of that heart, she recognizes it as her husband's. When the man invites her to come again, she replies that it will not be necessary for her to do so. She has been healed.

This is one of my own favorite stories—castrated by a damned fool who changed the title to "Follow Your Heart" when he published it in a magazine.

*

The oak trees around the house are teeming with warblers. I heard the black-poll, the yellow, the black-throated blue, and also the scarlet tanager. I cannot see them, as my vision has deteriorated and I do not have my sons to point to the birds.

*

October—and Janet is still rooting in the garden. Myself, I would let the weeds have their way. Their disorder is natural. To discipline the members of the vegetable kingdom is perverse.

All this I told her from the lawn chair into which I had sunk six inches deep. But then, there is the clamor of the daylilies and the ardent desire of the clematis for the trellis and the lumps of clear gum on the bark of the apricot tree.

*

In Leviticus xi.6 the hare is included among the ruminants. If someone could tell me why, I might be less staunch in my disbelief. The ruminitia is a division of even-toed mammals including those that chew the cud—oxen, sheep, goats, antelope, giraffes, deer, camels, and chevrotains. The hare is NOT a ruminant; it is a lagomorph, a gnawing mammal that feeds on herbage, bark, and other forage. This casts a small shadow on the OT as divinely inspired.

*

Asked in a letter from a loyal reader if I still considered myself an atheist. He expressed the hope that I had converted. I replied that although the gift of faith has not been given me, I am not an inveterate enemy to religion. I am, if the truth were known, envious of those in whom a belief in God is a great consolation and sustenance in time of need of such support. I have, at bottom, a conviction of the truth and a certainty of the usefulness of religion. I cannot acquiesce to the reader's wish that I have passed through an irreligious phase and emerged into the radiance of a Revelation. Sudden conversions are often superficial and transitory.

While I cannot believe in such things as the Virgin Birth, or the existence of a heaven where we shall all meet again, I do respect the beauty of those myths. Any reader of my works will come to the knowledge that, if not obsessed with the idea of God, I have a consuming interest in the idea of a higher power. Should I ever become seized by religious faith, of all the gods with whom I have some knowledge—Buddha, Allah, Jehovah, and Christ, I would hope to be able to worship the last-named. As for the lesser deities such as Asklepios, Mars, Eros and all the other *specialists*, I pay no attention whatsoever.

*

I am still mourning the loss of my beloved cane, gone now these past twelve months. No mere wooden stick it was, but an appendage of my body, no less necessary than either one of my other legs:

> Lines written on the loss of my favorite cane:
> No mere stick of wood for leaning and propulsion,
> But a friend whose absence triggers pain
> And instigates convulsion.

2011

Just before he left for a week in Maine, Doon showed my Wikipedia to me. I had no idea what such a thing was, but am now a bit educated: it's a kind of encyclopedia including every bit of news or falsities that pertain to the subject. I was dumbfounded to learn that there are 458,000 entries in my Wikipedia. Most of them, I'm sure, are insignificant, irrelevant and idiotic. Right after he had left, I found this handwritten note on my pillow:

> Dad—
> Aristolochia, swallowtail, small-eyed sphinx moth, sweet gum, Mill River. The list of wonders is endless, but only because you taught me how to see them. Thank you for that and, of course, for the shirts you didn't want, for Sabatini books and everything else. See you next weekend.
> I love you.
> Me

It is the finest love letter of my life. I read and re-read it with my pulse bounding and my eyes glistery. A bit of explanation: Aristolochia is the vine planted years ago by Jon across the chain-link fence separating us from Yale's Farnam Gardens. In and among the leaves of this vine, aswarm and aflutter, live dozens of black swallowtail butterflies. These are the pipestem black swallowtails, and aristolochia is known as the "pipestem" vine. I haven't seen another of its kind. The eggs of this butterfly are poisonous to birds and other predators, so that the butterflies thrive here.

The small-eyed sphinx moth refers to a double-winged insect of grand coloration—orange, gray and brown, that had affixed itself to the screen door at the front of the house. There it stayed for a day and a night until I touched it with one finger, at which it loosened its hold. Janet then released it and let it drop to the floor of the front porch. Was it in a middle state between life and death? Or in a state of self-hypnosis? But its beauty will live with us forever. Sweet gum is the name of a small tree we saw in the Water Company land on our memorable walk there. Jon is the family maven on plant life.

The Mill River is the lovely small stream that flows through East Rock Park on its way into the Long Island Sound. Its banks are a favorite walking site for the Selzer family. For me, these past few days with my sons was a preview of Paradise. For them, it was their childhood revisited. I need to say that while I did point out these treasures to them, the boys immediately attributed wisdom and knowledge of them when the truth is that each of them is far more knowledgeable and far wiser than I. It is love that bestows on me these honorary degrees.

*

It is forty-seven years ago that we purchased and moved into 6 St. Ronan Terrace. I was captured by the name of the street, and determined to find out who was Ronan. In fact, he was an ancient Celtic hermit who had mastered the art of miraculous healing. He lived alone, of course, in a cave that was too shallow for him so that his bare legs stuck out of the entry. I made an immediate personal connection with Ronan, so much so that we became one another in my mind.

The house is the third on the left of a dead-end steep offshoot of St. Ronan Street. It is a huge four-story white wooden structure, almost one hundred years old, previously occupied by a member of the Hooker family, one of whom was a Professor of Medicine in the nineteenth century, and another who became Governor of Connecticut. We bought the house from a branch of the Hooker family and paid a mere pittance, all we could then afford: $44,500. When I hesitated, Mr. Hooker said he'd throw in the Steinway piano in the living room at no extra charge. We have lived there all these years, raising our family.

It was within a short distance of the hospital where I worked as a surgeon, and of the Yale library to which I have walked every morning of the past twenty-five years since my retirement from Surgery and the beginning of my life as a writer. Over forty-seven years, the house has taken on the same ramshackle look as I myself have achieved. If something breaks down, the plumbing or garden wall, it is left to its destiny. No attempt at renewal or rejuvenation is made. In fact my whole identity has merged with that house. It is myself, expressed in architectural terms.

Now that the children have moved away, 6 St. Ronan Terrace has become a B&B. Within the big house, Janet and I roam, make excursions, hunt for lost objects, such as eyeglasses and notebooks, and generally do the best we can. At age 83 and 78, our best is not what it once was. But it is good enough.

*

The art thief who parked his van near the Louvre ran off with a famous painting, but he was nabbed when he couldn't start his van. How come? He didn't have the money to buy Degas to make the van Gogh.

(Awful joke sent to me by beloved son Jon. Shall I disinherit him?)

*

Last night attended the medical students' writing awards ceremony at the request of Professor Tom Duffy, head of the Medical Humanities department at Yale School of Medicine. The four winners (out of twenty-two submissions) read their work, some of it quite impressive. The ceremony attended by a number of faculty. The conversation was rather too much full of self-congratulations: "The Yale School of Medicine is the best in the world" and "The encouragement of student writing is unique and valuable in the making of a doctor."

I do agree with the latter claim, but I made the social mistake of asking what they do with submissions that are not worthy and show a lack of talent. The unanimous feeling was that no one should be discouraged, and there is always something to praise. I do not share that consolatory way of giving a measure of encouragement to those who ought not to spend their time chasing the rainbow of praise and publication. I turned out to be the villain of the evening, even though I spend hours each day reading the manuscripts of would-be writers who send them to me uninvited. I always reply, and try to mollify, but in the end must be honest. Finished the evening feeling that I did not fit in at all. I do seem to be cast in the role of curmudgeon lately. I must avoid attendance at any future such affair.

*

Finished reading a biography of Coleridge by Walter Jackson Bate. It left me deeply saddened by a sad life. Coleridge was a man afflicted by brilliance, for which he paid a most enormous price. He never achieved happiness or experienced love. He was addicted to laudanum for many years and thereafter suffered all the symptoms of withdrawal from this drug. He was naturally a hypochondriac. His greatest suffering was not physical, however, but had to do with his indecisiveness of mind and purpose.

He produced a gigantic tower of literary treasure, including such matchless poems as "Rime of the Ancient Mariner," which I have also just re-read. Then there are his letters, essays, and marginalia—all of which made Coleridge a legend in his time. But was it worth it? I think not. He himself would rather have been a farmer than a writer.

*

A peek into the long-ago occasioned by the news that an autograph notebook belonging to Julius Seltzer and dated in the year 1912 had been found among the papers left by George Allain, the last of my mother's husbands. A descendant of Allain decided that I should be the owner of this notebook, and with great determination initiated a search for my location. Her search finally led her to an old friend of mine, Don Faulkner, who gave her my e-mail address. I am now waiting to receive this relic of the past in the mail.

It was my father's dearest wish that one day I would become a surgeon. "Show me your hands," he would say, turning them over and back. "They are strong and gentle, the hands of a surgeon." His hope was not to be realized during his lifetime. He died at age 46 just as I turned 13.

The other motive for my decision to become a surgeon came from the general sense of surgery as the most manly of medical specialties. Frail and effeminate as I considered myself to be, I wanted more than anything to become a real man. Now almost four decades of my working life, spent in the practice and teaching of General Surgery, and twenty-five years after my retirement from medicine, I am led to wonder whether I was, in fact, temperamentally suited for the job. Unlike my fellow surgeons who were certain that they were to surgery born, I was never entirely confident, but more like that corporal who said before going into battle: "I tremble at the perils to which my profession will expose me."

But I did earn the respect of countless grateful patients, and to this day I am called "Doc" by everyone who knows what once I was. I confess here the pleasure it gives me to be known by this manly diminutive. I must also acknowledge that the subject of my early writings came directly from the experience of tending the sick: the characters of my stories were doctors, nurses, or patients. The "facts" are all there but, crafted into narrative by a retired sawbones, every one of those facts is transformed into a truth. Without first having become a surgeon, I would not have become a writer.

*

Read a small biography of John Ruskin and learned of his struggle with recurrent anxiety and despair, for which he was hospitalized several times. Also, there was the long, difficult relationship with his father, the loss of his religious faith, and the sexual impotence which brought about the nullification of his unconsummated marriage.

The more I read about the lives of the great writers, the less I feel myself to be pathologically strange. I am just one of the maladjusted, and an insignificant one at that.

*

Phone call from granddaughter Lucy who is writing an essay on two of Keats' odes: "Grecian Urn" and "Nightingale." She asked for my help in comparing them. I thought it might be easier to *contrast* the two, and show how Keats portrayed the ancient urn carved in the form of a woman as "unravished" (this is, never having experienced ecstasy) and utterly silent: the "bride of quietness." The word "still" in the first line has two possible intentions: one to suggest her long virginity after so many years, and also to stress her immobility. By contrast, the nightingale is nothing but ecstasy, as he pours himself out in song. Whereas the urn is dead, the nightingale is the epitome of life at its most intense.

In an e-mail this morning Lucy sent me her commentary, which describes the poet as trying to fend off death through the song of the nightingale, while in reality he is aware that his own death is nearing.

*

Just read a book of criticism by one Fred Inglis. He, like Matthew Arnold, deplores the "over-writing" of Keats, terms it "unmanly," and criticizes its emphasis on impressions and intuition rather than thought and reason. I could not disagree more. Keats was a genius second only to Shakespeare. But Keats was a boy of 25 when he died and had been sick with tuberculosis for a long time. To my way of thinking, Keats was manly and athletic, hampered only by the lethargy of consumption. It is those literary critics who are mannered and stylized, and full of shit!

*

Was told by a visiting OB-GYN that Quinnipiac University will open a new medical school in New Haven, and that it will not require the dissection of a human cadaver by the doctors-to-be. In its place, there will be plastic organs.

It is one more dehumanization of the profession of medicine. How will this affect my intention to donate my body for anatomical dissection by medical students?

*

Timing is everything. I am lucky to have left medicine twenty-five years ago before it became a cold, distant affair dehumanized by the avalanche of technology. I feel equally lucky to have left writing before the demise of the book and its replacement by the e-book.

Very little is being published nowadays, what with the publishers going out of business. I am glad to be taking refuge in an eloquent silence.

Soon literature, art and journalism may no longer be transmitted by the printed word. The time is approaching when printing will be replaced by other media—television and theatre. This I must say, despite my own life-long devotion to books. Writing is a perishable art. Too bad, but it does relieve an author of the delusion of enduring after death.

I recall the first time I heard my language uttered aloud. It was when I attended a staged reading of "Diary of an Infidel." It was electrifying for me to find that my words when spoken by the performers took on ten-fold their power on the page. There is no text so useful that a fine performer cannot make it more so. There is no operatic plot so trite and sentimental that a Caruso cannot make it moving.

*

Began reading "Travels with a Donkey" by Robert Louis Stevenson. From the first line, I loved it and identified with the author. Perhaps what warmed my early interest was a certain similarity between this journal in the mountains of South France, on foot with only a "mouse-colored she-ass the size of a dog" for companion, and my own stay in Venice where I knew no one and where I had never been before. In the end, I threw myself "on the kindness of strangers" à la Blanche Dubois, and announced myself to the gate-keeper monk of the monastery of San Giorgio Maggiore as an itinerant seeking shelter. There followed several weeks of my remarkable stay at the monastery where the monks and I became loving friends, as well as house-doctor and patients.

I cannot claim a rugged, adventurous experience such as that of RLS, but in a number of ways, our two selves were interchangeable. We both shared a skepticism, actually a disbelief in religion, yet found ourselves thanking God for the greatness of the human spirit.

*

No question that I am a clumsy butterfingers—I, who used to perform surgery. I am unable to master the mysteries of the computer and have to appeal to the young gents, Graham Sheriff and Morgan Swan, at Beinecke to dislodge me. They are invariably kind and patient with me.

*

Reading Nabokov, initially with great admiration and, as he would have appreciated, worship. But less and less so as my reading advances. In the end, I find him grotesquely clever, and even obnoxious. There is the tone of a show-off. (Ask me; I'm one of them.) There is a lack of human warmth, a cold, intellectual distancing from the pulsatile, vulnerable human being. I can stay with Nabokov only so far, and then have to put the book down. Perhaps it is more my shortcoming as a reader than his as a writer. I am incapable of distancing myself from my characters, even becoming them as I write. In the end, the transfiguration is complete. Call it sentimentality, if you wish. I do have a good deal of that.

*

Yesterday a sudden cloudburst afforded the rare opportunity for gallantry. I stepped quickly to the side of an umbrellaless woman of middle age or beyond, and exalted mine over her head. Arm in arm and side to side, we progressed to her destination. Best is that I did not know her, nor do I still. Second best was the chance to use the verb "exalt" in its literal sense—to raise up or lift.

*

So many years after its publication, I still get cranky letters from readers of my memoir *Down from Troy*—all having to do with my imperfect remembrance of facts. Why did I write that School 5 was a two-story building when it had three stories? Why did my father move the family from 45 Second Street to 2139 Fifth Avenue and then to 2145 Fifth Avenue? "If you have lived in New Haven for so many years, but your heart is still in Troy, why don't you stick with the facts?"—and questions of that ilk, all asked in a tone of reproach.

To each of these letters I reply with gentlemanly restraint that expresses my gratitude at having any readers at all, and confesses that at age 83 my memory is in tatters. It is the way in which I have tried to deflect anger all my life. Call me meek. But I can tell you that Jesus had it all wrong; it is not the meek who will inherit the earth; it is the presumptuous.

Besides, like many of my fellow forgetters, I am not interested in the facts. I am interested in the truth. The facts lie on the surface of life, while the truth lies hidden far below. You want the facts? Look them up in any of the new-fangled instruments—tweeter, blog, and facebook—none of which I have ever used. For the truth, you have only to gaze out the window for a long time and wait until it hoves into view. Upon my gravestone, it would be factual to have carved: "He told many lies." This too: "His unhappy childhood ended at age thirteen with the death of his father, and the onset of his unhappy adolescence. His adulthood has been fraught with a series of blunders for which he has paid in full, and then some. Now having 'distinguished' himself as a surgeon and a writer, he feels himself to have been no more than a failure and an impostor."

But any mention of this truth would be met with the accusation of false modesty, or an appeal for reassurance from the fact-seekers. (The reader will note that I have fled from the first person to the third. It is one of the cowardly devices of the autobiographer.)

*

Just finished re-reading *Down from Troy* and find myself in a slough of despond. The revived memories of the cobblestones and church steeples have unmanned me. My whole identity seems to be merged in the city of my birth. It is more than a town; it is a person.

*

Last evening Janet attended a city meeting that responded to the huge increase in property values and our taxes. It appears that we will not be able to keep our house, where we have lived for forty seven years. Too bad!

But it is an occasion for reassessment, not of our taxes but of our lives. For the major part of our family life, we have enjoyed the big old house on St. Ronan Terrace. But we must be philosophical. Next July, when the new tax is due, we will be 84 and 80, and ever more vulnerable to major upheavals such as health. Both of us are fortunate not to have any major ongoing illnesses such as have carried off some of our contemporaries. This upheaval is only in the place of our residence, and the worth of our savings. Neither of us has committed a crime that would put us in prison. We are free to adjust, to consolidate, and to go on partaking of the fruits of the earth. Such is what I have preached to Janet at breakfast this morning. I do believe that she will come to the same acquiescence, albeit with some reluctance at the beginning.

2012

Last evening in the Beaumont Room at the medical school, there was held the annual Richard Selzer Lecture in the "Humanities in Medicine" series. The talk was mostly a reading of his poems by Rafael Blanco, a jolly, pudgy attractive physician of perhaps 45. The poems were mostly case histories of his patients, sufferers from AIDS, and gay lesbian transgender and other members of the "queer" population, of whom he is proudly one. After the reading, the audience repaired to the graduates' club for dinner. I was lucky to be seated next to Rafael. Throughout the evening I was celebrated as the "Founding Father of Literature and Medicine." It was Richard-this and Richard-that. I was made uncomfortable at being on display, and would have preferred a dimly lit alcove. I was looked after with immense care and concern, transported everywhere by kind souls, without whom I would not have survived. After dinner, I was brought to my door by Ashgar Rastigar, Professor of Humanities at the Medical School, a truly lovable man. Lay awake all night regretting the exposure of my mental and physical deterioration.

Asked to "say a few words" about how and why and when I began to write, I spoke of the time when, at age 12, I was asked by my General Practitioner father to hold a man still while he sutured and dressed a wound of the thigh. I remember pressing the man's leg down with all my strength and bringing the wound so close to my face that I could smell the stench of the infection and pleading with the struggling man to "hold still." Father's office was on the ground floor of the house. The family lived upstairs. Mother had a lovely soprano voice that sounded as if a white mouse were ringing a tiny silver bell. From earliest days, I heard her practicing her scales upstairs, and the moans and cries of the patients downstairs. I was midway between Art and Medicine.

Over the years, journeying in a world of medicine that has become saturated with the technical at the expense of the humane, I have tried to remind the practitioners of that profession of its ancient origins, and to provide it the lore and the literature that it deserves. Just when it occurred to me that this was my mission, I could not say—only that I was elected to do it in accordance with a will other than my own. That I have succeeded in part was evident by the presence of so many doctors and nurses, each one engaged in writing. I had to accept the adulation, if only to satisfy these young writers. But I am glad that the event is in the past.

*

The house on St. Ronan Terrace is now one hundred years old. We have lived here for forty-seven years. Every room and every object is bound together by sacred ties of love and nostalgia. So many are the malfunctions of the house that the prospect of restoring it is risible. Cold drafts penetrate the so-called storm windows. We are always too cold or too hot.

The noose seems to be slowly tightening on our ownership of the house. With the taxes set to rise, the B&B has slowed to a crawl. I have approached the Divinity School, the Greenberg Conference Center, and the Beinecke in an effort to drum up some business. It will not be easy to keep things going, but neither would selling the house and relocating be.

*

I am reading the last letters of John Keats, those to his sister Fanny and to his sweetheart Fanny Brawne. In doing so, I do no kind service to my own mental health. His terrifying hemoptysis that he tries hard to minimize—but his friends know better. And so does the reader. He says "Thank God there is such a thing as a grave," and wishes to be in it as soon as possible rather than live without the companionship of Fanny Brawne. He is acutely aware of the imminence of death, which produces a natural bitterness toward those who are in good health. At last he is about to set off for Italy with that angelic Severn to care for him. He must go, as he knows that another winter in England would kill him. But he leaves with reluctance. I have just put the book down as I cannot bear the pressure in my chest from repressed sobs.

*

Finished reading *The Tenants of Moonbloom* by Edward Lewis Wallant, given to me by Kevin Kerrane, who found the novel "both touching and funny." I found it touching, all right, but not a bit funny; to me it was sad to the point of tragedy. The book is powerfully written. Wallant was another great artist who died young.

*

Yesterday I attended the writing awards ceremony of the Yale School of Nursing, of which I was one of the judges. The New Haven Lawn Club packed with nurses and students and their families. The three winners read their works, which were admirably brief. All three told of the experience of nursing a cancer-ridden child until he/she died.

The only dry eye in the place was mine. Either I am hard-hearted or I have read too many of these sorrowful accounts and have grown impervious. My single hesitation was that all of the finalists were women. Not a man in sight. This I shall protest to Linda Pellico, the faculty nurse in charge of creative writing.

I met many good-looking women who have been reading my own work for some time. I was treated with every sort of homage and it went to my head, I have to admit. An hour or two of it persuaded me that I was quite good-looking myself instead of the old spavined cart-horse who arrived. I struck a Great Writer Pose to blushful effect. I was home before ten o'clock and discovered that I had brought with me, not my own jacket, but someone else's.

This morning, I walked to the Lawn Club to return the jacket with my apologies, but was immediately absolved. "No. No! It was *our* fault, not yours." I am not allowed to commit any sin, no matter how slight. I remain an old man at the most trying time of life—mid-eighties—with an immense social popularity and no serious work to do, degenerating into a "good" fellow. I would much rather fling the gauntlet to society and join up with some brave bandits to rob a stagecoach or two on the highway. But such was not given to me, and so I am a goody two-shoes, as we used to call the teacher's pet at School 5 in Troy, New York.

*

Stopped at the box-office to acquire two tickets to the film of Verdi's *Un ballo en maschera*, which we will attend on Saturday afternoon. Janet delighted. Another cause of her approbation was yesterday's culinary concoction: sauteed cabbage with sliced green apple and sour cream plus brown sugar. I felt my way through it, fearing that it would have to be thrown out, but Janet tasted the mess and declared it delicious. This was reiterated at supper when it was joined by a baked potato and roasted chicken. I had to agree with her. Modesty can go only so far, and vanity is ever so much more pleasurable.

*

Today I began reading *Our Lady of the Flowers*, said to be Jean Genet's masterpiece. I first tried to read it at age 13, but soon discovered that I was too young. Now, approaching age 84, I find that I am too old. Just so has a "masterpiece" slipped away between adolescence and old age, leaving me unedified.

*

A surprise visit from RM after many years of non-communication. He had been an intern in surgery, and I was one of his mentors. We had become close friends. He was, and still is, a large well-built man with a somewhat tense manner, but most congenial. He had dropped out of Medicine after the internship, and embarked on a hugely successful nationwide construction business. He had also become a zealous member of a Christian sect, possibly Jehovah's Witnesses. I recall that he had been pressuring me in that direction and that I had severed the friendship which had become tiresome. But what had triggered this long-delayed reunion, I cannot imagine.

He had brought along his younger daughter, a beautiful, very bright and observant young lady who works in set design for films. Several hours into the reunion, he handed me two books, *What the Bible Teaches Us* and *The Holy Bible* (the latter a version). It quickly became apparent that he was still in pursuit of my soul. He *must* have it! And I became just as determined that he would not succeed. It seemed to me an obsessive pursuit by a man who is not accustomed to fail. It is also just possible that it was an act of love: He wanted me to be secure in belief in a hereafter.

Not long after his departure, the feeling grew on me that could not let go of me but was driven to have me in the palm of his hand. It was the same feeling I experienced at age 13, shortly after the sudden death of my father. I had taken an afterschool job at St. Peter's Church on the next block, setting chairs in the vestry on Friday, taking them down on Sunday, and washing the floor. The priest came upon me sitting on a bench under a great weeping beech tree in the field in back of our house. I too was weeping.

"I will make you feel better," he said, and drew me up on his knee. Next thing you know, his hand was under my shirt, then under my pants.

"Father," I whispered. It was not the priest I addressed, but my own newly dead father. I wished for him to come and help me, tell me what to do, extricate me from this predicament. But minutes later it was too late, I remember the pain of sodomy and the concurrent orgasm, my first. I wanted to die, but could not.

It was the same sort of encounter as with my former student. Here was another handsome adult man intent upon his own agenda, and I the object of his desire. It happened once, and never again. I quit my job and avoided the priest's presence, although he continued to present himself beneath that weeping beech tree—in high hopes, I was sure. This marked the end of any religious belief I had.

*

Went to the Yale Art Gallery to see van Gogh's "Cypresses" and "Starry Night," both on loan here. Wild and unrestrained, they are on the very edge of psychotic beauty. Here is an excerpt from the van Gogh's notebook:

> In the midst of an artistic life, there arises again and again the yearning for a real life which remains an unrealizable ideal. One feels exactly like an old cab horse who knows that he must return to the same old shafts, when all the while, one would so love to live in the fields, in the sun, near the river, in the country, with other horses also free, and have the right to procreate my kind. . . . One offers no resistance; neither does one resign himself.

And so he went mad, cut off his ear. With all my heart, I wish that I had been there with him, baking a bread to lift his spirits even as it rose in the oven, or creating a chicken carcass soup such as to raise the dead bird to exultant life.

Van Gogh's seemingly perverse distortions of reality are not distortions at all, but his perceptions of what is real—the way it affects him. He is drawn to find beauty and truth in the abnormal: for example, the node on the trunk of a tree that changes its shape. To some, this would be a sign of disease or ugliness, but to van Gogh it was precisely there that he located truth. I have tried to do something of the same in my descriptions of the lesions of the sick. It has to do with imagination and intuition, not reason. It surpasses mere fact. It is creativity through verbal magic, not so much a conscious manipulation of facts. It is a kind of "angelism" of the intellect.

*

Of the esteemed doctor-writers of the past, I feel closely akin to Sir Thomas Browne because of the shared fellowship of medical experience, which no other professional relationship can match, let alone exceed. What distinguishes me from Sir Thomas is his genius, his persevering curiosity in many areas of science and art, and his deep religious faith.

Compared to Browne, I can admit to ignorance and laziness. I spent some thirty-five years in the practice and teaching of General Surgery, all of it at Yale University—at the end of which, and still in my late fifties, I found myself standing at bay with my formerly beloved profession, and afflicted with an ennui that prevented me from continuing in it. In short, I had a strong revulsion to the act of cutting open the bodies of my patients, then rummaging among their cavities in search of what had gone wrong, and taking steps to right those wrongs to the best of my ability. I did not want to take out another gallbladder, repair another hernia or perform any of the *-ectomies* (splenectomy, gastrectomy, colonectomy, pneumonectomy, and so forth) which had for so many years been the reason for my existence. Suddenly I had the intense desire to set down my scalpel, and take up my pen. I would become a writer . . . and so I did. For the next twenty-five years, I wrote short stories, essays, memoirs, and plays, as well as keeping a daily diary. Most of this writing is contained in thirteen published volumes, but now, at the advanced age of 84, I have experienced the fading of creativity.

And so I have retired from the profession of writing as well, although I confess to still keep a daily diary, a most congenial form of literature that is free of the need to adhere to a plot or to advance a philosophical position. A diary is hardly more than a self-portrait. It should tell the truth about the "keeper" as he sees it.

*

Learned from Sir Thomas Browne that a *quincunx* consists of five objects arranged in a square with one at all four corners, and the fifth in the center. Mostly, I love the word itself, no matter what its meaning. From Browne I also learned that a daw's claw is shaped like a fig leaf, a fact that I sent to Doon, who in today's e-mail described a huge flock of crows overhead at dawn. He had never seen so many at once. Had they assembled out of fear of predators? But what kind of creature would eat crow, either in the flesh or metaphorically?

*

It is the morning of my four-monthly haircut, administered by Carl, that most accomplished barbarian, at Phil's barbershop on Wall St. No fewer than twelve persons have convinced me that I am, although not gorgeous, no longer a sight for sore eyes. As you can see, I have reversed the accepted meaning of that clumsy adage, which was supposed to be a compliment, but is just as likely to be taken as its opposite.

*

As an assistant innkeeper, I have enjoyed the leisure time to acquaint myself with a bit of facility in other languages—including Italian, Japanese, German, and Yiddish. I hasten to add that I am completely illiterate in most of these languages, and cannot read or write a single word. But the ability to exchange pleasantries in them has come to be rather useful—and once word got about that I was fluent in many languages, we became a minor-league international inn. It is an imposturage that I haven't disclaimed, to Janet's approval.

*

This morning at breakfast I was made aware that I am a relic of the nineteenth century. The man at the kitchen table is a frequent guest at Janet's B&B, which provides the means by which we are able to remain in the house where we have lived for forty-seven years. He and I could not be more different from one another. Among my options the only civilized one is to fall silent, to offer no riposte, and to evacuate the premises as soon as possible. In French "to swallow a toad" means to pocket an insult.

But enough of this morose self-pity! Instead of counting up my maladjustments and failures of fulfillment, I shall count my blessings—among which is that at age 84 I arise at five o'clock in the morning, wash hands and face and repair to the kitchen to make coffee for the family and the B&B guests. I then have a breakfast of one egg and a slice of home-made bread. I go out to retrieve the newspapers, pour another cup of coffee, and skim the front page of the *Times*. Now it is time for a shower and the walk to the library for a morning of reading and writing. To how many 84-year-olds is this given? I ask you.

*

I hardly ever intentionally read one of my early stories. It is always the result of idle fingering of a shelf in the scriptorium. Whenever I do, I am struck by a bit of airy persiflage that must have been written by someone other than the Richard Selzer I have become since then. I have only the faintest recollection of having done it, and I have no idea how it escaped my editorial discretion.

The few scholarly folks who have wasted their time in poring over my works have almost all seized upon the illegal phrase or sentence or paragraph as a window into my personal "keep," the deepest, darkest room of my character where my dirty little secrets are held. It is both to my credit and my embarrassment that I don't have any such dirty little secrets. Mine has been a long and colorless sojourn on earth which could not possibly attract the curiosity of anyone. But such are the nosy-Parkers of scholarship that a number of false hypotheses have sprung up likening me to Jekyll and Hyde. It is the reason that I no longer submit to interviews or analyses of my works, which are better left to shrivel up unexamined.

*

Last evening Janet and I partook of bowls of the Russian beet borsht I had made the previous day. Janet declared it delicious and a treat, and I experienced the pleasure of a chef. Here's the recipe—

> Plunge two large beets into two quarts of boiling water. Brush them with a sponge to remove the skin. Then return them to the boiling water along with two well-beaten eggs, one large chopped onion, the juice of a lemon with a tablespoon of sugar (sweet and sour), a teaspoon of salt, and a sprinkle of black pepper. Leave to simmer for an hour and a half or two, and then remove to cool. Then put in the fridge overnight. The next day, after stirring in a tablespoon of sour cream so as to turn it "pink velvet" in color, serve over diced scallion and diced cucumber.

*

I have now lost so much memory of the past, and thus am deprived of that most pleasant of pastimes—nostalgia. Memory is what distinguishes us from other creatures: most of them have instinct instead. Loss of instinct is one of the prices we paid for the ability to reason. Instinct causes the butterfly to lay its eggs on a cabbage leaf. The butterfly doesn't eat cabbage leaves, but its larvae do. How does the butterfly know this when it will have died before the eggs are hatched?

If given the choice between instinct and memory, give me memory any time. Instinct is devoid of the nostalgic love that gives life its sweetest dimension. So much for today's lesson in psychobiology.

*

Just finished reading "The Weaver's Grave," one of two stories by Seumas O'Kelly in a small volume entitled *The Golden Barque*, published in 1919. It is one of the best pieces of Irish literature I have ever read—very humorous and life-affirming. I learned of the book by reading the letters of James Stephens, whom I also admire. Stephens praised it unreservedly, and so do I. Some day, when my work falls into obscurity, I would hope that a living writer will do the same for me.

*

The readers of this diary will by now have discovered what a stupid person I am, and one who has nothing better to write about than these trivial fleeting thoughts. There it is no sense in my trying to cover up my stupidity, as so much is evident from my previous books. But if said readers knew in what utter ignorance of events and persons I dwell, they might soften their contempt a bit.

I do not own a computer; I do not use a cell phone; I have no idea what a Facebook or a Twitter are; I do not watch television or go to the movies; and I have little interest in politics. My main interchange with others is in the form of correspondence with readers of my work who want to know what I meant when I wrote whatever it was that mystified them. I do answer every letter promptly, which persuades said correspondents that I want to begin a correspondence worthy of that genre. Therefore I do not answer the second or third letter promptly, or at all. From this, the reader will doubtless assume that I am both faithless and cranky—to both of which diagnoses, I confess. If I were one of my own readers, I would eschew petulance and simply give me the go-by as just another "raughty tinker"—an Irish expression of contempt used in a letter by James Joyce, and nowhere else that I could find.

*

POSTSCRIPT

March 13, 2013:

Janet and I have made the decision to discontinue the B&B and sell the house where we have lived for 48 years. She wants us to settle in an assisted-living facility. Larry reassured us that we can afford to do this, even phoning our financial adviser to confer.

For me, it will be a huge adjustment, but it must be done. We are both too old to keep on here. Yesterday we visited the assisted-living place, Evergreen Woods, which Janet loved. And so it shall be done.

Part VIII

Two Unfinished Stories

Most of Richard Selzer's writing after 2008 exists in the form of diary entries. But there are two intriguing exceptions, and each is a study in psychological self-portraiture. Neither story has been published previously, and in fact neither was given a final form before the author's death.

In "Half Moon," a narrative of Henry Hudson's third voyage to North America in 1609, the main character is Kees Nooteboom, a sixteen-year-old Dutch orphan who joins the ship as a cabin boy and then uses his medical knowledge and intuition to assist Hudson and the crew. The story has a second protagonist: the river that would later be named for the ship's captain. Selzer's opening paragraphs echo poetic tributes to the Hudson in his memoir, *Down from Troy*, and in the PBS documentary *America's First River*, produced by Bill Moyers: "For those who live on its banks," Selzer says, "the river is time itself, approaching, surging past, vanishing, never to be called back. You can tell your secrets to a river. It just carries them away."[1]

Kees Nooteboom's reveries tend toward a pure contemplation of this environment—perhaps like the Dutch sailors mentioned on the final page of *The Great Gatsby*, who looked in wonder at "the fresh, green breast of the new world." In his journal, Kees describes the happiness of being alone on the river, with or without Captain Hudson's permission: "In the act of paddling the canoe, I am as near to Nirvana as can be." On board the ship, Kees is like a shamanistic healer, and some of his observations (such as the notion that a wound gives off its own light) are drawn from the author's memories of his father, Julius Selzer. In Holland, Kees had left the home of his foster father, a devout Jewish surgeon, because he could not share his benefactor's religious belief. In America, after contracting fever, Kees experiences a return of "long dormant faith," and ultimately the voyage of the Half Moon becomes "a spiritual adventure instead of a geographical exploration."

"Half Moon" has a double point of view, with the boy's journal balancing the author's omniscient voice. "Mister Stitches" is split in a different way. The story is conveyed entirely in the first person by a narrator, also named Richard Selzer, who tells of his lifelong friendship with the enigmatic Reuben Schneider. But Reuben is also Richard's alter ego: He is a surgeon who leaves his profession, and his doctor father and singer mother are described and quoted precisely as the author often portrayed his own parents. (Schneider was the maiden name of Selzer's mother.) "The one way in which Reuben and I differed," the narrator says, "was in the matter of religious belief. I am an infidel; Reuben was god-struck."

In "Half Moon," the division between doubt and faith is temporal, as Kees abandons and recovers religious belief. In "Mister Stitches," the division is deeper, resulting in the presentation of two characters as psychological twins, and the conflict remains unresolved. Selzer's concluding "Commentary" can only hint at some indistinct possibility beyond death.

In those final paragraphs, the author discusses his difficulty in finishing "Mister Stitches," and in fact his papers include more than a dozen variant manuscripts of the piece.[2] Richard Selzer finally chose the version presented here—not because he considered it definitive, but because he prized its very open-endedness.

NOTES

1. Richard Selzer, *Down from Troy: A Doctor Comes of Age* (New York: William Morrow, 1992), 52. In Part 1 of Moyers' documentary, "Stories from the River" (broadcast April 23, 2002), Selzer read this passage and others about growing up in Troy, New York. The full transcript is available online at http://billmoyers.com/content/bill-moyers-hudson/.
2. All of these variants are now part of the Richard Selzer Archive in the Moody Medical Library at the University of Texas Medical Branch in Galveston.

Half Moon

First, the river:

There are certain words that reverberate in the mind long after they are spoken. One such is "river," the way it is always flowing between its banks—called *rives* in French. The very word "river" evokes a rich correspondence between the actual stream and the imagination. Then too, there is its unpunctuated, on-and-on speech, the way it murmurs and chatters in the jargon of which it is sole master.

"Repeat after me . . ." the river says to the boatman but he cannot; he has the wrong-shaped lips and larynx. No, the river is water made word, word made water.

It is hard on September in the year 1609, some weeks since the Half Moon entered the estuary of this great river that is brother to the Ganges, sister to the Nile, and that gleams like the blade of a cutlass as it flows over the greenish light of an aqualune.

Now, the Half Moon:

Such a clunky, thick-hipped old Dutch *hausfrau*, waddling up the river in her wooden shoes. On board, she is all ladders, coils of rope, hammocks, boatcloaks and narrow passages. There is no mizzenmast, only a topmast and a bowsprit rigged with gaffs and staysails. There is a dory attached by ropes to the stern. It seats six men who do the rowing when dispatched to the shore to engage in trade with the Indians or to reconnoiter.

There is a third vessel, if such a grand term can be applied to a coracle. This is nothing more than a round deep wicker basket covered with deerskin. It is big enough for only one man to huddle at the bottom, bailing as fast as he can, and occasionally reaching out with a paddle to keep some command of his course. The little vessel is entirely at the mercy of the water and the wind. It is hardly more than a leaf in the current.

Henry Hudson commands the ship, makes it perform according to his will. He does so without the least affection for the vessel. He is like the driver of a donkey cart; his purpose—to accomplish a task, complete a journey. His passion is for discovery of the elusive Passage. For Kees, the sixteen-year-old Dutch youth taken on board as a cabin boy, Half Moon is a beloved and gallant beast for whose comfort and ease he would make every effort. It is the same feeling of a shepherd for his flock. He relishes the acreage of white sailcloth and the creaking of the timbers. Nothing is more deserving of his homage.

For the rest of the crew, the Half Moon has become their home; they know no other, never speak of family or friends. For them, the voyage and the ship is all there is. They are sleepwalkers, lost in a world unknown to others.

What, I am asked, prompted me to re-tell a story already familiar to generations of American schoolchildren? Perhaps it is a feeling of like-mindedness with Herman Melville. Melville was born in 1819 on Pearl Street in Lower Manhattan only a few yards from the New York harbor. It was only natural that he would write about the sea. I was born in 1928 in the city of Troy only a few yards from the Hudson River. It is only natural that I would write about the river. It was precisely at what is now called Troy where Henry Hudson abandoned his Third Voyage, having observed that the river above this level was not navigable by the Half Moon. Then too, Herman Melville had lived in Troy for a number of years. There he proposed to his future wife, and wrote a number of his stories. With *Billy Budd* not yet completed, Melville died in 1891. Perhaps it was a deep-seated wish to pay homage to a fellow Trojan, as I prefer to think of him, that I began to emulate the Master, and tell what *might* have happened aboard the Half Moon. In this re-invention of the voyage, I have told it from the point of view of Kees Nooteboom, a sixteen-year-old Dutch boy who, along with other homeless ragamuffins, haunted the port of Amsterdam, hoping to be chosen to go on a sea voyage.

About Kees:

At age seven, he was removed from the orphanage that had been his home from birth, and brought to the house of Mijnheer Nooteboom, a childless Jewish surgeon in the hope that he would become his assistant in surgery, as well as his son and heir. For the next nine years, he was trained in surgery and medicine, learned the plants from which to extract healing salves and ointments. In addition, he became fluent in the English language, and studied Hebrew to prepare for his bar mitzvah and ultimate conversion to Judaism. The doctor tried and tried to plant faith in the orphan boy of whom he had become inordinately fond, but was baffled by the resistance of the boy's soul. To his mentor's great disappointment, Kees could not accept Judaism, and so was expelled from the household to make his own way in the world.

"It is terrible for one's greatest hopes to be rejected out of hand," the surgeon moaned.

"But Master, I appreciate all you have done for me, given me a beautiful home and taught me so much. You have been the father I never had." When Mijnheer Nooteboom began to cry, Kees fled the house, never to return. It was at the port of Amsterdam where Henry Hudson had called out to the clamoring crowd of potential cabin boys.

"Does anyone here speak English?" Only Kees raised his hand.

"You are the one, then."

Shortly after setting sail, it became apparent that Kees was gifted in a number of ways. There was his knowledge of medicine. During his years of apprenticeship, in addition to the technique of surgery, and the suturing of wounds, he had learned how to distill the roots and leaves of plants to make healing decoctions and ointments. This he augmented with amulets that were useful in predicting the outcome of a treatment, and in foretelling the future. His mentor had further instructed him that he must not hurry into surgery, but to delay the use of the scalpel until there was no other recourse. "So long as a diseased limb is still attached to the body, there is hope that it can be saved," said the doctor. "But once amputated, it is gone, and there is no hope." All this Kees brought with him when he set foot aboard the Half Moon. Within the first month at sea, he set the fractured arm of one of the crew, drained pus from an infected wound, and sutured a lacerated scalp, this last after nightfall.

"But can you do it in the dark?" asked the sailor who held an oil lamp over the injured man's head.

"A wound is like a lamp," Kees told him. "You can dress a wound by the light it gives off." A week later, he removed the stitches and the man returned to full duty. By now, he had become the *de facto* Ship's Surgeon. Now and then, he thought of the Dutch surgeon who had been his mentor. Faced with an abdomen that was rigid enough to bounce a coin, he regretted that he had not accepted the singsong prayers of the Jewish faith. He had need of them now. But he could not pray. He had forgotten how and continued to suffer from a kind of spiritual amnesia. Instead, he looked off in the distance and asked the ghost of Nooteboom for the diagnosis.

"Pus," said the ghost. "You'll have to cut into him, low down on the right side, to let the pus run out." Kees then steeled himself for the ordeal while at the same time, pouring whiskey into the open mouth of the sick man, and talking him to sleep. No sooner had sleep been induced, he stabbed through the thickness of the belly wall, low down and on the right side. All at once, a fountain of gray-green, foul-smelling pus erupted under pressure. When it subsided, Kees kept the wound open with a hollow reed. Hours later, the gasped breathing finally eased, and the too-rapid pulse slowed and become regular.

Soon rumors were muttered among the men that the boy was possessed of supernatural powers. Once, he had pressed his ear against the naked chest of one of the crew, listening to his breath sounds and heartbeats, shushing the man with his fingers. When at last he lifted away his head from the chest, the man reported to the others that he continued to feel the boy's touch long afterwards. To the sick and injured men, he was a god, one who had escaped from the sky and was lent to them for the duration of the voyage. To his discomfort, from this exalted pedestal, he was unable to make friends with any of the crew. His instinct for diagnosis and treatment was a barrier that neither he nor the others could surmount. His encounters with the men took place only when his medical advice was solicited. "Feel this, will you, Doc; what do you think it is?" He would palpate a cervical lymph node, look off in the distance for a long moment, then return with an answer. The very touch of his hand seemed to ease pain and anxiety. He loved it when the men would sing their rowdy chanties. Two of the crew were Egyptians who had brought a tambour, flute and castanets. The music they played was wild, passionate. Caught up in it, some of the men clapped their hands and swiveled their hips. The lonely boy longed to join in.

In addition to doctoring, it was his duty to climb the rigging at the prow of the ship, from which he had a view of the river from on high. Cramming his mouth with Dutch, he would call down to the helmsman words of warning.

"*Zandbank!*" (shoal)

"*Ondiepe plaats*" (shallow place)

"*Gezanken boomstam!*" (sunken log)—whereupon the wheel would be turned accordingly, or the rowboat dispatched with half a dozen men to clear the path for the Half Moon. It soon became remarked that Kees was a natural navigator, observant and alert. Henry Hudson came to trust his calculations and estimates, his prediction of the time of moonrise and sunset, the presence of a mudflat that must be crossed by sheer manpower pulling on ropes.

For a boy who had never climbed a tree or seen a bird in its nest, the mast was a miraculous tower that rose from the water to the sky. The very act of climbing had something of the heroic about it. Kees felt valiant and vigorous. After attaining the highest bowsprit, he was rewarded with a feeling of purity. It was Henry Hudson's greatest pleasure to watch him spring up the mizzen shrouds, climb rung upon rung until he was sitting on the uppermost cross-tree. Kees was made equally of boyish excitement and preternatural calm. It did not occur to him to be afraid. The next moment, he would send a flat stone skipping on the surface of the river. Slowly, imperceptibly, there grew a mutual fondness between the Captain and the cabin boy that deepened into the love of a son for a father, a father for a son.

"My nestling," thought the Captain, "my sparrow."

Both Master and cabin boy, each at his post, was held there by the tentacular bonds of duty, and the passion for exploration, further strengthened by mutual affection. For his part, the Master delighted in the way that Kees *conducted* the river from his podium on high, suffering the tide to roll and circulate through his body. Once, when the Master had lain down on his cot for the night, Kees went to the chair from which he had moments before risen. On sudden impulse, he pressed his palms down upon the seat, and felt the warmth of his Master's body. Such, such were the feelings of the youth aboard this, the ship of his dreams. How wonderful it was to stand in the rigging of a boat pointed north toward the unknown. Nor was the magic lost on the others of the crew. At dusk the boy was indistinct to those below, soon to melt into darkness. The air was burdened with the fragrance of cedar. Along the banks, elms had lined themselves up, shedding the last of the light trapped in their leaves. More than once Kees felt the irrepressible urge to sing. Far below, the men would listen to his frail warbling, not quite music so much as a sound that rose up from his longing, an eloquence of his ripening body.

"Ever been with a woman?" Jouet, the First Mate asked him in the presence of others. Kees lowered his gaze and shook his head. Jouet could not repress a crafty smile. "A virgin, are you?" The youth was grateful for the night that concealed his blush. He stood up and moved out of range of hearing, but not before he heard Jouet telling the others: "He's a virgin; never been with a woman, and that's a fact."

It was this same Jouet who sought attention for a large boil on his neck. Kees bade him stay where he was, then left. When he returned, it was with a poultice of river water, sugar and soap which he applied to the boil, rubbing it in. The next morning, the boil had burst, discharging its foul cargo into a dressing of leaves. For this, Kees gave silent thanks to the surgeon in Amsterdam who had been his mentor. Jouet, up to this time, while not openly hostile, had been distinctly cool toward the boy. For minutes after the wound had been dressed, patient and doctor sat looking and not looking at each other. At last, it was Jouet who first lowered his gaze lest his gratitude rollick over into something warmer, more palpable. Kees too, roused himself from the enchantment he always felt at having been the instrument of healing. As if by mutual consent, they each retired to the remotest corner of their relationship and agreed not to speak.

At the sight of Kees descending from the rigging enveloped in white sailcloth that fluttered about his head, a sailor would fall silent at the transformation of someone he had taken to be human until just then. In the evening, Kees would sit at the desk of his Captain and write his own account of the voyage. It fulfilled him to set one word down after another on a page, suturing them together, as it were, and then ponder at the meaning of them, take pleasure in what they evoked in his imagination. Sometimes, he would fall asleep with the quill in his hand, the notebook on his knees. Once he woke up just as the candle was about to go out. He stood up to extinguish the flickering flame. But he was astonished to see that the light continued. Soon enough, he realized that the light emanated from himself!

He walked around the cabin, then up and down the deck, and saw that the light had indeed remained with him. Even when he went back to his cot and covered his eyes, the light was with him. What could this mean?

In keeping this log, Kees did not give any of the men a name, save for the First Mate Jouet. He preferred to identify them by description, as in the following entry:

> I have been treating one of the men for Dutch fever. He is short of breath and his pulse is weak and irregular. He bleeds from his gums. I believe it is caused by the lack of fresh fruit or vegetables. The men have returned from the forest with a sack of freshly harvested apples. Already, his heartbeat is more regular and he is no longer short of breath. He has hard black eyes and black hair. He has, no doubt, some Spanish blood in his veins. He wears drops of silver in his ears. They were given to him by a girl in Antwerp who loved him, he told me. Yesterday when I visited his hammock, he drew forth from his shirt pocket a little mouse, and invited it to run up and down his arm.

And these:

> We have come to a place where the river is absolutely calm and silent. Perhaps it is gathering its thoughts? From somewhere in the forest comes the intermittent liquid song of the woodthrush. Only the woodthrush with its tremulous melody can converse with the river. Ah! Listen! There it is! Sometimes I catch sight of one of the ruffians on the crew as he gazes down into the water. The sound passes into his uncouth face turning it into a countenance. The same thing happens to me. I lean my head on the railing of the foredeck and see the full moon making a broken column, an aqualune, in the black water that has seized it and holds it prisoner. How the river twists it back and forth, shaking the moon exultantly. I listen to the murmur and moan of the sunken creature, and I wonder which is the real moon—the one in the sky? Or the one submerged?

*

> Three canoes each containing five people came aboard. They sold us deerskins and various trinkets. Together with Captain Hudson, I rode to the shore in one of the Indian canoes. We were met by the elderly Chief of the tribe consisting of forty men and seventeen women. These women we saw in a circular house well-constructed of oak bark, with an arched roof. It is called a wigwam. It

contained a large quantity of maize and Indian corn and beans of last year's growth. Near the wigwam there lay drying enough of these crops to load three ships, aside from what is growing in the fields. On our entering the house, two mats were spread for us to sit upon, and immediately some food served in well-made red wooden bowls. Two men were dispatched with bow and arrows in quest of game. They returned with a pair of pigeons which they had shot. They likewise killed a fat dog and skinned it in great haste with shells they had got out of the water. After we had feasted, they made me to understand by signs that they wished me to tell their futures. (My reputation as a seer had preceded us to the village.) This I did, and in their own language. The Indians were astonished by this. How had I learned it? Who had instructed me? In fact, I cannot myself explain how I came to know their language. Perhaps, it happened when I placed my hands on them that I *understood.* Perhaps it was the *texture* of their skin beneath my palpating fingers that transcended the barrier of language, making the skin the organ of translation. And why not? The skin is the true organ of perception, sensing, as it does, the world in which one lives—the heat or cold of it, the dry or damp, the way it shivers or blushes. But I have no wish to dissect the phenomenon any further. Best simply to accept.

Our hosts supposed that we would remain with them for the night, but we returned to our ship after a short time. The land is of the finest for cultivation that the Captain has ever set foot upon, he said. It abounds in trees of every description. The Master always speaks in a kindly manner to and about the Indians and his kindness is rewarded by their friendship, something that cannot be said of the rest of the crew whose behavior toward the natives is harsh and insulting. Jouet has spread it about that the Indians are the descendants of the Ten Lost Tribes of Israel who had lived sinfully and whom God punished by darkening their skin and sending them into exile. It was Jouet who raised his spyglass and peered at something he had noticed in the foliage along the river—at most, it was an animal; at least, a leaf. The next moment he had aimed his musket. The Indian staggered to the edge of the river, blood streaming from his mouth. It was a fated act of thoughtless cruelty that was to initiate the war that would slaughter so many Indians. The natives are indeed very good people, for when they saw we would not remain, they supposed that we were afraid of their bows and arrows. Taking their arrows, they broke them in pieces and threw them into the fire. At the close of the visit, I drained an abscess on the neck of the old chieftain. Certainly, they are not the "lewd monkeys" described by some of the Christian clergy. Their tattoos give them the appearance of savagery, but it is the appearance only.

*

We have come to a place where the river has broadened into what amounts to a lake. Perhaps half a mile to the north there is a flat island in the middle of the stream. It appears to be uninhabited, and to be composed of a rocky ledge that supports only wild and primitive vegetation.

To the other voyagers, it was an uninviting, sterile patch, but to Kees it was a place of utter enchantment. Before long, the little islet had become the very Indies that was the goal and purpose of the voyage. The more he gazed at it, the more his fantasy was exercised. Its rocky beauty was to him seductive and irresistible. In his mind, he enlarged it, sculpted hills and valleys, a canyon with a torrent racing down to the river, high plains where sheep and goats grazed, fields of Indian corn. And he would be the king of the island ruling over the tribe of Indians who had fled there to escape warfare and famine.

It was this that induced the youth to hoist the coracle to the railing, then down a ladder into the river. He lowered himself into it; a single push carried him into the headlong, emphatic tide aimed toward the island of his dreams. From then on, he had only to huddle and surrender to wind and wave until he would come within a scramble to the shore of the island. A stroll along the shore in either direction confirmed that the island was uninhabited. The only living creatures were an abundance of fish in the water, and a species of migrating bird that had stopped to rest before continuing on.

Unbeknownst to Kees, Henry Hudson had been informed of his disobedient act. Mutinous, he called it, as he stood on the deck and trained his spyglass on the boy. At once, he ordered the First Mate to take four men in the dory and take the youth prisoner.

"The Master is furious," Jouet told him. "You are going to get the lash, for sure." There was more than a hint of satisfaction in his voice.

"I'll take it," said Kees. "It will have been worth it." The dory was greeted with cold fury by the Captain who directed that the boy be brought to his cabin. There his anger was in full force.

"Of course, you deserve the lash. The men expect you to be punished. What do have to say for yourself?"

"I accept my punishment." He would not apologize or beg for mercy. The man chosen to administer it was ruddy and hefty of trunk and arms. He was also hairless. *Alopecia totalis* thought Kees. The lashing was to be carried out within the hour. But Fate ruled otherwise. One of the seamen had fallen from the rigging and sustained a severe wound of the scalp. It would be necessary to delay the lashing while Kees repaired the lacerated scalp. Even as he was being stitched, the wounded man whispered.

"I will take the lashing for you."

"No man pays for my sins," muttered Kees. Just then, Henry Hudson came to where the surgery was in progress.

"Please, sir," began the sailor, "let me suffer the lash in his place. It was just a boyish prank, is all."

"It was not just a boyish prank. It was an act of mutiny for which he must be punished."

"I would not have it otherwise, Master," said Kees.

"I regret that the lashing must be postponed until your services are not immediately needed for the welfare of the crew." A moment later, Hudson had turned on his heel, and was gone. That night, Kees wrote in his log:

> Lest I present myself to the reader of this log, if any there will be, as being fearless and intrepid, I must confess to my abject terror while huddled in the coracle. All at once, the river unleashed its fury. What would I do when the wind sent a great billow to engulf me? What if I drown? But to have survived! What a prop to the ego! What better proof that one is braver than he thought. In this bit of brisk living, I have realized my potential as a man. To my sorrow, the coracle was lost and never retrieved.
>
> *
>
> To the Indians, I am sure we are strange and picturesque intruders, to be stared at and followed.
>
> *
>
> Standing by the hour in my little alcove high on the mast, I have fallen into a state of river madness in which the mind closes down. Then, by force of will, I must force it back to attention.
>
> *
>
> The long voyage has put kinks in the sexual practices of several of the men. They give themselves leeway, and excuse it by noting the prolonged absence from the company of women. It is not the disgraceful behavior it would have been on dry land. I have received a number of such propositions myself and try not to be offended by the vulgarity of it.
>
> One of the men, a roughneck brawler with hardly any teeth to speak of, has brought back from the Indian village a small white dog, hardly more than a puppy. He has given it the name Daleeta. He is almost never seen without the little dog in his lap with his arm encircling her. He speaks to the dog in long tender vowels and throat-clearing expressions of intimacy to which the dog responds by licking his face. His transformation from sadistic bully to tender parent is nothing short of miraculous. With what gentleness and affection he fondles the dog who in her turn is utterly content in the lap of her master. I have the premonition that no good will come from the presence of this animal on board. There is sure to come the day when another sailor whom he had bested in a fight will take out his revenge on the dog whose master will defend his darling to the death of one or the other.

*

I have acquired a measure of proficiency at the canoe. I know the proper inclination to dip the paddle, first on one side, then the other, so as to keep the canoe midstream. In the act of paddling the canoe, I am as near to Nirvana as can be.

In the evening, I think to see boats moving on the river. I know there are none. Still, their sails are to me like wings that awaken the old ache to know who I was before the Doctor, before the orphanage, even. Perhaps that is why I love every wound that is brought to me—each one is an opportunity to realize myself. This means more to me than all the rest of my experience. In the presence of a wound I come to life. I *am.*

*

Jouet is disturbed by the behavior of the ship's cat which "ranne crying from one side of the ship to the other." It is widely believed that these grimalkins with their slit eyes and prick-ears are in league with the powers of darkness, and are minions of the devil. Their actions are watched with great interest.

*

September 30, 1609

The name of this place is Schenedtadea, "the place you reach by traveling through pine woods." Henry Hudson sent First Mate Jouet and men in the ship's boat to explore farther upriver. At nightfall they returned with the bad news that above this latitude the river becomes a thin brown trickle unsuitable for shipping of any kind. As Jouet delivered this report, the Captain who had been lowered into the small boat, smote the water again and again with his cane, as if to scold it for not being cooperative. The reflection of his face in the water was more ferocious than his actual face. Later that evening, in his cabin, I was surprised to see him tilt a bottle of rum and take a huge swallow. His open mouth glistening with rum was a self-inflicted wound. He then unleashed a stream of curses in both English and Dutch. They sounded more fierce in Dutch.

"I see that I have shocked you," he said.

"It is easier to curse in Dutch," I replied.

"The Strait of Magellan," he remarked, "is narrower and shallower in places than this river, and even so, led the Spaniards beyond any expectation into the South Pacific." I made no comment, seeming to busy myself with the log book.

For two days we lay, sails reefed and fully anchored, letting the river have its way with us until such time as the expeditionary force in the dory returned with news that the upper stream could not be navigated. The boredom was hard to bear. Anyone who knows anything about sailors knows that they love murder, corpses and blood on the deck. This afternoon, two of the men stripped to the waist and began to fight. The rest formed a circle about the combatants, cheering on one or the other. There is much pride involved in these fights. The reason for them is not important; it is the fight itself that matters. A fight is good because it is a fight. Even if one of them is killed by the other, there would be no punishment other than a severe lashing, and no judgment upon the killer. Murder broke up the boredom. Today I watched as a man knelt astride his fallen opponent, grasping him by the ears, and pounding his head against the deck until the man lost consciousness. Then, taking a knife from his belt, the victor sliced off an ear of the defeated man. Later he jettisoned it with a flourish. Several of the others nodded, giving recognition of the right of passion to end in violence. Later Henry Hudson ordered the unrepentant victor to be brought to him. He studied the man's hands. They were the paws of a great animal, a bear perhaps, made for predation. There was black blood under the fingernails. I myself was shocked, silent.

When the man was dismissed from the cabin, the Master told me about the Australian Bulldog ant. On a previous voyage to the South Seas, he had seen such a creature that had been caught by one of the Maoris who had placed it in a small arena, then cut it in half. In short order, the two halves of the ant found each other and began to fight. Head seized Tail in its jaws; Tail stung Head. Back and forth the battle raged until both halves lay dead.

"With such violence as this in Nature," said the Master, "we cannot expect mankind to be free of it."

*

The weather has turned hot and still. The men are bathing in the river, half the crew at a time, their white bodies gleaming as they wrestle each other beneath the surface. There is laughter, shouting. Now one, now another looks up to where I am standing, high above the deck. They call out to me to come down, come down, and raise their fond and fondling hands. I pretend not to hear, and gaze upstream. When, at last, I look down and shake my fist at them, they roar with laughter.

*

It happened that soon after the decision was made to abandon the voyage and return to England, Henry Hudson came down with a sickness that almost carried him off, and surely would have, had it not been for the devotion and loyalty of Kees. The youth sat by his bedside, night and day, tending to his bodily needs, warming and cooling him as the fever waxed and waned. The most unappetizing acts of nursing he performed with a blend of grace and steadfastness. He massaged the feet of his patient, dripped water between his parched lips, and when the Captain could not breathe, the boy bent above him, pressed his lips upon those of his Master, and blew his sweet, cool breath into the sick man's chest, at the same time sucking the poisons from it, taking them into his own body.

"You will get well . . ." he murmured to his beloved Master. And so it happened. Soon Henry Hudson was able to cross the cabin with seven steps, six short ones, and the longer drag of his lame leg.

Through some weakness of character or, more likely, due to his illness, Henry Hudson was incapable of keeping his insubordinate crew under control. It was even more likely due to the large amount of grog they drank every day. On one such occasion the sailors went ashore to the Indian village and drove the natives from their houses and "took spoile of them." Another lapse took place during a visit by the Indians to the Half Moon for the purpose of trading. Instead, the men antagonized the Indians, then got them drunk.

But now, it became apparent that Kees had contracted the fever. The price for saving the life of the Captain would be his own. Within days, the boy was to a great extent already released, his temples hollowed, his eyelids opaque, but exalted by wave after wave of fever until only the thinnest veil separated him from death. What the others did not know is that for some weeks, a long dormant faith had stirred and fluttered like a child in the womb, until with the onset of the fever it was born again. Through the rapture of fever, he had seen again his guardian Nooteboom with the striped prayer shawl, the *talith*, and the phylacteries, the *t'fillin*, the one affixed to his forehead, and the other that wound down the left arm to his hand. He saw him reaching up to touch the mezuzah attached to the doorpost of the house, and he remembered hearing, or rather watching the ancient prayers as they emerged singsong from his lips.

"*Boruch atah Adonai Elohenu melech ha 'ohm*" (Blessed art Thou O Lord, King of the universe)

"*Shemah Yisroel, Adonai Elohen* . . ." (Hear O Israel, the Lord our God is One)

It was at this time that the Third Voyage of Henry Hudson became a spiritual adventure instead of a geographical exploration. Now, so many years after Mijnheer Nooteboom's failed struggle to convert the boy to Judaism, a moment of febrile rapture had flooded him with faith. Now it was Henry Hudson, sitting beside the cot where Kees Nooteboom lay dying who heard, or rather watched, the ancient prayers emerge from the boy's mouth. And so died the Jew, Kees Nooteboom.

It had been Hudson's intention to bury Kees along the eastern bank of the river and raise a pile of stones at the site. But a glance through the spyglass revealed a great number of the now hostile Indians in the nearby forest. They dared not bring the dory in to land. As one day led into the next, and the one after that, it was decided to consign Kees to the river. And so Henry Hudson in a dry and tremulous voice performed the office for which life at sea ought to have steeled him, but in this instance did not.

". . . man that is born of woman . . ." he read aloud. "Thou knowest, Lord, the secrets of our hearts . . ." Again and again the voice of the Captain broke apart, and must be mended with a long silence in order to resume after a clenched pause.

"... our vile body ..."

"... to subdue all things to Himself ..." The words of the service reached into the tortured silence that followed each phrase.

"Amen." After which there came to every ear the small splash from beyond the gunwale. The waters of Babylon had not sounded sadder. The caps that had been doffed were resettled. No man looked at anyone else, lest his grief be witnessed. Even from the eyes of Jouet, tears streamed. Who would have thought that the man had so much feeling in him? Now here he was, his mouth contorted in sorrow. And Henry Hudson himself, wondering would he ever be able to command the respect and obedience of these men who had seen him weeping.

The next day, the Half Moon sailed south on the great river until it reached the island called Manahatta, then into the harbor that brought them to the great sea. It was midway across this body of water that the crew became openly mutinous. The Half Moon that arrived on the coast of England was a ship from which all vestiges of seafaring discipline had departed.

So ended the Third Voyage of Henry Hudson in search of a direct route to the Indies.

Mister Stitches

I used to have a friend, Reuben Schneider. We were born three months apart (I was the elder) and lived on the same block of Second Street in the fabled town of Troy in upstate New York. From the beginning, we were inseparable companions. Besides sharing the same age and the same initials, we came to resemble one another to the extent that he was often taken for me, and I for him. But this might have been due to mutual imitation. He gave forth my laughter, I his sighs.

It is time to portray Reuben as I remember him. I have only to close my eyes and there he is—small and spare, almost translucent, hardly what might have been expected to emerge from the lower streets of Troy, settled as it had been by the matter-of-fact Dutch, although it was widely rumored that apparitions and "strange appearances" were more common in Troy than anywhere else along the upper Hudson river. Delicate he was in manner too, with no suggestion of the hearty, ebullient, self-confident temperament of his future colleagues in the profession of surgery. And then there was the faint odor of him—indescribable but if you think of balsamic vinegar, you will come close.

Even as a youth he never looked robust, always pale and thin and subject to colds. He ate little and slept badly. One glass of wine went straight to his head. His inhibitions kept him from making close attachments. Of women and love, he spoke to me shyly, admitting that he had never been in love. His innate delicacy and integrity inspired kindness and sympathy rather than ardor in women. They were content to wait on him. For not a few, he was the epitome of manly achievement.

He had a way of compressing his lips and, at the same time, wrinkling his chin when he wanted to be left alone. Most of the time it didn't work. Myself excepted, he preferred solitude. "Beata Solitudo" he called it. Was he a changeling? I don't know about that, but I do know that he was drawn to the ascetic life.

The one way in which Reuben and I differed was in the matter of religious belief. I am an infidel; Reuben was god-struck. More than once he voiced sympathy for my disbelief.

"You are missing out on the most beautiful part of life," he admonished. For my part, I found him naive and, to my regret, the object of gentle drollery. It is to our credit that we never let this dampen our affection for one another. When he was ten years old, his father contracted lockjaw from having stepped on a rusty nail. Within days, the man was febrile and delirious, and the doctors had given up hope for his recovery. Whereupon, Reuben went to St. Peter's church and recited the "Hail Mary" one hundred times. The next day, his father's fever had lysed and he quickly returned to normal. The news of his cure resulted in a religious revival within a six-block perimeter of Second Street. Was Reuben a saint?

From early childhood, his manual dexterity attracted the notice of his parents and teachers. He could assemble and take apart the most complex structure of blocks and pegs within minutes. By age eight, he was building miniature cars that were propelled by the ingenious use of wind and rubber bands. His father, a Family Doctor, was understandably proud. He had a special affinity for cloth and was often seen cutting and stitching material, a further bond between us—my grandfather had been a tailor, thus earning the family name Schneider.

"Show me your hands," he said to his son. Reuben held them out for his father's inspection. Over and back, over and back, he turned them, palpating each finger and the palms, and announced the prediction. "Oh, he'll be a great surgeon in due course. Just look at those hands, they are strong and gentle, the hands of a surgeon." His mother, a singer with a lovely soprano that sounded as if a white mouse were ringing a tiny silver bell, demurred.

"Nonsense!" she retorted. "Just look at his eyes. They have a yonderly look. They are the eyes of someone who has already departed for somewhere else. He'll be a poet." Just so was the Second Trojan War fought, only this time there was no hollow wooden horse filled with Greek warriors, only the old nag that pulled Freihofer's wagon through the streets delivering bread to the Trojan citizens, until one day he stumbled and fell to the cobblestones, never to stand up.

Alas, the father's hopes were not to be realized during his lifetime. When Reuben turned thirteen, his beloved father suddenly died of a coronary thrombosis. His mother had just returned from the hospital where it had happened. She drew the boy Reuben onto her lap and informed him of his loss.

"Your Daddy is no more," she intoned in that melodramatic way she had, not so much speaking as making utterance. Then and there, the grief-stricken boy vowed that he would fulfill his father's wishes; he would become a surgeon. From early childhood, Reuben was considered a "mother's boy." Years later, he gave his mother her due. He set down his scalpel and took up his pen. He became a writer, not a poet, as she had wished, but the next thing to it. He became a storyteller.

Orphaned at thirteen, Reuben was apprenticed to a tailor and found to his pleasure that the creation of clothing was what he liked to do best. Stitchery, he decided was his *métier*. Still, it happened that both of us gravitated toward the study of medicine and attended the same medical college in nearby Albany. It was in the fourth year of medical school that our interests diverged. He elected to fulfill his father's hopes and became a surgeon, more specifically a Plastic and Reconstructive surgeon, while I opted for Family Practice. By the end of our training at the Samaritan Hospital in Troy we were both still bachelors, and so were inclined to seek our each other's company. It was no time at all before the professors of Anatomy and Surgery became aware of Reuben's innate manual dexterity. It all looked effortless, as though his hands themselves had devised the operations they were performing. More, as though the scalpel and forceps drove his fingers to their own purpose rather than the other way around.

Within several years, his reputation soared. No sooner had he begun to practice, than patients were referred to him from far and wide. It came to pass that the sixteen-year-old Pirkko arrived from a Finnish island north of the Arctic Circle. She had been under the care of Carmelite nuns and had been sent by an unknown benefactor who had heard of the prowess of our great surgeon. The unfortunate Pirkko had been born with a number of congenital deformities—harelip, crossed eyes, macroglossia and others. To the French nuns who had brought her to Reuben, Pirkko was "laide comme un chenille" (ugly as a caterpillar). Her appearance in Reuben's office was a fated incident. Immediately, he accepted the girl as his patient, even took her into his home to live, and began a series of reconstructive operations, some dozen of them, that he would perform over the next three years. In addition to the immense satisfaction of meeting this surgical challenge, Pirkko became Reuben's *raison d'être.* Slowly, imperceptibly, what had been a preoccupation became an obsession. Even below the level of conscious thought, he fell deeply in love with her. It was no wonder. Over the three years of the treatment, she had been transformed into a beautiful young woman—grace and delicacy personified. It was not too much to call it a transfiguration.

It was widely whispered among the medical community that what he had fallen in love with was not Pirkko, but his own work. Eminent surgeon that he was, he never revealed his feelings to her. It would have been, he thought, a violation of the proprieties of the doctor/patient relationship. It was Pirkko herself who released him from that restraint. It was on the day of her final surgical procedure, the revision of a scar of her cheek. She lay on the operating table in a state of partial sedation, but still conscious. Reuben stood beside the operating table looking down at her. All at once, she reached up one hand and touched his lips just as the anesthetic was administered. It was by this gesture that she acknowledged and accepted his love. Minutes later, the anesthesiologist announced that he could not obtain a heartbeat or a blood pressure. Pirkko, it seemed, had suffered a massive cerebrovascular accident, so called.

All efforts at resuscitation were unsuccessful. "This girl is dead," pronounced the anesthesiologist. In the silence that followed, Reuben stepped back from the operating table, stripped off his gown and gloves, and left the world of surgery for good. He would never operate again. That evening he did not light his lamp but lay awake the entire night brooding over what had happened.

"It was my arrogance," he told me later. He would spend the rest of his life atoning for having been the instrument of her death.

It was shortly thereafter that Reuben bought a big old brownstone house on a dead-end street in Sycaway, a hillside suburb of Troy. There were no other houses on the street, which provided the silence and solitude that were to his taste. Facing west, the upper windows caught the red glow of sunset. It had been built at the end of the eighteenth century by a wealthy merchant, but had been then vacant for a long time. Over the years, additions had been made—walkways, a colonnade, a solarium, chimneys, and a verandah, all without the least concern for architectural unity. There was a steep descent to the river at the bottom of the hill. In the eaves countless swallows twittered. A bell tower dominated the hillside. It was in a large attic room at the foot of the bell tower turned by a skylight into a luminous egg where Reuben spent his days in seclusion attended by a former patient of his, Giovanni, whose duties included marketing, preparing food and taking care of the grounds. Reuben seldom emerged from what he called his prison. Indeed, it was a house worthy of Piranesi. More than once Reuben referred to the house as himself. He *was* his house. There was a steep descent to the river at the bottom of the hill. While I have long since misplaced the exact layout of the rooms and could not reconstruct it, I still have installed in my mind the garden where Reuben and I strolled arm in arm in absolute silence. His taciturnity, it seemed, was contagious.

"How do you stand it?" I asked him. "The silence."

"I know what to do with silence," he replied. "There can never be too much silence for me."

"You need to have an occupation," I urged.

Several years went by. By this time, I too had retired from Medicine to take up the profession of writing. I used myself as an example of changing careers. One day, I received a message from Reuben asking me to come up to the house. There was a note of urgency. "Unless you are afraid of nettles, take the narrow path through the orchard."

I hurried over. It was autumn and the untended vineyards were laden with grapes and plums. There was the sticky-sweet smell of decaying fruit and the sound of apples thudding to the ground. It was in the attic room at the foot of the bell tower where I found him. When I entered the room, I saw Reuben sitting in the traditional tailor's position as produced by the *sartorius* muscles. The word *sartor* is Latin for tailor. The *sartorius* is the longest muscle in the body. It arises on the antero-lateral aspect of each iliac crest, then crosses in front of the thigh to insert on the tibia well below the knee. With the contraction of both of these muscles, one is enabled to sit cross-legged with the knees widely apart and touching the floor, the ankles apposed and the soles of the feet pressed together. What was he doing? He was sitting, or rather squatting on a woven carpet, engaged in cutting and stitching. On and on he stitched, the needle rising to the same height with each pass before plunging back into the cloth to be pulled through. There was something hypnotic about it, not unlike a religious ritual repeatedly performed. For some minutes, he was not aware of my presence. At last he looked up to see me standing nearby.

"What are you staring at?" he asked.

"Your hands," I told him. "They have lost none of the dexterity of surgery."

"One minute," he said and lay down his needle and began the painful attempt to stand up. I realized that he had been sitting thus for many hours until he had lost all feeling in his lower extremities. Forming his hands into fists, he pummeled and squeezed the muscles of his numb calves and thighs as though they were lumps of dough to bring back the flow of blood into the arteries and veins from which it had for a long time been forbidden entrance. His body curled up now like scorched paper, his head bent toward his lap, his right ear cocked and listening for the return of the blood flow, at first a whisper, then a clamor. From the mask of pain that flowed over his lips and cheeks like a beard, and from his groans, I know that the process of reclaiming his legs was agonizing. In the struggle he was like the stub of a candle sputtering at the bottom of a sconce, almost spent and no longer giving light or warmth. A minute more and *pfft* it would go out. But that was not meant to be. From some extracorporeal source came the strength to rise. At last! At last Reuben stood, his lean body bent slightly forward, expressing relief and exhaustion at the struggle. His right hand lay open showing the palm, with the raised ridge of scar tissue extending from the base of the fourth finger almost to the wrist, while the left hand was raised, palm upward in an attitude of supplication. If not for his chest heaving for breath, he could be an antique statue.

It was then that he told me that he would become a tailor, and furthermore that he had changed his name from Reuben Schneider to Reuben Sartorius.

"No one calls me 'Doctor' anymore, nor does anyone remember that once I was a surgeon. That way, I will keep my same initials, and at the same time, declare my new profession."

And now it is my sad duty to report the death of Reuben Sartorius. It took place months ago, but something kept me from accepting the fact of it. He died in a fire at the house that he loved. In one letter to me he had written "the house and myself." It seems to me now, months later, wise and just that he and his house perished together. For a long time I could not bring myself to visit the ruins of his house. I had an almost morbid need to know how he died. Had he suffered? Was anyone with him at the time? Did dying offer him as much relief as anguish? It was on my last visit to Troy that I had the impulse to go to the house on the hilltop. By now, the steep ascent from lower Troy taxed my strength and breath. Upon reaching the summit of the hill, I saw that the house was no more than a strew of fire-blackened boards and a stone foundation.

COMMENTARY

For the past year and a half, I have been trying to write a piece entitled "Mister Stitches" to commemorate the life of my friend. It is neither fact nor fiction. Nor is it a story with a beginning, middle and end. It is more a convoluted sketch of an enigmatic surgeon who left the world of medicine to practice a craft in which cutting and stitching were necessary. The other character in the piece is myself, the author who becomes a kind of *doppelganger* of Reuben, his alter ego. Neither the tailor nor the narrator is given much action. The fragments of plot are presented as recollections of the narrator. Like many of the stories of Edgar Allan Poe, it has a perverse quality that lies outside the pale of human experience but which takes on a certain rationale. Day after day for over a year, I have rummaged among my endless notes trying to write *finis* to "Mister Stitches," without success. For all that time, I have been like a drooping flag awaiting the one gust that would unfurl and show itself. I have come to the conclusion that it is Reuben himself who will not let me have done with him. Were I to let Reuben escape from my pen and paper, it would be an act of literary suicide. If Reuben Sartorius is not to go on existing, then neither am I.

Reuben Sartorius dead? Perhaps, but I have seen him twice since his death was reported. The first apparition, I call it, took place by the Hudson River in Troy. He was alone and gazing down into the stream. On that occasion he did not see me. The second appearance took place in the Oakwood Cemetery, also in Troy, where I used to walk. I had only just passed through the cemetery gate when I saw him about to leave through that same gate. He paused and turned to look at me. We exchanged a look of recognition, as if he were trying to convey a thought. I saw that his face had aged much more than his body, which kept the old erect posture. The gray eyebrows seemed to have inched toward one another like caterpillars. There was the sunken tragedy of his eyes. In his hand, what looked like flowers. When he had disappeared from view, I continued into the graveyard where I came upon a gravestone upon which lay a bouquet of fresh flowers—red poppies they were, and just below them was the name Pirkko. He had been visiting her grave.

After a few minutes, I made my way back toward the gate. On a bench nearby sat a lone woman. As I watched, she reached into a bag and took out a small bottle of what looked like gin or vodka, and two long-stem wine glasses into which she poured the contents of the bottle. With a formal gesture, she raised one glass aloft and uttered a toast. And I so close, I could hear what she said.

"A votre santé, mon cher," she said, then brought the glass to her lips. The other glass she poured on the fresh grave at her feet. She was sharing a drink with the man buried there! For me, it was a moment of revelation that provided me with the ending of "Mister Stitches." If for this woman there is no death, then why not for me?

From then on, I have had the intuition that Reuben Sartorius is still alive and fully in command of his senses, and that, should I cease to write "Mister Stitches," he would vanish forever. It is not as though I have only imagined him; I have re-created him. And so I *must* go on with this so-called work of fiction. But with each stroke of the pen, the story becomes less coherent, more obscure and even contaminated, if you will, with the mystical, the surreal. Faster and faster goes the pen back and forth across the page, as though my life depends upon it. And perhaps it does.

Two years after beginning this story, I am no closer to finding a realistic ending to the story. Why did I persist so long in trying to tell the story of Reuben Sartorius? Precisely because it was my own story I was attempting to tell. It is what comes of creating a character like Reuben who is, a self-portrait, and with whom I have come to identify to the extent that my hand simply cannot write *FINIS.* To put an end to him would be no less than an act of suicide. There came the day when it is so that I did put him to death by setting fire to the house that he, in turn, considered *his* other self. "The house is me," he said to me. It seemed artistically right to have them die together. But that was before I encountered him twice as an apparition so life-like as to convince me that Reuben was not dead. He lives, not in the narrow realistic sense of someone within arm's reach who could be drawn close and embraced, but in the wider sense of the unrealistic, the possible—one who can be conjured, or imagined in a world that, in the words of John Keats, is "the vale of soul-making." It is a world where what is unreal or telepathic, dreamt or the stuff of what others might call delusion, takes on the sense of what *is*, or what may be. I concede that this constitutes a break with all of my earlier work in which the rational prevailed and the natural laws were obeyed. I have the sense that, were I to discontinue writing "Mister Stitches," he would cease to exist altogether. I cannot let that happen, and so I have ended the story by not ending it.

About the Editor

Kevin Kerrane, Professor of English at the University of Delaware, received his bachelor's degree from Wheeling Jesuit University and graduate degrees from the University of North Carolina at Chapel Hill. His research has focused on journalism, drama, and Irish literature. He is the author of *Dollar Sign on the Muscle: The World of Baseball Scouting*, and coeditor of *Classical and Medieval Literary Criticism: Texts and Interpretations* and *The Art of Fact: A Historical Anthology of Literary Journalism*. His work has appeared in such journals as *Sports Illustrated* and *Literature and Medicine*, and online at salon.com.

Marie Borroff is Sterling Professor of English Emeritus at Yale University. She earned bachelor's and master's degrees from the University of Chicago and a doctorate from Yale, where she taught for 35 years. Among her scholarly books are *Sir Gawain and the Green Knight: A Stylistic and Metrical Study* and *Language and the Poet: Verbal Artistry in Frost, Stevens, and Moore*. Her own poetry is collected in *Stars and Other Signs*. In 1991, she became the first woman at Yale ever to be named a Sterling Professor, the highest honor bestowed on university faculty. An endowed chair at Yale has since been named for her.

www.ingramcontent.com/pod-product-compliance
Lightning Source LLC
LaVergne TN
LVHW101444200926
848483LV00001B/46